Janet M Schreiber PhD
HC 81 Box 631
Questa NM 87556-9705

D0045061

VOLUME 2

BEYOND THE INNOCENCE OF CHILDHOOD:

Helping Children and Adolescents Cope with Life-Threatening Illness and Dying

David W. Adams, M.S.W., C.S.W.
McMaster University
and
Eleanor J. Deveau, R.N., B.Sc.N.
McMaster University

Death, Value and Meaning Series
Series Editor: John D. Morgan

Baywood Publishing Company, Inc.
AMITYVILLE, NEW YORK

Library of Congress Catalog Number: 95-20406
ISBN: 0-89503-129-9 (Cloth)

Library of Congress Cataloging-in-Publication Data

Adams, David Walter, 1942-
    Helping children and adolescents cope with life-threatening
illness and dying / David W. Adams and Eleanor J. Deveau.
        p.   cm. - - (Beyond the innocence of childhood ; v. 2)
    Includes bibliographical references and index.
    ISBN 0-89503-129-9 (cloth)
    1. Children- -Death- -Psychological aspects. 2. Terminally ill
children- -Psychology. 3. Critically ill children. 4. Child
psychotherapy. 5. Children and death. I. Deveau, Eleanor J.
II. Title. III. Series: adams, David Walter, 1942-. Beyond the
innocence of childhood ; v. 2.
    BF723.D3A33 1995 vol. 2
    155.9'37'083 s- -dc20
    [155.9'37'083]   95-20406
                                                          CIP

DEDICATION

*To Ellie's brother, **Edward Anthony Gzik,** who will always be remembered for his encouragement, support, friendship, and profound belief and pride in close family ties.*

Foreword

In a culture in which one has little personal exposure to death and bereavement prior to one's thirties, the idea that children can be subject to life-threatening illness and even die, is considered absurd. While it is true that the infant and childhood mortality rate is significantly less than it was one-hundred, or even fifty years ago, children come with no more guarantees than do the rest of humanity.

The question that the authors of this, the second volume in Professor David Adams and Mrs. Eleanor Deveau's *Beyond the Innocence of Childhood: Helping Children and Adolescents Cope with Life-Threatening Illness and Dying* is how we might help children and their families achieve fulfillment in life, no matter how shortened or compromised their lives might be. Death today is more technological, isolating, and ambiguous than it has been in the past. In prolonging life, medical technology has separated the chronically ill and the dying persons from their families and other sources of meaning. Meaningfulness will be found only in open communication, in superb symptom management, and in spiritual and emotional support.

Caregivers are called upon to show children and their families that their lives can have meaning in spite of adversity. There are many ways of implementing such care. The school can be a source of support and meaning. Art, music, play, and story, normal parts of a child's day, can be used for teaching and as expressive therapies. The limits of our aid to threatened children are only the limits of our imagination and our commitment.

It is an honor to be invited to write a foreword to the second volume of this series in which the need for, and aspects of care for seriously ill and dying children are explored. The editors of this volume and the other authors of the chapters constitute a "who's who" of teachers, researchers, and clinicians who care for children. There could be no single person or group more qualified to bring together a number of experts than Professor Adams and Mrs. Deveau.

John D. Morgan

Acknowledgments

We owe a debt of gratitude to the contributing authors for sharing their time, effort, and expertise in producing the chapters which appear in the three volumes of this book.

We are indebted to Dr. J. D. (Jack) Morgan who provided support and encouragement at each phase of the development of this project and to Stuart Cohen, President of Baywood Publishing Company and his staff for making this publication a reality.

A special thank you is extended to Dr. Phyllis Blumberg, Professor, Family Medicine and Director, Geriatric Educational Development Unit, Educational Centre for Aging and Health, Faculty of Health Sciences, McMaster University, for her encouragement, understanding, and patience. Our appreciation is extended to R. E. (Ted) Capstick, Chair, Board of Trustees, Greater Hamilton Employee Assistance Consortium and Vice President, Human Resources, Chedoke-McMaster Hospitals; Dr. Nick Kates, Past Chair, Department of Psychiatry, Faculty of Health Sciences, McMaster University; and Dr. Michael Stevens, Senior Staff Specialist and Head, Oncology Unit, Royal Alexandra Hospital for Children, Camperdown NSW, Australia, for their encouragement and continuing support.

We wish to thank J. Richard Small, M.S.W., C.S.W. for his suggestions and advice; Trudy Leask for typing parts of the manuscripts and helping to communicate with the authors; and Lois Wyndam and her staff at Chedoke-McMaster Hospitals Library for their bibliographical assistance.

Finally, we are most grateful to our spouses, J. Paul Deveau and M. Anne Adams, for their **patience**, advice, and assistance. With continual support, understanding, and encouragement from Paul, Anne, and our children we were able to immerse ourselves in the thousands of pages of manuscripts and complete a challenging, interesting and, at times, monumental task!

Table of Contents

Introduction

The first volume of this series, **Beyond the Innocence of Childhood**, focused on issues related to how children and adolescents acquire a mature understanding of death and then examined how influences in today's society, such as the media, political conflict, and AIDS affect children and adolescents' attitudes toward death. Other topics included the impact of a country's culture on the management of childhood cancer and the role of traditional death rituals on children and adolescents' understanding of, and adjustment to, death.

The first part of this volume contains chapters that focus on: therapeutic techniques and adjuncts for children with life-threatening illness; camps; interventions for potentially suicidal adolescents; and challenges for alleviating the pain and suffering of seriously ill children and adolescents. The second part of this volume includes: the palliative care of dying children; dying adolescents; therapeutic imagery; truth-telling; spirituality; the development of a pediatric hospice; and an annotated resource of relevant stories and reading materials.

VOLUME 2–PART A:
Helping Children and Adolescents Cope with Life-Threatening Illness and Threat to their Lives

The world of seriously ill children and adolescents is filled with uncertainty and lack of control. Expressive techniques such as art, story, music, and play provide non-threatening mediums through which children can reveal difficult feelings, incorporate problem-solving skills, and release their emotions.

Robert Stevenson begins by describing a drawing as a lens which can help us to "see" what a child may be thinking or feeling. Children and adolescents facing life-threatening illness seek ways to express their inner feelings. The use of artwork may permit the translation of their hopes and fears into spontaneous drawings. Stevenson stresses

1

the importance of avoiding the overanalyses of drawings and encourages their use as a focal point for discussion and to facilitate communication.

Donna O'Toole introduces the use of *story* as a multifaceted approach which "may mend us when we are broken (and) heal us when we are sick." Story provides seriously ill children and their families with the potential to gain insight, release internalized or repressed feelings, piece together their "brokenness," and restore their lives.

Petra Hinderer describes music therapy as a technique which has similar restorative and healing capabilities to those of *story*. Music provides another medium through which children's moods, feelings, and tensions are transformed into sound thus allowing them to build a bridge to the external world. She suggests that music may offer a sanctuary where difficult feelings can be more easily expressed when disguised in a melody.

As a child life specialist, Ruth Snider believes that play is the "unique language of children." Therapeutic play provides opportunities for seriously ill children to manipulate medical equipment, act out procedures and treatments, express intense anxiety, and gain control over difficult situations in a safe environment.

Humor and laughter are cathartic processes which may provide much needed release when emotions are strained and tensions are high. As Gerry Cox and associates explain, humor and laughter allow seriously ill children and their families to escape, if only for a very short time, to a world where illness, pain, suffering, and impending loss do not exist.

Additional therapeutic benefits may be derived from pets who provide unconditional sources of love, comfort, and acceptance when children and adolescents' lives are severely compromised. Sharon McMahon supports the belief that pets are "restorative agents" and "milieu enhancers" that empower children to face and overcome the difficult challenges of life-threatening illness.

Increasing survival rates, long-term remissions, and cures emphasize the importance of addressing the psychosocial and developmental needs of children with cancer and their siblings. John Maher provides extensive insight into the establishment, operation, and therapeutic value of camp as a special place away from the hospital where children and teens can develop friendships, and acquire new coping skills, independence, and self-confidence. In addition, Maher focuses on the growing population of children with HIV/AIDS who would also benefit from camp experiences, but unfortunately are denied access to regular camps. He believes that when professionals incorporate adequate precautions, protect confidentiality, and maintain sensitivity to these children's particular needs, they will provide a milieu in which children with HIV/AIDS can share common bonds and receive support in a camp setting.

The greater number of adolescents who think about suicide and the higher number of suicide attempts in this age group emphasize the need to pay particular attention to the work of Antoon Leenaars and Susanne Wenckstern. They stress that there is a lack of understanding of suicide itself, an underestimation of the pain of these young people, and an oversimplification of their treatment needs. Suicidal adolescents must have long-term treatment to cope with their hurt, anguish, depression, helplessness, and hopelessness.

We must not ignore the fact that many children and teens experience pain and suffering from the sequelae of life-threatening illness. We know that children are very resilient but we also know that suffering consumes their energy, weakens their tenacity, interferes with their ability to cope, and increases their dependence on others. David Adams discusses the intellectual, instrumental, physical, emotional, social, and existential challenges faced by suffering children and teens. He suggests that caregivers must work with children and their families to find ways to control, decrease, and preferably eliminate, their suffering.

VOLUME 2–PART B:
Helping Dying Children and Adolescents

Dying children and adolescents have the right to receive palliative care that is carefully planned and implemented by staff whose mandate is to maintain children's quality of life rather than unrealistically continue aggressive treatment. They are also entitled to honesty regarding their illness and should be included when planning their care. Such care must be flexible enough to accommodate children and their families in the familiar surroundings of their home, at the hospital, or at times, in both settings.

Michael Stevens emphasizes the need to establish a foundation for effective palliative care during the early management of childhood cancer, should such care become necessary. From diagnosis on, families require open and honest communication, ongoing support, and continuity of caregivers. Stevens provides valuable guidelines for working with dying children, parents, and siblings. He underscores the need to preserve hope at all stages of the child's illness including the terminal phase.

Mark Greenberg defines hospitals as bureaucratic systems which may lack the flexibility to accommodate the needs of terminally ill children and their parents. He graphically illustrates the challenges faced by parents in their 'cocooning' role as protectors, monitors, gatekeepers, and controllers. Greenberg suggests that caregivers shed the standard image of the dying child as one of sadness, misery, pain, and distress because "children are as variable in their dying as they are in their living."

For adolescents, impending death destroys personal goals, threatens and alters their body integrity, gradually erodes their independence, and forecasts the inevitable loss of friends and family. From her experience as a clinical social worker, Joan Auden provides several useful guidelines which address the thoughts, beliefs, feelings, concerns, and needs of dying adolescents.

Leora Kuttner and Cindy Stutzer describe imagery as a nonintrusive, gentle, yet powerful way to join with children and adolescents in managing serious illness and coping with dying. Imagery helps to sustain children's inner strength and self-esteem by providing diversion from fear, anxiety, tension, and pain. They believe that imagery is a link with the child's inner process which can release the kind of energy that "lifts the spirit" even as death approaches.

A recurring theme throughout this series is the need to be open and honest with children and adolescents. When death is imminent does telling the truth burden children with unnecessary anxiety and grief? Do children have a right to know that they are dying? John Maher and Eleanor Pask bring us face to face with the challenges that confront parents and professionals when they must decide if they should tell the truth to dying children.

According to Barrie deVeber: "The problem is not in determining whether or not children are spiritual but whether or not they are given a chance to develop their spirituality." His chapter identifies spirituality as a vital component in an holistic approach to the care of dying children and their families. deVeber challenges professionals to examine their own spirituality and to interact with children to address their spiritual questions, concerns, and needs.

The step-by-step challenges of developing the first free standing children's hospice in North America are delineated by Betty Davies and Brenda Eng. They believe that a children's hospice can make a significant difference in the lives of dying children and their families. Hospice provides a home-like environment in which parents remain the primary caregivers and all family members are encouraged to be part of the decision-making process regarding terminal care.

The final chapter in this volume by Donna O'Toole is an adjunct to her previous chapter which discussed how story and active imagination help seriously ill children and their families. She provides an extensive annotated bibliography of current storytelling and reading materials including therapeutic story resources, stories to read aloud and to tell, stories written by and about seriously ill or bereaved children, and books which address feelings.

VOLUME 3

The third volume of this series, *Beyond the Innocence of Childhood,* takes the reader into the world of bereaved children and adolescents. The death of someone close forces these young people to face intense feelings and contend with many changes. Their grief is an ongoing process which is gradually integrated and becomes a part of their lives. Grief during childhood and adolescence goes on for a long time and may, in fact, be timeless.

This volume begins by addressing the phenomenon of anticipatory grief, considers what is required to respect bereaved children and adolescents, and reflects upon the role of religion and spirituality during bereavement. The long-term implications of the death of a brother, sister, or parent are discussed, followed by sensitive accounts of the traumatic impact of the death of a family member from AIDS and suicide. Losses accumulated as a result of domestic violence render an additional dimension to the grief experienced by some children and adolescents. Attention then turns to the critical role that the school plays in helping students deal with the death of a friend or classmate. This volume closes with a final section on the structure and benefits of support groups for bereaved children and adolescents.

VOLUME 2–PART A

Helping Children and Adolescents Cope with Life-Threatening Illness and Threat to their Lives

CHAPTER 1

The Use of Art in Helping Children Cope with Life-Threatening Illness

Robert G. Stevenson

What can I do to help this child cope with this situation? This question is one asked by many caring adults. It has often been asked by parents of a sick child. When a child is facing a life-threatening illness, the question takes on even greater urgency. If we could know what the child is thinking and feeling at this time, an answer to the question might be clearer. However, children often cannot find a way to express those thoughts or feelings. They may not be able to find the words, or they may simply feel too overwhelmed to even try to communicate. One way of finding possible answers to the questions we ask is to use the child's artwork, spontaneous drawings, as a lens to help us "see" what a child may be thinking or feeling.

Death and the emotions it inspires have long been topics for the world's artists. A trip to almost any art museum will provide numerous examples of such pictures. These artists have used their talents to illustrate universal themes, to share their thoughts and feelings with others, and to reexamine the topic for themselves. The collected work of an artist is a body of information. This information has been used as a lens through which information about these artists, their lives and personalities can be examined. Such examination of art is not limited to the dusty work of long-dead artists. People of all ages create art on a daily basis, everything from formal paintings to personal doodles. It may be hard to think of the crayons in the basic "Crayola 8" as tools with which to examine personal thoughts and feelings, but through a method of art interpretation they can be just that. For older children, art interpretation can be a way to know more about their own personalities. For parents, health care professionals, educators, and other caring adults who work with children facing life-threatening illness, the lens provided by these works of art can be a valuable tool indeed, since it can help young children express thoughts and feelings for which they might not be able to find the words.

The spontaneous artwork of children can serve as a focal point for discussion and can help others to understand the thoughts, fears and hopes of those children. The work of Furth [1, 2], Buck [3], DiLeo [4, 5], Burns and Kaufman [6, 7], and Bach [8] have shown the valuable role that the spontaneous drawings of children can play. There are two basic ways of looking at such artwork: the quantitative approach and the qualitative approach.

QUANTITATIVE EVALUATION

An example of the quantitative approach can be found in *The House Tree Person Technique: Revised Manual* by Buck [3]. Detail, proportion and perspective in a subject's drawings are assigned numerical values and these are used to classify the intelligence and developmental level of the artist. There is some controversy concerning the validity of the quantitative method of scoring. There is disagreement over whether these quantitative evaluations can be deceived by someone who knows of particular symbols and their meaning. Even if this method is useful for professionals, it would be difficult or impossible for parents or any non-professionals to gain anything from this system.

QUALITATIVE SCORING

The quantitative evaluation of art does require detailed knowledge, but a qualitative approach does not require the same type of detailed knowledge to be useful. The approach developed by Furth has been shown to be a method of facilitating communication between artists and children, on the one hand, and parents, teachers or other adults who are seeking to better understand them [2]. The method is simple to describe, but becomes more effective with time and experience. It also gives an active role to both the artist, the child, and to the caring adult. The child's picture is looked at by the adult, who then asks himself and the child a series of questions about the artwork. These questions are designed to have the viewer look at the drawing from more than one perspective, and to look at the artist and the artist's life in the same way. Furth tells the viewer to begin by asking himself/herself, "What do you see in this drawing?" [2]. This basic question is then followed by more specific questions, such as:

- What is present?
- What is missing?
- What is odd or unusual?
- What features stand out? How do they stand out?
- If you were "in" this picture, how would you feel?
- If colors are used, what do these colors suggest?
- What numbers are repeated?

The uses of colors and numbers are based on the work of Carl Jung [9]. He identified special importance for these symbols. His work with symbols has been summarized and explained by Jacobi [10] and expanded by Furth [2].

The details of each drawing are examined by looking at such points as the placement of figures or objects, movement, or unusual details. The placement of figures and direction of any movement can be important. For example, a drawing made with the paper in a vertical position may be said to "make a statement" while a horizontal position often "tells a story." The top half of the paper can be said to represent the mind (or spiritual aspects) of the artist, while the lower half relates to the body (or physical functioning) of the artist. Things depicted in the center of the page may describe an issue of "central importance" [2].

The child is then asked to describe the picture in his or her own words, beginning a discussion of the picture. "Tell me about your picture," may seem to be the obvious starting point, but it is sometimes overlooked by adults who are "sure" they already know what a picture means. The child does not cease to be an active participant, merely because the drawing is completed to his or her satisfaction. They should be active in looking at what it *may* represent. The adult listening to the child's description of the drawing must try his/her best to be non-judgmental. Issues should not be addressed with labels such as "good/bad." Reactions to the child's description should be neutral so as not to influence the child to tell a story we hope to hear instead of one they actually drew. The picture is simply a "lens." Through this lens the child and the adult can each have a better understanding of the thoughts and feelings which may be expressed in this picture.

THE CHILD AND LIFE-THREATENING
ILLNESS

While the techniques for drawing interpretation developed by Furth and others can be used with anyone, there are some special benefits which can be gained when they are used with a child trying to cope with a life-threatening illness. Children facing such an illness may experience helplessness, loneliness, anger, sadness, guilt, fear or any combination of these feelings. They are seeking ways to express their feelings, to let off some of the pressures that can be building up inside.

Helplessness

Creating a picture is a first step in getting out some of those thoughts and feelings that are building up "inside." Just putting them "outside," in this way, is a first step in regaining a feeling of control at a time when so many things can seem out of control.

Loneliness

If a child can put his/her thoughts and feelings in a picture (even unconsciously) and then share them with someone else, it is a type of communication. Sharing feelings in this way can strengthen the good feelings and help cope with the ones that hurt. My wise Irish grandmother often said, "When happiness and love are shared, they are multiplied. When sorrow and pain are shared they are divided." A child's drawing can be a means for just such sharing.

Anger

It is not fair when life, or fate, or God, forces a child to face the circumstance of a life-threatening illness. When children see unfairness, they get angry. They may be angry at God, at "life," or at the people in their lives. Their drawing can be a way to vent this anger. Once it is expressed on paper, they can show it to other people and talk about it.

Sadness

The sadness of children comes from several possible sources. They may be sad at the possibility of losing those that they love. The sadness may come from the inevitability of change, since change is something which young children do not always welcome. There are many losses that accompany the course of a life-threatening illness. These may include loss of strength, loss of body image through amputation or the side effects of chemotherapy, loss of the ability to do things such as run, throw, play or go to school. Children may be sad at their inability to enjoy a life that may soon end. They may also be sad because they believe that when they are gone, they will have left nothing behind by which they can be remembered. Drawings can help to identify the cause of the sadness. The drawings themselves can be a legacy to others. The way in which people react to, and appreciate, the drawings can show young people that they are special and that they still have the ability to create things which make people happy.

Guilt

A life-threatening illness is felt, by some children, to be a punishment for past misdeeds, real or imaginary, or for bad thoughts. If the illness is *really* bad, then their actions or thoughts must have been *really* bad as well. Drawing can offer ways to identify feelings of guilt and may also be a form of catharsis.

Fear

Drawings can once again provide a means of identifying the things that children fear. They can also be a tool for children to find ways of coping with those fears. Drawing gives a child an outlet to represent personified fears, such as the fear of death or dying.

An example of the way in which children translate their fears (and hopes) into drawings can be seen in a picture drawn by Sean when he was starting school (Figure 1). This picture was found on a small piece of paper in one of his school books. When asked what it was, he said it was a "friendly monster." This friendly monster would protect him from "bad monsters." If they came near Sean, his friendly monster would bite them on the leg and make them go away.

The friendly monster could not be hurt because, as you can see, it had no legs that could be bitten. Sean often took his fears and translated them into a drawing. On his own he had also begun to construct *defenses* against his fears. His picture of a "friendly monster" was an amulet to help keep bad things ("monsters") away . . . an amulet of his own creation.

Like Sean, Grant, who was an older adolescent facing metastatic cancer, drew pictures which reflected his fears and coping. In every picture he drew there was a person or a house. That person or house was turned to the side, never facing the viewer. This repeated type of portrayal is often seen when there is some issue that the artist does not wish to confront directly. Talks with Grant, and knowledge of his intelligence and his behavior, confirmed that these pictures showed the way in which Grant was coping with his illness. He knew the illness was there and what the ultimate consequences would be. He spoke to college classes for nurses about his condition including his reactions to the treatments he had received and to the caregivers who had provided them. However, in his day-to-day activities, he wanted to concentrate

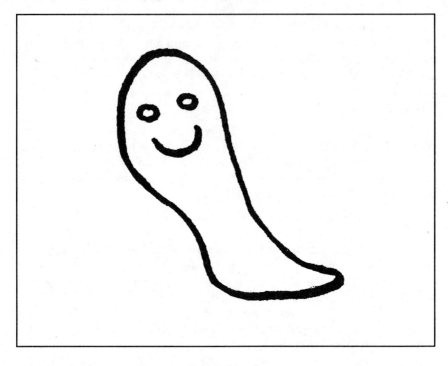

Figure 1. Sean's friendly monster.

on life and chose not to speak of death. In a picture drawn close to his death, he was asked to draw his favorite place. He drew a small black cabin (turned to the side) standing alone on a wide open plain. The ground and sky were colored with pale yellow, some gold and a great deal of orange. Orange is a color which may indicate a situation which needs to be resolved or one which is life threatening. His house was alone. There were no roads, no mountains or buildings in the distance, no animals or birds. Shortly after drawing this picture, he had his three private duty nurses replaced. They believed that it was to spare them from being there when he died. Throughout his illness he almost never spoke of it with family or friends, but he said a great deal about it through his pictures.

THE USE OF COLOR

It is important not to overanalyze these drawings. However, we can examine a number of factors and ask ourselves and, where appropriate, ask the child, "Could this be true?" The use of color is such an area.

Colors set a tone in a drawing, as does an absence of color. However, for this to be an important factor, the child must have a variety of colors. It is preferable if all of the colors of the spectrum are available to the child. Then colors can give added dimension to a drawing by looking at the ones that were chosen and at those that were omitted.

. Those who use a Jungian approach to drawing interpretation have developed a set of basic information about color in drawings. The following information is **not** exhaustive, but it can give an indication of information which can be revealed through an examination of the use of color in Western psychology.

Red

The color red may be used to portray an issue of "burning" importance, surging emotions, or danger. Pink sometimes suggests an illness just past, as in feeling "in the pink."

Orange

This is often used with a situation which needs to be resolved. It may reflect a suspenseful situation, especially a life and death struggle. It may represent rescue from a threatening situation (or the desire for such a rescue). It may even symbolize *courage* in the face of such a situation.

Yellow

Golden yellow may suggest an emphasis on things of a spiritual or intuitive nature, something of great value, or a life-giving source of energy (such as the sun). Pale yellow can indicate a precarious life situation.

Green

Yellow (pale) green may relate to psychological or physical weakness, a fading out of life or a coming back to life (with the aid of treatment). Dark green may reflect good health, growth, or newness of life (as in a healing process).

Blue

Pale blue may represent distance, as in the far-away pale blue sky, a fading away or distancing, or a period of contemplation or even depression. Bright blue is often connected to health, the vital flow of life, or energy.

Brown

Dark brown may indicate nourishment, health, or a person who is "in touch" with nature or the earth. Pale brown may denote rot or decay, or a struggle to overcome destructive forces and return to a healthy state.

Purple

This is a color related to *control*. It may indicate a need to feel more in control, to have more control/support from others, or the feeling of being controlled. It may be connected to some burden or responsibility (a "cross to bear"). It may depict a controlling situation, sovereignty, or even supreme power (physical or emotional).

Black

Black often symbolizes the "unknown." It can be connected with "dark" thoughts, a threat, a fear, or an uncertain future.

White

In drawings, white may be represented by uncolored paper. This indicates an absence of color and is associated with repressed feelings. If colored in after all other colors have been used, it can sometimes indicate thoughts of the end of life.

There are those who believe that physical (somatic) health can be seen in drawings. One noted surgeon uses the drawings of patients as part of his diagnostic process. However, there are themes which reoccur frequently enough to deserve mention. Leukemic children use the colors red and white as a recurring theme in their drawings. This use of color in drawings as part of a diagnostic process may be of value to the medical community but it is best left to them. This sort of drawing interpretation is not of real value to family members or other concerned adults and may lead to undue anxiety on the part of all concerned.

One of the most common errors in drawing interpretation is "over-interpreting" the content of drawings. Looking at the colors used is, perhaps, the most common way in which people overinterpret. Such mistakes occur most frequently when the artist is left out of the process. A good example of "overinterpretation" can be seen in one episode of *The Dick Van Dyke Show*. Rob and Laura Petrie are called to their son's school by the school psychologist. He informs them that Richie is "depressed" and that this can be seen by his use of black in painting all his pictures in art class. The opinion of this professional is that Richie should be in therapy. However, Rob and Laura insist on speaking to Richie first. They ask him why his pictures are all black and he says, "because I'm short." The psychologist smiles smugly. They ask Richie to explain further and he says that when it is time to paint, he cannot reach the shelf where the paint jars are stored. By the time he gets a chair, all of the colors are gone except black. It seems that he is a happy, well adjusted child who is painting with the only color available.

A different result can be expected when the artist's insights are included along with the drawing. When he was in second grade, Sean drew the picture reproduced in Figure 2. He had all colors available, but drew the picture entirely in orange. When asked to tell us about the drawing, he said it was a picture of him, that the circle represented the sun and on the side was a table. The reversal of person and sun showed that, in this drawing, things were out of their traditional place. One object was still unexplained. When asked what was on the table, Sean replied, "It's a dead body." That statement gave the clue that opened up the meaning of the drawing.

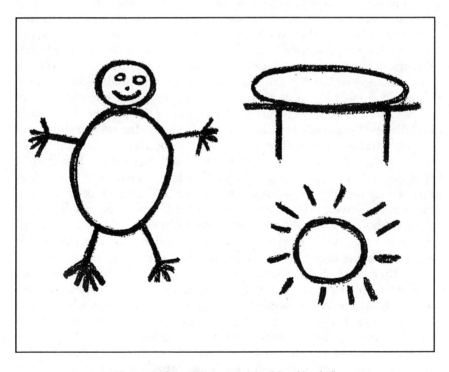

Figure 2. Sean, the sun and a "dead body."

A former student had died several weeks before, following a long battle with bone cancer. Early in his bout with the illness one of his legs had been amputated. During his treatments, Sean and I had visited him at his home. He had shared candy and stories with Sean and his death had been one of the saddest days of Sean's young life. Sean had not spoken of it since the young man died. However, his drawing showed how he was trying to understand what had happened, and how he was trying to explain it to himself. To many young children, the term "body" means "torso." Sean knew his friend had a leg amputated and he was still alive. In Sean's mind, as his friend got sicker, he must have lost his other leg, then his arms and, finally, his head . . . so he died. Until we saw his drawing, Sean, at age six, had been pondering questions of life and death on his own. When he could not speak about his feelings, his drawing allowed him to express his concerns to others. With the lines of communication open, help and healing could begin.

ART AS A LENS

This sort of communication is not limited to young children. Young people of all ages can use drawings as a lens through which they and others can look at the events in their lives. Ellen was a high school senior who felt pressured because her life seemed to be out of control. When she tried to speak about her feelings she would cry for the entire time, sobbing so heavily she could not speak. She produced two drawings and was finally able to speak as she described her pictures. In both, she and her father were in the center of the picture. Her father had died two years earlier. She now had to choose the college she would attend. That decision involved selecting the country, the United States or her father's country, where she would build her future. She wished that her father could help her decide. She had been unable to speak to anyone in her family because, when her father had died, a well-meaning relative said that she must not cry but must be strong for her family. She added that it was "what your father would have wanted." She was now unable to speak to her family about the decision which she must make because she was afraid that she would cry . . . and let her father down. She took the two drawings home and spoke to her mother about them. Speaking about her drawings allowed her to open a discussion about her pent-up feelings and the decision she felt she had to make. Feelings were released, the situation was resolved and the two drawings had provided the starting point.

Ellen and the people she loved cared for each other. They held in their feelings because they did not want others to worry or to share their pain. Young people facing life-threatening illness sometimes hold in their feelings for similar reasons. They do so to *protect* the people they love. The intent is good, but the effect is to isolate everyone. Fear, isolation, and anxiety grow in such a lonely atmosphere. Any technique which facilitates communication and sharing can help both the young person and the others in their lives.

AN INVITATION TO DRAW

It is not difficult to have young children draw. They seem to do it as a natural part of life. They need not draw about a particular theme, or follow specific instructions. Their pictures simply spill out onto paper and those pictures provide a starting point for looking at their lives. Adolescents, however, must sometimes be encouraged, and their fears addressed, before they are willing to draw. They want to be sure that they will not be embarrassed. They may be so critical of their own work that they are afraid others will "judge" their drawings in a similar manner. They may be afraid of revealing "too much." It is important that young people feel that they are "in control" through this experience. The drawing is theirs. The meaning is theirs. It is their decision whether or not to share it with others. The way in which the idea of drawing is suggested can be central in helping an adolescent decide whether or not they wish to cooperate by drawing. A simple introduction can help to clarify the role of this drawing. The following scripts are samples of how this introduction can be accomplished.

Script

> Everyone has feelings. These feelings can be exciting, happy, scary, or confusing. Sometimes it is hard to tell other people about these feelings. We may not even be sure ourselves. One way to show these feelings to other people or to ourselves is to put them on paper. Drawing, and talking with someone about the drawing, can make these feelings clearer. I would like you to draw a picture of . . . (insert topic).

When the young person is finished, ask him or her to tell you about their picture. The topic can be a general one (a favorite place, doing something with others) or a more directed theme (a self-portrait, a picture of the child's illness, or a picture which shows the child's plans/hopes for the future). The topic should be appropriate to the feelings and attitude of the young person involved.

The topic portrayed by these drawings will not necessarily be about the young people themselves. Many young people use these drawings to present honest and touching responses to the death of people they loved, perhaps in an attempt to strengthen themselves as they confront their own mortality. These were not bitter revelations; for the most part they were very moving outpourings of sorrow for the loss of a grandparent, a father taken by cancer, a child, a mother, a friend. Other comments revealed a sentiment of kinship with animals and a parallel anger that some people remain indifferent to the killing of whales, or seals, or deer. Death is often a theme, but it may not be presented as directly affecting the young person.

A parallel theme is that of relationships. Drawings depict the relationships important to the artist, showing the people in the life of this young person. It is these relationships which may be lost in the face of life-threatening illness. The drawings allow the young person to speak about the important roles played by others.

These drawings have also served as the basis for a discussion of the artist's "view" of death. Something in the drawing may be said to represent "death." It has been found through examination of spontaneous drawings that an abstract representation of death is produced by those who view death as an abstract concept. More concrete representations indicate concern about a particular death or type of death (sometimes based on past losses) [11]. Young people who are aware that they are battling a life-threatening illness typically view death in a very concrete way.

The most common illustrations of a concrete "death" followed those of traditional Western artists: the dark, hooded form of the "grim reaper" (often complete with scythe), a "grinning" skull, or a human form (in the classic "kneeling-running" position of one about to die, in repose in a casket, or as a seductive, beckoning figure).

CONCLUSION

When a young person faces a life-threatening illness, it has an impact on every aspect of that young person's life. The medical community has developed treatment protocols for treating the physical impact of the illness. The emotional, psychological and social effects must also be addressed. The spontaneous drawings of these young people can be helpful to those who wish to understand and to help them cope with these other dimensions of life-threatening illness. The drawings can also assist these young people toward a better understanding of themselves. Such an understanding may give them stronger feelings of self-control at a difficult time in their lives.

The interpretation of the artwork of these young people is both an art and a science. Knowledge of symbols and psychological studies of *children* must be accompanied by care and concern for *this child* in this situation. Art can be a method of uniting knowledge and caring and, as such, merits further study by those who are providing care for a child facing life-threatening illness.

REFERENCES

1. G. Furth, The Use of Drawings Made at Significant Times in One's Life, in *Living with Death and Dying*, E. Kübler-Ross (ed.), Macmillan, New York, 1981.
2. G. Furth, *The Secret World of Drawings: Healing Through Art*, Sigo Press, Boston, Massachusetts, 1988.
3. J. N. Buck, *The House-Tree-Person Technique: Revised Manual*, Western Psychological Services, Los Angeles, California, 1981.
4. J. H. DiLeo, *Interpretation of Children's Drawings*, Brunner/Mazel, New York, 1983.
5. J. H. DiLeo, *Young Children and Their Drawings*, Brunner/Mazel, New York, 1970.
6. R. C. Burns and S. H. Kaufman, *Actions, Styles and Symbols in Kinetic Family Drawings*, Brunner/Mazel, New York, 1972.
7. R. C. Burns and S. H. Kaufman, *Kinetic Family Drawings*, Brunner/Mazel, New York, 1970.
8. S. R. Bach, *Spontaneous Pictures of Leukemic Children as an Expression of the Total Personality, Mind and Body*, Schwabe and Co., New York, 1975.
9. C. G. Jung, *Man and His Symbols*, Doubleday and Company, Garden City, New York, 1964.
10. J. Jacobi, *The Psychology of C. G. Jung*, Yale University Press, New Haven, 1973.
11. R. G. Stevenson, *Draw What You See: An Exercise To Explore Student Views of Death,* paper presented at the Association for Death Education and Counseling 11th Annual Conference, Baltimore, Maryland, 1989.

BIBLIOGRAPHY

Bettelheim, B., *The Uses of Enchantment: The Meaning and Importance of Fairy Tales*, Vintage Books, New York, 1976.

Dennis, W., *Group Values Through Children's Drawings*, John Wiley & Sons, New York, 1966.

Edwards, B., *Drawing on the Right Side of the Brain*, J. P. Tarcher, New York, 1979.

Favat, F. A., *Child and Tale: The Origins of Interest,* National Council of Teachers of English, Urbana, Illinois, 1977.

Kellogg, R., *The Psychology of Children's Art*, CRM Inc., Chicago, Illinois, 1967.

Schildkrout, M. S., Shenker, I. R. and Sonnenblick, M., *Human Figure Drawings in Adolescence*, Brunner/Mazel, New York, 1970.

Von Franz, M. L., *The Feminine In Fairytales*, Spring Publications, Irving, Texas, 1972.

Von Franz, M. L., *Interpretation of Fairy Tales*, Spring Publications, Zurich, 1975.

CHAPTER 2

Re-storying Brokenness: Using Story and Active Imagination to Help Seriously Ill Children and Their Families

Donna O'Toole

> Everything is story. Break the pattern that connects and you destroy all quality. Restore the pattern that connects and you enter into all kinds of evolutionary options [1].

The diagnosis of a life-threatening illness or the death of a loved one can be a break, even a gaping hole, in the fabric of life. These losses represent the unfinished sentences, paragraphs, and chapters in the life story of individuals and families.

Yet many who have processed great losses know that brokenness can be only part of the story. These people have navigated the pain of loss and have emerged feeling connected and restored. They have recognized their losses and have reckoned with them. They have rewoven the fabric. They have written new chapters. Having experienced their losses fully, they report personal stories of healing and growth. Rather than being diminished by brokenness, they have been expanded.

The thesis of this chapter is that restoration of a broken story has at its heart the connective power of narrative thought—the world of story. Unlike scientific paradigms that use logical proof and tightly reasoned analysis to predict and control reality, the narrative approach to life relies on interactive or internal experiences. Narrative approaches do not rely on theories which tend to suggest the way things should be. Instead, narrative thought welcomes subjective realities and encourages creativity and flexibility. This allows children, or adults who are already challenged by change, to be nourished by possibilities rather than impoverished by existing structures that no longer fit their life situation.

Let us explore the practice of story together. This chapter will discuss principles that undergird and guide the use of story as a therapeutic practice. Suggestions for specific ways that story can be used to reweave or "re-story" brokenness for seriously ill and dying children and their families will be offered.

STORY:
THE NATURAL LANGUAGE OF CHILDREN

> Responding spontaneously is what most children do best. They do not try to figure out the story being presented; they simply enter into it with the full force of their imaginative powers. These imaginative powers are the critical substance of change and healing once they are activated. The metaphor can act as flame to candle, igniting the child's imagination to it's brightest valence of strength, self knowledge, and transformation [2, p. xxi].

Story is the natural language of children. At an early age children know what is and is not story [3, p. 24]. Story researcher, Gussin Paley explains how preschool children play and think as follows:

> Children are born knowing how to put every thought and feeling into story form. If they worry about being lost, they become the parents who search; if angry, they find a hot hippopotamus to impose his will upon the world. Even happiness has its plot and characters: "Pretend I'm the baby and you can love only me and you don't talk on the telephone" [4, p. 20].

For children the actual story, and the playing out of the story, can be resolution in itself. Further, it is the images in stories, not the stories themselves, that children appropriate to suit their immediate personal wishes and desires. McAdams suggests that children "make the image do what they want it to do, even in ways that seem strange and illogical to adults" [3, p. 55].

Children often resist or avoid all efforts to verbally analyze or gain conscious awareness of the stories they so naturally engage in [3, p. 2]. Indeed, children are surprised and embarrassed if references are made to anything overheard when they are in the dreamlike state of story and play [4, p. 22]. One explanation for this reservation may be that many children below the age of ten or eleven have not yet mastered rational thinking. Be that as it may, even bright children who abstract and analyze information at an early age usually prefer to solve problems and order meaning through a process of subjective realities [3, pp. 24-27].

Story comes in many forms and is used for many purposes. In some instances, the stories we tell ourselves and the stories others tell us may mend us when we are broken, heal us when we are sick, and move us toward psychological wholeness and maturity. Stories that heal often exude some measure of optimism and hope [3, pp. 31-33, 47-49]. This healing can happen in spite of the adversity of ill health or the reality of grievous loss. Such is the story I am about to tell.

A Personal Story

Although he was pale and thin, nine-year-old Matthew Schmidt knew himself in another way—he was "Super Cystic." "Super Cystic" had many powerful friends and cohorts. There was an inventive nurse named "Fabulous Fran Fibrosis," as well as "IV Man," "Bob The Breather," "Carol Capsule," "Polly Pounder," "Ralph Respiratory," and "Erving Enzyme." Together "Super Cystic" and his mighty, wise friends would battle the powerful bad guys—the bugs—"Boris Bacteria" and "Nasty Pneumonia." It was from "Super Cystic" that I first realized the power of story and imagination in dealing with emotionally charged and life-threatening experiences.

In real life "Super Cystic" was my son, Matt. Matt was born with cystic fibrosis, a hereditary disease that adversely affects the inward secreting functions of the body, primarily the lungs and the digestive system. Matt died when he was twenty-one years old. But I prefer to say it this way—"My son, Matt, lived well for twenty-one years." His life was rarely easy, but it was good; I heard him say this many times. Although ultimately he could not stave off the infections that gradually limited his physical abilities, he was anything but a victim. I watched Matt's creative spirit blossom and then bear fruit even in the midst of physical decay.

In his imagination, Matt could and did experience many things that he could not experience in the ways most people call "real." He once told me about an exceptional experience he had in relationship to his brother, Steven. The event happened just months before Matt's death. Matt was twenty years old at the time and very physically limited by his disease. His poor oxygen exchange allowed him to walk only the briefest distance on the wooded paths he so loved, at a very slow pace. Steven was then a senior in high school and an excellent gymnast.

Although Matt's physical limitations made it difficult for Steven to feel good about excelling in sports, he had, against many odds, worked hard in his gymnastic endeavors. Matt and I were proud of Steven's perseverance and abilities.

There was awe in Matt's voice when he told me that the night before, as he sat in the gym watching his brother perform his floor routine at a regional gymnastic meet, he had actually experienced being in his brother's body. He explained:

> It's hard to talk about, Mom. It's hard to put into words. I don't think other people could believe this, but it really happened.
>
> I was watching Steven come up to the floor mat and I just filled up with love for him. I was so proud of how he moved and how hard he had worked to learn his routine. I could feel his nervousness too—his uncertainty. And then I felt the determination come into his body like a great rush of strength.
>
> Then all of a sudden I had this incredible feeling of sadness. I wanted to feel my body work as freely as Steven's could. I wanted to feel my legs lift my body off the ground—wanted to feel myself somersaulting through the air. Then it happened. I was in the air. I was somehow inside Steven's body, but at the same time it was my body. I felt my legs push up. Then there I was in space. I felt the hard jolt as I came out of the spin, landing firmly on the mat. My breath came easy and strong as I extended my legs, gathered momentum, and ran across the mat before I flew once again into the air. My flip was high. What a feeling!
>
> It happened, Mom, it really happened! I felt it. It was not just my imagination. When the routine was over I was in Steven's body for a while longer—and also in his mind. I knew I had done a great routine. We had done a great job together.

After he told me this, Matt cried for some time. "How will I ever be able to thank Steven for what he gave me last night?" he said. "There was more love in that experience than I could ever give words to." Steven's immediate reward was the high score he received from the judges. Much later he learned the rest of the story.

Matt's imaginative capacities allowed him choices and control that would have otherwise been lost in the circumstances of his disease and the regimen of treatment. When the going became especially rough he could often call forth a larger story, an experience of his own making. With this larger story activated, he was no longer powerless or alone. Those, who have experienced serious illness and grief, know how debilitating powerlessness and loneliness can be if they are not somehow transformed into a sense of mastery and affinity. I watched Matt gradually gain confidence. I, too, was changed. Although his body was wasted, I came to see him as whole. As his parent, I was and continue to be deeply moved and comforted by what I witnessed.

As Matt grew older he gained a deeper compassion for others. He called up the images and experiences he had as a young boy and drew them out in cartoon characters that spoke for themselves. In this way, Matt developed an educational book to help children and families with cystic fibrosis understand and cope with the disease. Through a grant from a pharmaceutical company, his book *Super Cystic and Fabulous Fran Fibrosis* was published and distributed. There have been many stories of how Matt's book helped others whom he was never able to meet. But the helpfulness of Matt's book was not limited to strangers. In printed form, Matt's family and friends were able to witness the experiences of Matt's life in a more imaginative, less painful, and even playful way. Matt had found a way to give his story away to those who needed it most.

UNDERLYING ASSUMPTIONS

> Healing means, first of all, the creation of an empty but friendly space where those who suffer can tell their story to someone who can listen with real attention. Healers are hosts who patiently and carefully listen to the story of the suffering stranger. Patients are guests who rediscover their selves by telling their story to the one who offers them a place to stay [5, pp. 67-68].

Before turning to some of the many ways in which story and imagination can be used as therapeutic practice, a survey of some of the assumptions and principles that serve as a foundation for practice may be helpful.

1. Loss defined: Loss can be defined as the actual or expected deprivation of anyone or anything that is valued, needed, or desired. It is assumed that many actual and expected losses are shadowing the lives of adults, children, and their families who have received a life-threatening diagnosis. This is also assumed to be true if a death has already occurred.

2. Grief is a natural reactionary process to loss: Grief accommodates the realities of physical, spiritual, and existential changes so that the person's unique developmental and spiritual needs can be furthered.

3. Grief is a highly individualized experience: No two people will experience a loss in exactly the same way.

4. Grief affects the whole person: Grief is more than an emotional experience. It also impacts the physical, mental, emotional, social, spiritual, and evolutionary aspects of self.

5. Processing grief involves mastery: Grief is processed as the bereaved person is able to tolerate and safely navigate the pain and dissonance created by the loss. For many, mastery is realized as people gain their own unique balance between facing and avoiding an awareness of the loss.

6. Loss is processed over time: A storied view of life proposes that human development is continual and that loss and grief are likewise processed over time and often across the life span.

7. Processing grief affirms continuity and connectedness: The processing of loss through grief assists people in remembering, integrating, and transforming the loss. Children, siblings, and parents can come to recognize that love and caring transcend death. There is an infinite comfort in knowing that a life will not be forgotten.

8. Children and parents are capable of resilience: Adults and children alike have demonstrated the ability to master cycles of disruption and integration as they deal with the emotional and spiritual pain related to loss, threat to life, and dying [6, 7].

9. Healing is possible in the midst of illness, death, grief and existential tension: In the context of this writing, healing is an expression of being at peace with the self and with the situation. This definition does not imply the absence of illness or grief. Neither does healing necessitate the absence of tension. Existential tension can be understood as a natural state that occurs when a person is simultaneously realizing two basic human needs: the need to be separate and autonomous and the need to lose separateness by merging with someone or something larger than the self [8].

DEFINITIONS, GOALS AND PRINCIPLES TO GUIDE THE USE OF "STORY" FOR THERAPEUTIC MEANS

Externalization is an approach to therapy that encourages persons to objectify and, at times, to personify the problems that they experience as oppressive. In this process, the problem becomes a separate entity and thus external to the person or relationship that was ascribed as the problem [9, p. 38].

Story Defined

Story as therapeutic practice is most commonly spoken of as bibliotherapy [10, p. 12]. However, because the term bibliotherapy is often thought of as related to books, I prefer to describe narrative therapeutic practice as *story*. Story refers to the use of narrative expression in the broadest sense. Story is any narrative form that orders a person's understanding of life and can be used to communicate and express thoughts and feelings. This includes oral presentations, all forms of literature or written presentation, and narrative presentations including plays, audiovisuals, and cartoons. Story material, or story forms, involve language and some degree of internal coherence [10, p. 13]. In the context of this chapter the term story and narrative are used interchangeably.

The Goals of Therapeutic Story

Practitioners of therapeutic story have identified the following goals related to the use of therapeutic story with adults and children:

1. To improve the capacity to respond by stimulating and enriching mental images and concepts and by helping the feelings about these images to surface.
2. To increase self-understanding by helping individuals value their own personhood and become more knowledgeable and more accurate about self-perceptions.
3. To increase awareness of interpersonal relationships.
4. To improve reality orientation.

These goals serve one comprehensive purpose—to improve the participants self-esteem and morale. Toward this intent, therapeutic story materials are chosen to help individuals:

- have a kindly regard for themselves
- find ways to develop themselves more gracefully
- deal more creatively with what cannot be changed [10, p. 24].

Subjective Experience and Inner Strengths

Two hallmarks of story as therapy are worth noting. First, the therapeutic goals of story are based in subjective experience and thought. The wisdom that comes from narrative therapeutic practice specifically addresses an understanding of the self rather than a grasp of the nature of the world at large [10, p. 43].

Second, therapeutic story as practice assumes there is an inner strength inherent in each child and adult. This is the belief that the locus of control is from within—that even young children can access inner strengths for problem-solving and self-healing. Therefore, story as therapy makes a special appeal to make use of a child's unique experience of life and is "directed more to the encouragement and reinforcement of strengths than to the diagnosis of problem areas" [10, p. 17]. The therapeutic effect of any narrative interaction relies on the non-coercive qualities of the story form that is being used. The most effective narrative forms are those that avoid prescription and moralization. Such story forms are rich with all kinds and levels of meaning. They invite subjective interpretation allowing the participant to either reflect on a problem area or to affirm a strength. Either way, the solution to the problem comes from within.

The Role of Insight

Story as therapy often involves an observable complementary process of analysis and synthesis. However, there is evidence in the practice of story as metaphor, that insight is supplemental, even irrelevant to change [11, p. 19]. Therefore, while self-disclosure and discourse may aid people in validating and realizing insights and internal shifts, it is not essential. The very fact that children and adults can utilize a story privately, even without admitting to having had a problem, is one of its stellar qualities.

STORY PRACTICE

> Stories go in circles. They don't go in straight lines. So it helps if you listen in circles because there are stories inside stories and stories between stories and finding your way through them is as easy and as hard as finding your way home. And part of the finding is the getting lost. If you are lost you really start to look around and to listen [12, p. 104].

In this section, I will present a variety of story "forms" that can be used therapeutically with seriously ill children and their families. These include storytelling, cartooning, personal bookmaking as artistic metaphor, story books, and personal story practices. Developing categories for this section has been challenging, since in practice there is considerable overlap. Also, while there is ample information in the literature regarding the therapeutic benefits of particular story forms, there has been little effort to formulate their use with seriously ill, dying, and grieving children and their families.

Therefore, I encourage you to use these ideas more as a catalyst than as a guide. The therapeutic use of story rests strongly in the story leader's ability to match the story content with the listener's personality, circumstances, and present needs, and in many cases to do so in ways that allow for what Milton Erickson termed *indirection*. The use of indirection means presenting story in metaphorical and symbolic terms so that the listener can interact with the material not only through cognition but through unconscious, nonverbal, and indirect channels. One does not have to be a child to know that when it comes to dealing with painful and frightening situations, the safest route may not be the most direct [11, pp. 19-26, 68].

Additionally, there are abundant opportunities for the direct transmission of information from books in the use of therapeutic story by the novice or seasoned story-practitioner. These books, coupled with desire, empathy, astute nonjudgmental observation, and the intractable belief that others are capable of self-healing, will undoubtedly lead you to satisfying and meaningful story experiences.

1. STORYTELLING

The storyteller is one who uses the oral tradition to carry seeds of life that are both actual and mythological [13, p. xi]. Storytelling is a unique and ancient oral art that has been vastly neglected, and in many cases almost lost, in modern life. Stories can be told in all kinds of settings, to people of all ages. All that is required is a teller and a listener.

For its therapeutic value, storytelling is perhaps the most compelling medium of all the story forms. In the past several years, I have had many opportunities to perform stories about loss and grief, and death and dying, to audiences both large and small. It has been a remarkable experience to witness the depth and breadth of the learning that people extract and create from the telling.

Brett, a seasoned Australian psychologist and practitioner of therapeutic storytelling, has effectively used this technique to help children deal with fear, pain, hospitalization and death [14]. Brett gives the following suggestions for therapeutic storytelling with children:

1. Model the story character after the child. This assists the child in using the story through identifying with the character.
2. Make the problems and conflicts echo those of the child. This means that the narrative tone of the story should match how the

child sees the conflict, not how you see it. Again, this assists identity fixation with the story character. The idea is to have the child think, "Yes, that's exactly how I feel." After the child has identified with the character, you introduce the way the story character comes to shift their thinking as they first struggle with, and then resolve, their concern.

3. Keep things simple. Use concepts and language the child can understand. Tailor the length of the story to the child's attention span.

4. Have the story honestly portray real conflict, uncertainty, and struggle. Children have internal experiences of these feelings that need to be matched by the story characters if the story is to be believable.

5. Remember to identify the strengths of the child and weave them into the story. This helps children recognize these traits in themselves and to increase their sense of worth and potency.

6. Use humor whenever possible. Like story, laughter can be good medicine. It too, allows for psychic shifts to take place and helps to release tension.

7. When the child is tense use your voice to encourage relaxation.

8. As you tell your story watch the child for cues. If the child is engaged, you are on target. If children are disinterested, you might be on the wrong track or the content may be something they are not ready to hear.

9. If you are unsure of where to go next, ask the child—"What do you think Tommy did then?" Encourage responses by engaging a guessing game until you have enough direction to continue.

10. Give the child hope by ending in a way that brings relief to the story character's distress. Brett suggests that these positive endings should be honest and possible—-an idea the child can use [15, pp. 15-19].

The Mutual Storytelling Technique

Gardner, a child psychiatrist, has also been an enthusiastic user of story. His numerous books, audio and video tapes provide copious examples of the successful practice of therapeutic story. Central to his work with children ages five through eleven, is a technique Gardner calls mutual storytelling [16]. Like Brett, Gardner believes an essential benefit of the storytelling technique is that its symbolic language avoids direct, anxiety-provoking confrontations [16, p. 5]. Gardner also agrees that the majority of children have little interest in analyzing stories and that this does not adversely affect the child's ability to use the story's problem-solving properties [16, pp. 2-3].

Using the mutual storytelling technique, the story leader elicits a self-created story from the child. The story leader listens intently to the child's story to surmise its psychodynamic meaning and then tells a personal story in response. The story told back to the child uses the same characters, setting, and initial situation as the child's story. However, the catalyst for change comes as the story quickly evolves in a different direction, providing alternatives to respond to the dilemmas of the original story. This technique graphically illustrates the potential of story as a conduit for healing the wound by means of itself. In other words, restoration of the self comes through "re-story-ation."

Storytelling in Psychotherapy With Children, offers many case examples of Gardner's work with storytelling [16]. Besides providing specific methods in the practice of mutual storytelling, Gardner also outlines his use of many other story techniques. These include the uses of dramatized storytelling and storytelling games.

Therapeutic Storytelling as Metaphorical Process

Psychologists, Mills and Crowley, have taken therapeutic storytelling in another direction. Trained in Ericksonian metaphor and story modalities, Mills and Crowley have used storytelling in their work with both children and their parents. While they began by using Gardner's mutual storytelling techniques, they gradually shifted their focus from psychodynamic meanings to the subtleties of the behaviors actually taking place within the therapeutic session. From this they began to create original metaphors using a tiered communication process that includes interspersed suggestions and "sensory interweaving" into an engaging storyline [2, pp. 42-43].

Mills and Crowley favor the story process, rather than story content, as the factor that optimizes the child's ability to respond. They found that by using their method the story listener is able to dissociate further from the problem area and is better able to respond "without the interference of conscious mental acts" [2, p. 43]. Mills and Crowley parallel the situation of the child with less closely related metaphors than Gardner. Their stories introduce an entirely different name for the main character in the story. They change the storyline so that only through disguise does it depict the concrete events in a child's life.

Luckily, story practitioners can benefit from the ground-breaking work of Mills and Crowley. Their book, *Therapeutic Metaphors for Children and The Child Within,* carefully weaves theory, technique, and examples that are as instructive as they are readable. Readers will find many therapeutic storytelling techniques that they can put to practical and immediate use. Moreover, there are instructive chapters that illustrate how they have increased the value of storytelling by adding the multidimensional approach of artistic metaphors [2, p. 161]. The use of several such artistic practices are provided in the next section.

2. CARTOONING, BOOKMAKING AND ARTISTIC METAPHOR

The artistic metaphor uses strategies such as drawings, board games, puppet shows, and healing books that are all conceived and created by the child. The concept of artistic metaphor makes use of storytelling by expanding it into multi-sensory and three-dimensional forms. It is especially helpful "as a means of externalizing pent up feelings as well as the simultaneous activation of inner resources and strengths" [2, p. 166]. Like the storytelling technique, artistic metaphor has as its goal the recognition of the ability of the self for healing and problem-solving. However, artistic metaphor allows the symbolism of the metaphor to be transformed into a tangible, physical form that can be witnessed and validated by the creator of the work as well as by others. In other words, artistic metaphor opens "still another door through which the unconscious mind can express and resolve the child's problem by way of conscious representation" [2, p. 161]. Cartooning and bookmaking are two artistic endeavors that can be easily used with seriously ill children and their families.

Cartooning

Super Cystic and Fabulous Fran Fibrosis, the cartoon book conceived and illustrated by my son, Matt, is a good example of the way a seriously ill child can make use of art and metaphor in the shaping of a story. Once Matt drew his imaginative symbolic characters to deal with the treatment and dangers of his disease, he and others could more easily validate his personal strengths and creative ability to solve problems from within.

Cartoon characters are by nature powerful symbols for many children [2, p. 209]. In *Cartoon Magic,* Crowley and Mills teach parents how they can use modern day cartoon characters for therapeutic home remedies [17]. These cartoon characters and their adventures are seen as fully developed metaphors to which a child has ready access. Parents are taught how to help their child introduce and incorporate cartoon characters into the child's story so they can suggest solutions and alternatives to help the child deal with conflict, pain, and issues related to loss and grief. Parents are also given methods to evaluate cartoon characters for therapeutic value.

Cartoon images help children on both conscious and unconscious levels. On a conscious level, cartoon characters can become important imaginary friends, to help them deal with difficult situations such as accompanying children to the doctor's office. On an unconscious level, cartoon helpers are symbolic images of the children's own inner strengths and resources. In choosing cartoon helpers, children are learning to resonate with their own abilities to help themselves modulate and even master distress [2, p. 210].

Bookmaking

Bookmaking has recently emerged as an easy-to-learn therapeutic technique that can be used by parents and professionals alike. In the past, it was possible to find published stories by adults about their experiences with loss and bereavement, but it was rare to find books written by children. Today, it is possible to find many such selections.

One of these, *When I Die, Will I Get Better?*, is the story created by five-and-a-half-year-old Joeri after the death of his only brother, Remi, aged two years and eight months [18]. Remi died after a brief struggle with meningitis. The two boys had shared a bedroom and they had been very close. After the funeral, Joeri was sad, withdrawn, and often angry. Yet he could not talk about Remi's death or his illness. His parents were at a loss as to how to help their young son. Because they had always used storytelling and story reading with their young sons, they looked for children's books on death, but few appealed to them.

To his dismay, Joeri's father discovered that the characters he had invented for making up bedtime stories to comfort and instruct his sons, "Joe Rabbit" and "Fred Rabbit," were no longer acceptable to Joeri. Joeri knew that he was really "Fred Rabbit" and that "Joe Rabbit" represented Remi. Joeri said that it was impossible to make up stories about "Joe Rabbit" now, since Remi was dead. Intuitively, Joeri's father suggested making up a story in which "Joe Rabbit" would die. That was fine with Joeri.

The story was a healing process that took about four weeks to write and illustrate. The book uses animal characters to describe Joeri's own experiences, including how Remi became ill, how he died, the funeral, the loss, and coming to terms with the sadness. Joeri enlisted his father's help in writing the story and drawing the illustrations. Joeri was clearly in charge of the bookmaking process, telling his father what to write and what images could be used for illustrations. Joeri even censored drawings that did not clearly, or correctly represent his experiences. Once the book was completed, Joeri was very proud of the result. At first, he told his teacher he had made a story about rabbits. Later, he told her it was about his brother. He then took the book to school and was very, very proud when his teacher read it aloud to him and his classmates.

The technique of bookmaking as a therapeutic process is carefully outlined in *Homemade Books To Help Kids Cope,* by Ziegler [19]. In this informative book, Ziegler, a child psychiatrist, highlights his successes and shares his easy-to-learn techniques so they can be used by parents and professionals alike.

The *Pain Getting Better Book* is another resource that demonstrates the value of self-created story books as artistic metaphors of healing [2, p. 178]. Mills and Crowley created this method to help sick children create their own home-made healing metaphors. They have had considerable success using this technique as an adjunct treatment that assists children who are dealing with physical pain. They believe the bookmaking story technique works for several reasons. First, it allows children to dissociate themselves from the pain. Second, it helps "decatastrophize" the pain. By putting the pain into a tangible image the children are more effectively able to obtain a measure of control. Mills and Crowley argue that their approach helps children release sensory focus from the pain and to symbolically realize that it is possible for the pain to actually become "all better." This three step process involves having each child draw three separate pictures:

Drawing #1—How the pain looks right now.
Drawing #2—How the pain looks "all better."
Drawing #3—What will help picture one change into picture two.

This technique is not to be used to mask pain but rather to control, dilute, or dissociate from it. Naturally, they recommend that all pain symptoms be evaluated medically [2, pp. 178-179].

Journal writing and diary-making are additional applications of story that can be used to promote awareness and externalize feelings. Journals written by parents have often been used to create books that tell the larger story and can only be written after the crisis has passed or the child has died. Today, it is possible to find many blank journal books for adults, children, and teenagers. Additionally, many excellent how-to-books are available to guide the person in journal writing in ways that enhance self-awareness and personal growth.

3. USING BOOKS

Bibliotherapy is the term that has been used to describe the use of books in the therapeutic process. Like storytelling, written stories can be a powerful form of communication. Most people can remember a particular book received at just the right time—a book that gave them hope or courage to face adversity.

One such powerful story came to me as a complete and unexpected surprise. I was biking in Vermont with a group of friends who were considerably more physically fit than myself. The hills were especially steep, and although we had traveled only five miles out of a planned forty-seven mile tour, I was falling behind and becoming exhausted. Just as I was saying to myself, "I will never make it, I'm going to have to turn back," I began to hear a song inside my head. "I think I can, I think I can, I think I have a plan . . . and I can do most anything if I just think I can." It was a song from a story-book of my childhood, *The Little Engine That Could*. Singing the song over and over again in my head (I was too out of breath to sing it out loud), I made my way up the steep hill, caught up with the others, and completed the tour.

Years later, I read an account of how *The Little Engine That Could* had performed an even more amazing feat. The story was of an elementary school child who had pulled his mother from a wrecked car and dragged her up an incline to safety. Unable to move, the mother reported she had heard her son say over and over, as he struggled and pulled her, "I think I can, I think I can, I think I can!" Because of the story, *The Little Engine That Could*, a young child and an aging woman were able to respond to difficulties with extraordinary actions [20, p. 9]. Both of us benefited from the power of a good story.

Books can be used in many ways as a therapeutic choice. In *From Wonder To Wisdom*, psychologist Charles Smith suggests that good stories contain both surface and deep meaning. "Surface meaning" is the obvious story line, the explicit message. This is often a factual description. "Deep meaning" is found in the less obvious messages, from the mythical or symbolic dimensions of the story. These deeper meanings are what enables children and adults to link their personal situation with the story possibilities [20, p. 14].

In *Storytelling in Psychotherapy With Children*, Gardner agrees with Smith. He puts therapeutic stories into four categories: 1) expository, 2) reality oriented, 3) fables, and 4) fairy tales [16, p. 232]. Gardner believes that books that are primarily expository and reality-oriented have important therapeutic value in their ability to educate, as long as they are appropriately matched to the reader or listener's intellectual and maturation levels. However, it is the story that uses fable and fairy tale that is the least anxiety producing and the most effective for bringing about inner change.

Fables and Fairy Tales

Both fables and fairy tales use symbolism in order to transmit and disguise information. By using stories about things that happened to others, messages are made more palatable. Additionally, their hidden messages allow the listener to search for meaning and to be the actual meaning-maker or problem-solver.

The fable, one of the purest forms of allegory, uses animals as its protagonists. However, the animals in fables have human characteristics. Animal characters allow us to look at our own situations while maintaining a safe distance.

In some cultures, the human characteristics of the animals are real, not imagined. Native American story teller, Johnny Moses says to his non-native audiences, "The stories of my people are the stories of the animal people. You call these animal people stories our myth and lore. We call them our true and real teachers" [21].

Usually the fable has one or more lessons or morals to teach. Children who often resist talking about themselves or their families can easily enter the make-believe world of story, listening and learning with animal characters. Adults too can make therapeutic use of fables and fairytales.

Aarvy Aardvark Finds Hope tells the story of an Aardvark that has become an orphan and is so sad he wishes he could die [22]. Another animal, "Ralphy Rabbit," who is imbued with all the mythical characteristics of the perfect therapist, befriends Aarvy. With Ralphy's help and by following his own instincts, Aarvy gradually regains hope that life could once again have meaning. As the author of *Aarvy Aardvark Finds Hope,* I have been privileged to receive many poignant letters from adults and children who tell me how they clung to the hope of the *Aarvy* story when they felt only despair and hopelessness. Repeatedly, these people have asserted that they were able to journey through great sorrow because of Aarvy Aardvark and Ralphy Rabbit. Of course this is only partly true. The healing power of a good story cannot be credited to the author alone since the value of the story can only be known when it is experienced by another. Healing through story is therefore a creative co-evolutionary process.

Fairy tales make use of human forms, animal forms, and imaginary creatures from the other world. As with fable, the therapeutic appeal and value of a fairy tale lies in the symbolic presentation of its message. Fairy tales are proven vehicles for enhancing visual imagery

[16, p. 255]. They often emphasize heroic action, risk, and sacrifice. Story writer and critic, Yolen warns us that good fairy tales should be gentle enough to touch a child's mind with insights, yet challenging enough to show children that heroic paths are difficult, that they require action and perseverance [23].

The choice of material is a critical factor in the success of the story experience. Those who would help seriously ill and bereaved children and their families can provide a great service by carefully screening books and making them readily available so that families can read them together. In many cases, book choices will include those that provide information and an orientation to reality, as well as those that are more imaginative and metaphorical.

When useful books are provided, many families can, with only brief coaching, immediately put them to use. Books empower parents and children and help them to gain control. Providers of books also gain indirectly as the selection process offers opportunities to introduce and discuss therapeutic issues that may also help the parents cope and grow.

Today, there are many resources to assist parents and professionals in choosing and using therapeutic story books. Although these materials may be difficult to find in local book stores and libraries, there are a number of organizations that provide them by mail-order. Chapter 17, at the end of this volume of *Beyond the Innocence of Childhood*, lists books according to topic, as well as information concerning mail-order suppliers of therapeutic books and audio and videotapes that relate to illness, dying, death, and bereavement.

4. PERSONAL STORY-SHARING AND LISTENING

No discussion of therapeutic story would be complete without highlighting the importance of personal story-sharing and story listening. Both have therapeutic properties.

Psychiatrist, Whitfield says, "While we can listen to the stories of others, and they can listen to ours, perhaps the most healing feature is that we, the storyteller, get to hear our own story" [24, p. 97].

Personal story-sharing allows us to externalize beliefs and release internalized or repressed feelings. This provides us with a mirror for self-reflection. By listening to our own words, we are better able to decide whether to appreciate and maintain the story as it is, or to take steps to rectify or reframe it.

Listening to the stories of others also provides opportunities for new insights about ourselves and others. Through listening, especially through the practice of benevolent listening, in which judgments are suspended and goodwill is protected, we are able to gather information, experience affinity, and enlarge our subjective and objective reality.

Likewise, there is a healing dimension to the experience of being heard. When we really listen to the stories of sick and grieving youngsters and their families, we are practicing a special style of healing touch. Metaphorically speaking, we are "laying ears on them" [25]. Anyone who has had the good fortune to have been really listened to in times of distress knows the solace of such a gentle touch.

Using Story as Ritual

The use of ritual story-sharing is ancient and has long been used in therapeutic practice with adults. Story rituals can also be used with seriously ill and grieving children, adolescents, and their families. Story rituals and ceremony are especially helpful to transmit values, validate a loss, explore individual and shared meanings, and experience affinity. While space does not allow an extensive exploration of these activities, I will outline a ceremonial story practice I have used with grieving adolescents and adults.

The Story Circle

The story circle makes use of ceremony and the inner wisdom and healing experiences of all participants. When facilitating a ceremonial story circle, it is important that everyone who joins the circle understands that the process is experiential. Each person should want to participate to some degree, either as an active participant or observer. This should be clearly stated before the circle begins. The story leader should also foster a caring approach that will enable anyone who is uncomfortable or unsure to leave.

In my work, I use an inner and outer circle, allowing participants the option of active or passive involvement. I also provide time for circle members to determine which role suits their present needs. In addition, participants are encouraged to modulate their involvement, trusting themselves to be the best judge of their unique needs for emotional safeguarding. Moments for silent contemplation and discernment are interjected at each phase of the ceremonial process.

Story circles can be used to focus on a specific issue. Topics I have used include: *About My Grief, About My Illness, About Death, About My Ability/Inability to Heal,* and *Sacred Stories That Have Influenced My Life.*

The story circle progresses through cycles of sharing—listening—echoing—contemplation—sharing. Usually the process develops through the following phases:

1. Trust building.
2. Ceremonial process and pacing the tempo of the process.
3. Forming a physical circle through the placement of chairs and people.
4. Giving story circle participants information about the structure of the ceremony and what is expected from participants.
5. Focusing.
6. Participants verbally name their fears and concerns and symbolically place them into the center of the circle.
7. Calling forth restorative wisdom stories from inner story circle participants to re-story some particular fear with hope.
8. A ceremonial acknowledgement of all that has not been restored (restoried).
9. A silent or verbal meditation of appreciation for the gifts received from the experience.
10. A ceremonial closure of the story circle and reentry into the larger space.
11. Individual processing in pairs, small groups, or by writing or drawing out the experience.
12. Group processing and closure with the inner and outer circle as one group.

SHAWN'S STORY—DARE WE FORGET?

When people are so caught up in their problems that they forget that other dimensions exist, it is particularly important for therapists to remember that people are a lot more than their problems [11, p. 6].

Shawn, a dear friend of mine, died on the eve of his twelfth birthday. Shortly before he died he told his mother this story:

I know you are very sad and unhappy, Mom. You think I am too young to die. Well you should know I'm not really eleven years old. I'm 77. Then looking directly into his mother's eyes and in a tone both strong and clear, Shawn asked her: "Mom, do you know how you can get to be 77 in just eleven years?" "No Shawn, I certainly don't," she replied, her voice trembling with despair. "Well," said Shawn, "You just get the bullshit out of your life."

Shawn's mother looked at her son. Then she began to laugh. She laughed until she cried and Shawn laughed and cried with her.

Weeks later at a formal Catholic funeral, Shawn's body was laid out in front of his family and friends. The casket he lay in was lined with blue denim fabric, the fabric Shawn had chosen for the purpose some weeks earlier. There in the church, Shawn's story was retold to all of us by their family priest. As we listened, the spirit of Shawn's story filled the church. Many of us laughed and many cried, sometimes we laughed and cried simultaneously.

I chose Shawn's story as the ending for this chapter because for me it represents the theme of this chapter in the clearest, deepest way. It provides a narrative representation of wholeness that is both real and profound.

Shawn's story to his mother—to all of us—is a larger story. It is a story that goes beyond brokenness—a story of unity and peace in the midst of disruption and sorrow. Those of us who have had the pain and the privilege of walking with families through the illness and death of their children know that not all stories have this same narrative tone. We cannot impose these larger stories on others, but neither can we forget them. They remind us of something bigger. They remind us that lives can be rewoven—that peace is possible. Dare we keep that a secret?

EPILOGUE

The stories people tell have a way of taking care of them. If stories come to you, care for them and learn to give them away where they are needed. Sometimes a person needs a story more than food to stay alive. That is why we put these stories in each other's memory. That is how people care for themselves [26, p. 48].

REFERENCES

1. J. Houston, *The Healing Power of Story*, taped speech, Lansing, Michigan, 1986.
2. J. C. Mills and R. J. Crowley, *Therapeutic Metaphors for Children and The Child Within,* Brunner/Mazel Publishers, New York, 1986.
3. D. P. McAdams, *Stories We Live By*, William Morrow and Company, New York, 1993.
4. V. Gussin Paley, Child's Play, *Storytelling Magazine,* Fall, pp. 20-22, 1990.
5. H. Nouwen, *Reaching Out: The Three Movements of the Spiritual Life,* Doubleday, New York, 1975.

6. F. Flack, *Resilience, Discovering a New Strength at Times of Stress*, Ballentine Books, New York, 1988.
7. R. Veninga, *A Gift of Hope: How We Survive Our Tragedies*, Little Brown and Company, New York, 1976.
8. D. Bakan, *The Duality of Human Existence: Isolation and Communion in Western Man*, Beacon Press, Boston, Massachusetts, 1966.
9. M. White and D. Epston, *Narrative Means to Therapeutic Ends*, W. W. Norton and Co., New York, 1990.
10. A. McCarty Hynes and M. Hynes-Beny, *Biblio/Poetry Therapy, The Interactive Process: A Handbook*, Westview Press, Boulder, Colorado, 1986.
11. G. Combs and J. Freedman, *Symbol, Story and Ceremony: Using Metaphor in Individual and Family Therapy*, W. W. Norton and Co., New York, 1990.
12. D. Metzger, Circle of Stones, *Parabola*, IV:4, pp. 104-105, 1979.
13. N. J. Livo and S. A. Rietz, *Storytelling: Process and Practice*, Libraries Unlimited, Inc., Littleton, Colorado, 1986.
14. D. Brett, *Annie Stories: A Special Kind of Storytelling*, Workman Publishing, New York, 1988.
15. D. Brett, *More Annie Stories: Therapeutic Storytelling Techniques*, Brunner/Mazel, Inc., New York, 1992.
16. R. Gardner, *Storytelling in Psychotherapy With Children*, Jason Aronson Inc., Northvale, New Jersey, 1993.
17. R. Crowley and J. Mills, *Cartoon Magic*, Brunner/Mazel, Inc., New York, 1989.
18. J. Breebaart and P. Breebaart, *When I Die, Will I Get Better?*, Peter Bedrick Books, New York, 1993.
19. R. Ziegler, *Homemade Books To Help Kids Cope*, Brunner/Mazel, Inc., New York, 1992.
20. C. A. Smith, *From Wonder To Wisdom: Using Stories To Help Children Grow*, Penquin Books, New York, 1989.
21. J. Moses, The National Storytelling Festival, speech, Jonesborough, Tennessee, 1992.
22. D. O. Toole, *Aarvy Aardvark Finds Hope*, Mountain Rainbow Publications, Burnsville, North Carolina, 1988.
23. J. Yolen, *Touch Magic: Fantasy, Faerie Tales and Folklore in the Literature of Childhood*, Putnam, New York, 1981.
24. C. L. Whitfield, *Healing The Child Within*, Health Communications, Inc., Deerfield Beach, Florida, 1987.
25. D. Manning, *A Minister Speaks About Funerals,* public address, 1978.
26. B. Lopez, *Crow and Weasel*, North Point Press, San Francisco, California, 1990.

CHAPTER 3

Music Therapy for Children with Cancer

Petra Hinderer

Pediatric oncology is a new frontier for music therapy. This chapter presents the preliminary observations of my work in the oncology ward of the Children's Hospital in St. Gallen, Switzerland. Music therapy in this clinic is anything but an independent discipline within a psychosocial concept of care. It is a program which is available to patients to help them come to terms with the side effects and end results of medical treatment. It is also meant to alleviate the impact of hospitalization.

Using case studies I will illustrate how music, as a means of therapy, is especially suited to children who have potentially fatal illnesses. I will describe the therapeutic music methods which I use in oncology, talk about instruments, explain the forms of music therapy, and briefly touch on my work with adolescent cancer patients. The chapter will close with a consideration of other possibilities for the use of music therapy in pediatric oncology.

Every physical ailment has psychological aspects. The task of music therapy is to give a voice to the psychological aspects of illness; to recognize the call for help; and at the same time, to support and nourish the patient's own potential for healing.

The success of music therapy is based on two phenomena: first, the qualities inherent in music itself, and second, the relationship between the therapist and the patient.

MUSIC MAKING

Music making in the context of music therapy means making oneself heard and expressing oneself through tones, sounds, or even noise, either with or without instruments. Moods, feelings, tensions, and relationships are transformed into sound. One becomes aware of one's own inner music, one's own rhythm, and builds a bridge to the external world. In this process there is no right or wrong. Music making is a matter of free and elementary life expression without any artistic aspiration.

MUSIC:
THE BENEFITS AND CHARACTERISTICS

What is it about music that justifies its use as a means of therapy? Music touches a person's emotions by penetrating and surrounding the body. It often by-passes consciousness and reaches the soul directly and immediately. Music is perceived at every level, including the level of bodily functions; it effects pulse, breathing, and muscle tone. Music can trigger both positive and negative emotional states and it can aid in relaxation. It stimulates powerful associations by awakening memories, emotions, moods, and wishes. It is difficult to protect oneself from these effects—a fact which, for example, is exploited by the psychology of advertising. In spite of these strong influences music is not normally considered to be threatening.

Music offers a sanctuary. Especially for children, negative feelings, such as rage or fear, can be more easily expressed when disguised in a melody. An example of this in the hospital is the way in which children, while singing, can curse their fate at length and in the most vulgar language without having a bad conscience.

Music, in contrast to other means, provides a forum in which many feelings, otherwise considered to be mutually exclusive, can be expressed simultaneously by one person. Through the polyphonic nature of music, tenderness and rage or feelings of isolation and union can be expressed at the same time and in such a manner that does not destroy an essential harmony—both in a musical mode and in a broader sense. Expressing emotions in this way, and hearing and experiencing the simultaneousness, has a strong effect on children with cancer. Such expression can be very beneficial for children in crises who are trying, often without success, to bring their contradictory feelings into some kind of accord. It is possible to express contrasting and changing emotions in rapid succession through music making. This presents many therapeutic possibilities, especially in the case of children whose abrupt emotional changes are often difficult for adults to follow.

What possibilities does music offer that other artistic activities, including drawing, working with clay, and theatre arts, do not? An important characteristic of music is that it cannot be destroyed. One can play the most delicate of tones at one moment, and at the next, break into a hard beating fortissimo without destroying the previous tender mood. Whereas in painting or working with clay the expression of a new emotion may cover or destroy what has gone before. Children are quick to paint over their own picture if its message is too charged for them or they do not wish to share it with others.

Music speaks directly to feelings, but music making is also an intellectual activity. Playing an instrument and repeating or composing a melody is a considerable intellectual accomplishment for children. This fact offers diagnostic as well as pedagogical and therapeutic possibilities.

Music, principally because of its rhythm, has a strong ordering function which can be exploited for therapeutic use. For example, a child who uses a drum to express a temper tantrum can be carefully encouraged by therapeutic intervention to find his or her rhythm in the chaos, thus turning the explosive discharge into an experience of stability. In this way music can have a cathartic effect.

A twelve-year-old boy with an amputated leg was sitting in his room, visibly upset, because his prosthesis was not functioning properly. As he tried to explain the problem to me, he stammered with rage and struck the table with his crutch. After a few heavy blows I started to answer him by knocking on a chair. This game quickly developed to the point where we found ourselves in a very complicated but stable percussion session striking the crutch, opening and slamming the drawers of the table, stomping our feet, clapping, and clicking our tongues. It was fun for both of us. It channelled his rage, left him proud and appeased, and we could refer back to this experience during future situations. This example demonstrates that where words fail, even feelings like rage, which are otherwise charged with fear and guilt, can still be expressed. Children with cancer, whose lives are very constrained by long hospitalizations, often take advantage of such opportunities.

In spite of its ordering function, rhythm does not have a limiting character. Diagnostically, it is always significant when a child cannot find a way out of his or her own static rhythm or is unable to adjust to changes in tempo when playing with others. This can indicate an inner numbness which should be observed further.

Another important aspect of music, as observed therapeutically, is its social character. In music making you make yourself heard; you present yourself to others. It is possible for a number of people to make music together, to hear each other, and to be in contact with one another without losing contact with oneself. For example, when playing in a group, you can enter the musical space without taking away the place of someone else. This self-actualization within a group strengthens the feeling of self-worth. When people play music together they enter into a relationship. These relationships are made audible, thus offering many possibilities to learn or reanimate social skills. Music making further encouraged social learning in the hospital setting, which is especially important for preschool children. It can also help diminish the threatening isolation and loneliness that children with cancer experience.

As a therapist, because I cannot hide behind my music, the children get to know me and, at the same time, I get to know them—building a relationship of trust. We all share a common experience. A successful musical contact can replace many verbal contacts. Closeness and intimacy arise in the musical context and so much happens that cannot be put into words; often a feeling of sharing a secret develops between myself and the children. Children tend to carry over this trust into non-musical contact with the therapist.

The experience of being accompanied, which music making affords, is an important and effective interpersonal experience. When a child plays an instrument the therapist has the possibility of accompanying him or her on another instrument. He can sustain or stabilize the music by giving the beat or elaborating on the beat that the child gives. He can try to interpret the child's mood or change it if the child is willing to accommodate his actions. He can act as a mirror or, if appropriate, share his own feelings with the child through the music. Children often try to see just how far the therapist can follow them.

A four-year-old girl, to whom I gave a Glockenspiel, was visibly moved by the delicate tones which seemed to come almost magically from the instrument. After awhile I began to accompany her on another Glockenspiel, trying to create a pleasing harmony to compliment her melody. She was astonished and stopped playing for a moment. Then she began to play again, with great concentration on the music that we were creating together. After we played for awhile in literal and figurative harmony she suddenly began to play very fast and then very slow, very softly and then very loudly. Finally, as she laughed, she threw the sticks onto the Glockenspiel. Again, she tried to imitate my playing and set the tone herself. During all of this time, she carefully observed me. She was quite surprised that I could follow her with my tones. In time she became braver, more open, and more cheerful. We were both having a good time. I did not have any contact with her before this encounter. I had frequently seen her on the ward, mostly with her mother, and noticed that she was usually shy and afraid. Now we have a close relationship which does not have to be constantly examined but on which we can build new experiences.

Though children's musical outbursts of emotion may be quite powerful, they are normally not accompanied by feelings of guilt. Music making usually has the characteristics of play rather than therapy and therefore, offer children a protected space where they really can express their difficult feelings.

Playing is an important aspect in music therapy. In playing, the strength which is focused on self-healing, self-realization, and growth, shows itself in its clearest form. Playing is an activity which engages the whole being. Making music and playing are closely related. In musical playing it is possible to be centered in on oneself and still be in active contact with the outside world through communication. Playing in music therapy involves sounds, tones, rhythms, noises, various dynamic levels, and pauses, as well as mimicking and signaling in a nonverbal and sometimes uncontrolled way. All this can serve the purpose of entertaining, without ulterior motives, as well as providing diagnostic information and suggesting therapeutic procedures.

The purpose of music therapy does not necessarily depend on concentrating on specific problems. Children with cancer are often concerned and preoccupied with the threats imposed by their illness. For this reason, it is often more helpful to work with them in a playful and, above all, in a musical way. Thus, these children can turn away from their inner problems for awhile, step into another sphere as it were, and tap another source.

THE USE OF INSTRUMENTS IN
MUSIC THERAPY

The close connection between playing per se and music making is also apparent when we consider playing an instrument. Instruments are, of course, important tools in music therapy. Many instruments are too complex for children because they demand considerable motoric and intellectual skills. Thus therapy with children calls for slightly different choices in instruments than therapy with adults. I prefer to use folk instruments from all parts of the world because they are usually simpler to handle and often made of natural materials. Also, they arouse the curiosity of children because of their unusual appearance and tone. The instruments developed in anthroposophic music therapy are well suited for children. But one can just as well use pots and pans or even infusion stands as instruments. Usually, I do not use the standard Western orchestral instruments unless a child expresses an interest in learning to play one of them. For example, one child in the ward wanted to play the flute. His goal set his energy free to learn this instrument and make plans for the future. But usually this type of instrument is too difficult to cope with and children may associate it with the pressure of achievement.

In their original meaning, instruments are an extension of the body. The instruments which are inherently a part of the body—specifically the voice—are especially important for my work. At the child's bedside usually there are no instruments at your disposal, however, you can still work effectively by using singing, clapping, shrieking, and stomping.

Instruments always initiate movement and are, therefore, very well suited to training specific bodily functions, without giving the feeling of mechanical practice. In this way musical activity can be helpful in overcoming certain handicaps, for instance, those resulting from brain tumors.

In music therapy, instruments are often disassociated from their original function. Because of their symbolic potential they can easily represent other things, be it members of the family, injection syringes, or a washing machine.

FORMS OF MUSIC THERAPY

Music therapy provides the possibility for individual or group therapy depending upon the indications and the facilities. In individual therapy the emphasis is on the conscious activation of creative energies rather than on focusing in on the psychological details of the child's history. In oncology, I usually work on an individual basis but sometimes other children join in spontaneously to form a group.

Group therapy is concerned with relationships, listening to each other, and setting common goals. It is valuable in overcoming difficulties with communication and in establishing contact with others.

In both individual and group settings music therapy is used passively or actively. Passive music therapy means that the patient himself is not involved in music making, but rather he listens to music played by the therapist or generated from another source. For example, music can be played in the background in order to create a comfortable atmosphere, stimulate learning, or encourage motion. Music can be the center of attention, in which case children concentrate on it, use it as a stimulus for their imagination, or lose themselves in it and are better able to relax. In specific cases I have tried to take advantage of music's relaxing character for palliative effects. Listening to appropriate music and entering into it can distract children from relentless pain and nausea.

In active music therapy patients play or sing by themselves. Improvisation, with its various forms, is the most important technique in music therapy. You can improvise with both highly talented children and those with no musical ability. No previous training is necessary. Improvising means "transforming into sound" without any preconceived scheme. The only limits that are imposed depend upon the amount of time at your disposal and the rules set up by the therapist to accommodate groups. For example, the rule "tutti-solo-tutti," allows each person to take a turn at being the soloist. Sometimes a theme evolves, for instance, "waking up from narcosis."

Apart from improvisation, working with songs is another very important method used in music therapy. Well-known children's songs are an excellent point of contact between the therapist and the children, as well as among patients within a group. As everyone knows, songs can take you back to better days. They can create a happy and carefree atmosphere, and thus they speak to children's need for freedom and security. I often use well-known songs, those with verses that the children can alter to fit their present situation, or we make up completely new songs using familiar tunes.

Children can easily accompany songs using simple instruments. The therapist influences the atmosphere of the song by catching onto the verbal and nonverbal expressions of the children and incorporating them into his accompaniment, without giving up the stable structure of the song.

Songs which involve gestures or movement can be adapted so that bedridden children can join in on the activity. These songs are especially helpful in developing a positive attitude toward the body when, for example, treatment has caused a mutilation. I often have children pick their own songs and I am always astonished as to how well their choice expresses their own personal situation.

One ten-year-old boy in the oncology ward wanted to sing a song from a book of camp songs. He had a wide variety to choose from, but chose a prayer that he sang again and again, similar to a canticle. The central message of the prayer was that a person has to do penance when his world falls apart. According to his mother the boy did not have a religious upbringing. He was sad, well-behaved, and always tried to be a model patient. On several occasions after his hair fell out completely, he mentioned that he wanted to become a monk. He frequently sang or recited this prayer. It became obvious that his inhibited aggression was caused by enormous feelings of guilt concerning his illness. He tried to rid himself of these feelings by doing penance, praying, and isolating himself—just like a monk. In our conversations I dwelt upon the positive sides of cloister life; I brought him wine bottles and different varieties of cheese with pictures of fat smiling monks. For centuries, the monks in Europe have been known as connoisseurs and producers of fine food and drink. We sang prayers and songs that celebrated the optimistic and sensual aspects of life and these gradually helped to relieve his inner tension. He even became amused by the aggressive outbursts of his room-mate, who underwent brain surgery and was always talking about wanting to beat everybody up. Together we all sang a song about a fellow who traveled around, picked fights in which he lost an arm, an eye, and a leg but still told his story in the refrain of what a good time he had.

ADOLESCENT CANCER PATIENTS

Everything we have touched upon also applies to adolescent patients. However, this age group is usually not quite so innocent, more inhibited (not just musically), and more likely to find playing an instrument or singing slightly ridiculous. Music can be a stepping stone to establishing contact and trust. Often a conversation about music—especially about their music—is a good beginning. Teenagers readily demonstrate their choice of music and declare what and with whom they wish to be identified or associated with. For teenagers with cancer, involvement in rock and pop music is an important point of contact with their peer group. It is, of course, a distinct advantage when the therapist is up-to-date and possibly even shares their musical taste. Today's bizarre rock scene with its array of personalities provides many topics to talk about, be it intimacy, self-presentation, singers' shaved heads, or cosmetic surgery. Talking about musical experiences at home, as a listener or a player, can provide insight into the family's interests and dynamics from the teenager's point of view.

In active music therapy, rhythm is always of utmost importance for this age-group. This should not be surprising since puberty is a time of rhythmic transformation, both physically and spiritually. In addition, the lives of cancer patients are burdened with the rigid rhythmical structure of their medical treatment, a burden which they understandably do not easily accept.

Individual work with percussion instruments helps them find their own rhythm and make it audible. In percussion groups, inner instability can be compensated for by accommodating themselves to a loud stabilizing group rhythm. Participating in the common beat alleviates, at least for a short period of time, the feeling of loneliness and lack of understanding that is characteristic of this age group, especially under circumstances of serious illness. Feelings of group identity and freedom are aroused, an effect which has always dominated music, be it disco, folk dances, marching songs, political songs, or military music.

MUSIC THERAPY: OTHER USES

Other possibilities exist for the use of music therapy in pediatric oncology. I believe that a parents' music therapy group can help them cope with the strain that serious illness imposes on families. Music therapy can provide parents with a means to deal with the common feelings of helplessness and the difficulties in expressing themselves verbally. Music therapy can also provide opportunities for these parents to relax.

Another field for music therapy can offer assistance to work groups of hospital and clinic staff. First, experiencing music therapy yourself is the only way to really understand what it can do. Secondly, nonverbal work is suited to a hierarchical institution. It is very difficult to verbalize problems in the presence of superiors, that is, in a team setting. Team music therapy sessions can offer a means of dealing with problems directly related to patients or to the dynamics of the team itself.

CONCLUSION

Some of the benefits and characteristics of music and the role of music making in the context of music therapy have been described. Music has the potential to touch a person's emotions and also facilitates the expression of both contrasting and changing feelings. The task of music therapy is to give voice to the psychological aspects of an illness and therefore, it is especially well suited for the treatment of chronically or potentially fatally ill children and adolescents.

BIBLIOGRAPHY

Alvin, J., *Music Therapy*, Hutchinson and Company, London, 1975.
Brückner, J., Mederacke, I., and Ulbrich, C., *Musiktherapie für Kinder*, 2. Auflage, Verlag Gesundheit, Berlin, 1991.
Evers, S., *Musiktherapie und Kinderheilkunde*, Heidelberger Schriften zur Musiktherapie, Band 5, Gustav Fischer Verlag, Stuttgart, 1991.

Hegi, F., *Improvisation und Musiktherapie. Möglichkeiten und Wirkungen von freier Musik*, 3. Auflage, Jungfermann, Paderborn, 1986.

Munroe, S. and Mount, B., Music Therapy in Palliative Care, *The Canadian Medical Association Journal, 119*, 1978.

Priestley, M., *Music Therapy in Action*, Constable and Company Ltd., London, 1975.

Timmermann, T., *Die Musen der Musik, Stimmig werden mit sich selbst*, 1. Auflage, Kreuz Verlag, Zürich, 1989.

CHAPTER 4

The Therapeutic Use of Play in Helping Children Whose Lives are Threatened

Ruth M. Snider

Play is the unique language of children. It is a complex activity which children spontaneously engage in that influences their stages of development from infancy to adolescence. Play is essential to the physical, emotional, cognitive, and social well-being of children. It is through play that children of all ages learn to problem solve, interact, and master the stages of normal development and critical experiences. The skills they learn in play continue into their adult lives.

Under the supervision of a trained professional child life specialist, hospitalized children can, through the use of therapeutic play, be empowered to understand the stresses that are imposed upon them.

PETER:
THE PERCEPTIONS OF A CHILD

Peter, age four years, was admitted to the hospital with severe burns to his legs caused by being immersed in very hot water by his mother's common-law partner. His mother, too distraught to visit, received counseling on a daily basis from the social worker until she could provide the necessary nurturing for her son. Due to his mother's distress, Peter had no family support during this critical period.

To assist Peter in coping with separation, painful dressing changes, and a strange environment, the health care team developed a routine to make his hospital stay as close as possible to his normal life. His routine involved nourishment, rest, peer interaction, and play.

As a child life specialist (CLS), my role with Peter was to communicate with other members of the team, provide diversion during dressing changes, and spend a quiet time each day with him in a play situation. My involvement encouraged Peter to relax, communicate, and trust me. On the third day, Peter said, "How come all you have to do is play?"

This was a very serious and perceptive question as Peter had observed the many different roles of the health care team members on the ward. We talked about how both children and grown ups played and how this made them feel.

MEDICAL PLAY AS THERAPEUTIC PLAY

In her description of new dimensions of medical play, McCue states, "Medical play is a form of play that always has, as part of its content, medical themes and/or use of medical equipment" [1, p. 158].

Thompson notes, "The research further suggests that play with stress-relevant materials may be beneficial to children, possibly resulting in reduced disturbance in the period following health care" [2, p. 225].

There is no question that, under the supervision of a trained professional, medical play can help children come to terms with their treatment. They are provided with the opportunity to handle equipment such as intravenous tubing, syringes, needles, and blood pressure cuffs. The manipulation of this equipment removes the mystique and enables children to control experiences that are often overwhelming. Initially, the CLS shows them the correct and safe way to handle the equipment and reiterates that doctors and nurses use such equipment to help make children better. Since safety is always a prime concern, needles and other potentially harmful equipment are not available to more than two children at a time.

In order to successfully engage children in medical play, the CLS must first establish rapport, understand their level of cognitive functioning, and be aware of the influence of previous experiences. Also, it must be recognized that anxiety created by the illness and hospitalization interferes with their ability to absorb new information.

Depending upon the health care setting and the availability and skill of the staff, there are a variety of approaches to medical play. In this chapter, I will refer to the approach utilized by child life staff at The Children's Hospital, Chedoke-McMaster Hospitals, Hamilton, Ontario, Canada. This program was established in 1972 and is well-integrated into the philosophy and approach to care for children in this university teaching facility.

MEDICAL PLAY:
A MODEL FOR PRACTICE

The benefits of the Chedoke-McMaster approach are seen most clearly in the work with children with cancer and their families, but can be adapted to benefit all children requiring health care treatment in in-patient, ambulatory, and community settings.

In the Chedoke-McMaster approach, children are presented with blank cloth dolls. These dolls, measuring approximately twelve to fourteen inches in length, are made of white or brown muslin with polyester stuffing. Children are encouraged to personalize the doll using assorted nontoxic markers. This process of creating the doll is individual to each child: some draw happy faces, others draw sad or angry faces. Clothes and hair may or may not be added as the child sees fit. Initially, some children are so distressed that they may be reluctant to participate. The CLS must be patient and sensitive to the feelings and needs of each child in order to carry out the child's carefully elicited instructions. Parents are encouraged to be involved in order to understand their child's feelings and the treatment process. Children often ask their parents to help them create their dolls.

In addition to the cloth dolls, there are many other tools used in medical play as illustrated in Figure 1. Syringes, intravenous equipment, and colored medicines may be introduced. This preliminary medical play is intended to increase the trust and comfort level of children, provide a release for their anxiety, and assist them in gaining control over their environment.

Having established this relationship, the CLS is then able to prepare the children for planned medical procedures such as surgery, Port-A-Cath™ insertion, lumbar punctures, bone marrow aspirations, CAT scans, MRIs, and radiation. For children, dolls become their surrogates and are used to rehearse procedures in a safe and non-threatening manner. The personalized doll often travels back and forth from home to hospital and in some cases, as treatment changes, several dolls may be created.

Susan, a ten-year-old with a central nervous system tumor, said, "My doll is like my twin. I do to her what has been done to me and it takes all the pain away."

Another approach to medical play involves children drawing "happy and sad" and "good and bad" cells or bumps that are not helpful to their body. In this way the disease is given a visual identity that children can understand. The children can help "get rid of" the disease by drawing pictures of the medicine obliterating the unwanted cells.

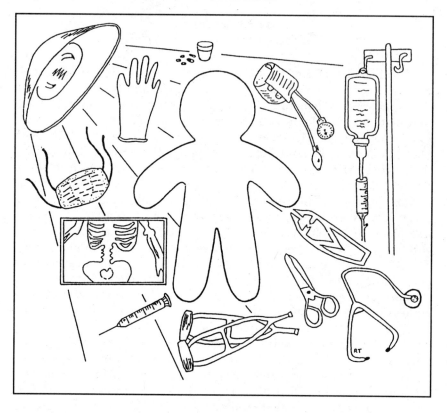

Figure 1. Tools used in medical play.

OTHER TYPES OF THERAPEUTIC PLAY

Recognizing that all play is therapeutic, medical play may be supplemented by creative or diversional play activities essential to normal growth and development. Play opportunities are provided for all hospitalized children and teens by the CLS, assisted by trained and supervised child life volunteers and students who offer additional consistent, daily interaction for patients and their families. Their outreach to children and teens who are confined to their rooms and the provision of group activities are important in helping pediatric patients adapt to illness and treatment. This is especially true when children are dealing with a serious or life-threatening illness.

Therapeutic play activities can pave the way to meeting the educational needs of all pediatric patients regardless of age. Once the emotional needs of children and adolescents are addressed and met, beneficial learning can take place.

Professional communication and collaboration must be maintained between the hospital classroom teachers and the child life staff. It is the responsibility of the teacher to provide an optimal educational experience for the children in the classroom, at the bedside, and in any other appropriate area within the hospital setting.

INITIAL CONTACT WITH THE HEALTH CARE TEAM

Families experience overwhelming feelings of shock, denial, and other intense reactions when their children are diagnosed with a life-threatening illness. Therefore, it is essential that the CLS, as an integral member of the health care team, initiate contact with the children as soon as possible in order to prepare them for hospital routines and treatments. This process must proceed slowly in order to give children time to adapt. It should also be tailored to the developmental stage of the child and be in tune with the needs and wishes of the parents. It is imperative, at all times, to respect and try to understand the influences of their cultural and religious beliefs, past experiences with illness, communication patterns, and social situation. Information that promotes this understanding may be offered directly by the parents or obtained and provided to the CLS by other members of the health care team. Child Life Specialists must negotiate with parents regarding their involvement in helping children, including establishing appropriate boundaries.

INFANTS UNDER SIX MONTHS

During the first six months of life, it is generally believed that infants are less at risk for psychological damage from hospitalization than older infants. However, it is also recognized that parental participation must be maximized to maintain the parent-child attachment. This can be accomplished by encouraging parents to bath, feed, change, and play with their infants. Schaffer and Callender suggest that:

> Separation from the mother as a traumatic event does not commence until after the middle of the first year of life, and that consequently in those cases where there is a choice, hospitalization should be arranged to occur before the crucial age is reached [3, p. 539].

At the Children's Hospital, an active cuddler's program was developed to provide stimulation for infants whose parents found it difficult to visit on a regular basis. Cuddlers are recruited from within the hospital and the local community. One cuddler is assigned on a consistent basis to each hospitalized infant. Training is provided by the child life specialist, nursing, and occupational therapy staff and focuses on stimulation, positioning, and feeding appropriate to the individual infant. Parents are introduced to their child's cuddler in advance in order to reassure them that the cuddler will help to meet both the physical and emotional needs of their infant. When infants are seriously ill or their lives are threatened and hospitalization is prolonged, this service becomes essential.

As part of the care of seriously or critically ill infants, it is important to recognize that the hospital ward environment is often noisy and busy. Lighting is frequently harsh and a combination of other disturbances may be disruptive to infants' sleep patterns. Therefore, it is advisable to keep the number of staff involved with infants to a minimum, to subdue the lighting, and to provide a calm, quiet atmosphere to encourage consistent sleep patterns at a time when the need for rest is so important.

The Importance of Stimulation

Several years ago, five seriously and critically ill infants, ranging in age from one to six months, were confined to their hospital rooms. On observation, it became apparent that the nursing staff took the opportunity during feeding times to sit quietly in the rocking chairs. Their sole purpose was to ensure that the required amount of formula was consumed by the infant and no other stimulation was provided. Although these infants were ill and more lethargic than normal infants, their decrease in eye contact, limited reflex response, and reduced verbal sounds were soon recorded and caused concern.

The ward staff met and reviewed the stages of growth and development for this age group and mutually agreed that a problem existed. They decided that the infants would be held so that they could visually interact with their nurse who would in turn talk, sing, and gently stroke their cheeks, hands, legs, or other exposed parts of their bodies. Within three days, despite their medical difficulties, the infants became less listless, responded with imitative facial movements, made soft cooing sounds, and increased their eye contact.

CHILDREN SIX TO EIGHTEEN MONTHS

When children are between six and eighteen months of age, separation from parents is of great concern. Although many children are accustomed to being briefly separated from their parents and attend day care centers or are left with sitters, the separation is temporary and most children adapt reasonably well. Hospitalization is more traumatic because they are taken from their familiar environment and exposed to strangers, the trauma of various forms of treatment, and extended absences from their parents. When they are seriously or critically ill, this trauma is often compounded.

Much of the knowledge of the effects of separation anxiety on children comes from the work of John Bowlby. He observed children ages fifteen to thirty months who were admitted to the hospital for investigation or elective surgery, or to a residential setting. The children were cared for in the usual manner by a variety of nurses, students, and other care providers and they spent very little time with their mothers. The separation from their mothers resulted in three predictable phases of behavior. These include:

1. Protest that lasts a minimum of a few hours and a maximum of more than a week. Children try during this time to use all of their limited abilities to recover their absent mothers and are in acute distress. Crying, shaking the crib, throwing themselves around, and being vigilant for sights and sounds of mother are all common behaviors. Children expect their mothers to reappear and substitutes are often rejected or the object of clinging behavior.
2. Despair is characterized by increased hopelessness. Children tend to withdraw, or monotonously cry and appear to be in a "state of deep mourning." This is sometimes mistaken as a reduction in their levels of distress.
3. Detachment follows despair and may be seen as a time of recovery. Care and caregivers become acceptable to children during this phase, but the relationship with their mother is often characterized by withdrawal, apathy, and loss of interest in her. After an extended period of institutionalization and loss of a series of surrogate mothers, children may focus on treats and toys, become unaffected by changes in personnel, and less afraid or concerned about adults, including their parents [4, p. 90].

Although parental participation at the Children's Hospital is encouraged, parents cannot always be present. Their absence and the impact of the separation necessitates an increase in stimulation to further encourage the development of mobility and socialization of children in this age group.

A special area in the playroom with safe, age-appropriate toys and activities is ideal. For some children, sitting on a volunteer's knee and watching the activities of the other children provides a sense of security similar to the home environment.

Lynn

When Lynn, age twelve months, was admitted to our ward with hydrocephalus, cleft lip, and congenital anomalies, it was observed that she slept for extended periods either on her back or her side. She was irritable when touched and rigid when held. She regarded toys passively, rarely touched them, and made no eye contact.

Lynn was taken to the playroom on a daily basis and assigned to Louise, a child life student. Each day Louise would hold her for brief periods, gradually increasing the frequency and duration. Toys were put within her reach and with time she became more aware of her surroundings, her body began to relax, and she was able to tolerate physical contact. Lynn began to reach out for the toys, roll over, and hold out her arms to be held. This was followed by smiles, sounds of laughter, squeals of delight, and much more eye contact.

Her response to the consistency of one caring adult, combined with age-appropriate stimulation, confirmed the diagnosis of deprivation and depression.

THE TODDLER

This age group, involving children from eighteen months to two years, is still susceptible to separation anxiety but has gained a new found independence through increased mobility and language. Parents have developed routines combined with limit setting to encourage autonomy, security, and self-esteem. Petrillo and Sanger state that:

> For the toddler and young three-year-old, hospitalization is less of a devastating event when medical personnel understand the need for 1) continuity of the mother child relationship, 2) the incorporation of familiar routines and rituals (when they are not in conflict with medical goals), 3) structure and limit setting, and 4) mastery and control [5, p. 143].

Debbie

Debbie was diagnosed at birth with an autoimmune deficiency and had difficulty absorbing food. She was treated with Total Parenteral Nutrition therapy (TPN) which provided all necessary nutrients by intravenous infusion (IV). An IV tube was inserted in her abdomen and each feeding required a fluid flow for up to eight hours. Since TPN would continue for the rest of her life, it was necessary to prepare a plan for Debbie's overall development.

Children like Debbie lack the normal oral stimulation provided by sucking and eating, resulting in a delay in the development of expressive language. In addition, the continuous attachment to an IV frequently impacts negatively on gross and fine motor skills, impedes peer interaction, and interferes with the development of socialization skills.

Debbie's mother played a strong and supportive role in her daughter's life and closely consulted with other team members in preparation for Debbie's future development.

Once discharged at six months, mother and child enrolled in an infant development program in the community and TPN was administered at home by her mother. Out-patient visits to the hospital were frequent and when complications such as infections arose, Debbie was hospitalized for periods of up to five weeks.

When the CLS was assigned to this case, careful plans were developed in consultation with the family to examine Debbie's needs and facilitate her optimum development.

Through games with age-appropriate toys, her verbal skills were enhanced so that two word phrases were achieved. Introduction to the playroom, very early in her hospitalization, soon became the highlight of her day. Once her TPN was capped, the magnetic attraction of the playroom motivated her to make the long slow walk to this exciting child-oriented area, thus improving her gross motor skills. Exposure to scissors, crayons, paper, and small challenging toys increased her fine motor co-ordination. Involvement with other children enhanced her social skills.

Since the IV tubing played a dominant role in her life and deprived her of running, climbing, feeding, and experimenting with new foods, it was important to introduce Debbie to medical play as soon as possible. In the beginning, she chose to put bandages and electrodes on her doll and then graduated to using the intravenous infusion apparatus (IV) and syringes. Using the syringes, she would add fluids to the tubing then retract them, counting the bubbles in the process of imitating her treatment. Innumerable needles were also given to her doll. Her voluntary attention span increased from fifteen to forty-five minutes and she would verbally request to "play doctor." Her enjoyment was reflected in her concentration and the brightness in her eyes.

A community special needs worker was assigned to Debbie's home and was oriented by the CLS to provide appropriate continuous stimulation in order to encourage autonomy, security, and self-esteem. With the ongoing support of Debbie's parents and the medical team, Debbie gradually approached the developmental level of her peers.

THE PRESCHOOLER

Between the ages from three to six years, children have established themselves as individuals and seek to discover the extent of their abilities. They observe and imitate the activities of adults and engage for long periods in imaginative play. At no other time of life do children learn so willingly. Consequently, their initiative should continually be fostered. Thompson and Stanford recognize that:

> Fantasies still abound for this age group, with fears of castration and mutilation common. The view of hospitalization as a form of punishment persists, accompanied by misconceptions about medical equipment and procedures [6, p. 33].

Although children in this age group usually are less dependent upon their parent(s) than younger children, separation from them continues to create anxiety when children are hospitalized. As a result, they also require assistance to adapt to the hospital.

The preschooler is able to comprehend the process of preparation for medical procedures or treatment if approached slowly and soon learns to handle the equipment with skill and enjoyment. This age group becomes more involved in personalizing their doll(s).

Linda

Linda, a five-year-old with aplastic anemia, a life-threatening blood disorder, had been hospitalized intermittently for many weeks during a period of two years. The treatment for her aplastic anemia involved both IV and oral medication.

When it became necessary for her to return to the hospital more often and for longer periods, there was a change in her happy, out-going personality. She would come to my office when she knew it was time for me to leave for the day, sit down and say, "Let's have a meeting." Linda then attempted to negotiate my company for the evening, or would suggest that I find a volunteer. Her feelings of loneliness, sadness, and anxiety were intensified because her mother, a single parent who was also feeling the stress, was visiting less often.

The intensity of the distress in both mother and child concerned the hematology team, and in light of Linda's uncertain prognosis, it was agreed that the consulting psychiatrist would meet with Linda's mother to explore her feelings and needs. I would provide individual therapeutic play sessions for Linda on a daily basis in an attempt to identify her fears, fantasies, and misconceptions, as well as help her re-establish her self-confidence. One day, she initiated the following conversation:

> I'd like to go to heaven.
> Why would you like to go to heaven, Linda?
> 'Cause I'd like to talk to God.
> Why would you like to talk to God?
> Because I would like him to make my sickness go away.
> Do you think it will go away?
> No, they gave me IVs and my bleeding didn't stop. They gave me pills and my bleeding didn't stop.

What was Linda really saying? Was she saying, "I'm afraid?", "Am I going to stay here for the rest of my life?", "Am I going to die?", "Am I going to live with my family again?", "Am I going to stop hurting?", or, "Who will help me?" This was Linda's way of asking for assistance from someone who, in her eyes, might answer her needs.

Due to her age she did not view this visit to heaven as permanent. Except for short clinic visits, Linda was able to spend the last two years of her life at home with her family, attend school, and play with her friends. On her final admission, it was necessary to insert a nasal gastric tube in preparation for emergency surgery. During this process Linda said to the nurse, "Johnny had one of these and he died. Am I going to die?" Although Johnny's death happened three years previously, Linda still remembered him.

SCHOOL AGE CHILDREN

The period from ages six to twelve years, is one of calm, steady growth. It is a time to learn a variety of new skills, including social skills. Consequently, children need to make real achievements in accordance with their own particular abilities. Their independence is increased as they move away from their families for longer periods of time and school assumes increased importance in their lives. Medical play for this age group may increase their knowledge and understanding of medical technology as well as helping them to regain some control over their lives when they are feeling ill.

John

John, a ten-year-old, was diagnosed with leukemia. He was very ill and his prognosis was doubtful. His parents were separated and he and his two siblings, Jane and Samantha, lived with their mother, Margaret.

His mother was extremely protective and unable to accept the fact that her son's life was in jeopardy. Consequently, she refused to allow any discussion to take place about the seriousness of his illness or the possibility that he might die. The anxiety and tension within the family made John extremely apprehensive and clinging. Rae points out that in situations like John's:

> Children have neither the energy to deal with the emotional upset of their parents, nor the emotional strength to deal with the illness itself [7, p. 61].

As part of her involvement, Margaret wished to prepare John for medical procedures and intense chemotherapy treatments or to be present during the preparation by staff. Although this involvement by parents may be supportive, in this case, Margaret's feeling of mistrust of the professional staff was soon relayed to John. Any form of treatment or investigation further increased his anxiety and resulted in crying and physical rejection of procedures.

When children are hospitalized with a life-threatening illness, parents are upset and feel sad, angry, and guilty. They grieve for losses created by changes in their child and the threat of their son's or daughter's death in the future. They also have difficulty in adjusting to a new role of heightened nurturing required to comfort and reassure the child in a new and threatening environment. When they are in distress, parents must be encouraged to accept the assistance and expertise offered by health care professionals to assist them in caring for their child. This will allow parents to concentrate on their changed role as part of their child's treatment team.

One day during a game of scrabble John asked, "Am I going to die?" My response was, "Do you think you are going to die?" After this brief interaction, John appeared pensive but quickly changed the subject and we returned to our game.

In sharing information about this interchange with his mother, she became both angry and frightened. She resisted any suggestion that this issue should be explored. However, Margaret did reveal that when John had tried to discuss his possible death with her, she became very upset. His response was, "But you have Jane and Samantha at home and you don't need me." In return, Margaret told him, "John, you are the one that gives me all the love I need."

My experience has shown that when parents, no matter how well intentioned, do not allow their children to express their fears concerning illness or death, they inadvertently force their child to take on the adult role of protector. Children must then assume the burden of meeting the emotional needs of their parent. They must face their illness and the possibility of their death with many questions unanswered and be denied the opportunity to discuss and understand what lies ahead.

ADOLESCENTS

The task of establishing their identity is of primary importance for adolescents. They are often preoccupied with what others think of them, and contemplate their appearance, relationships, and future.

Hospitalized adolescents are faced with many challenges resulting from decreased independence, less opportunity to interact with their peers, and body changes caused by the treatment and the illness, especially when their lives are threatened or they are dying. According to Plank:

> Helping older terminally ill children with their feelings is an especially difficult question. They generally know that they are not supposed to know, they tend to deny the severity of their illness so as to be able to live with it, and yet they desperately want our honesty [8, p. 37].

I believe that the same holds true for children who must face an uncertain prognosis when diagnosed with an illness such as cancer that may be potentially fatal.

James

At age fifteen, James was very ill when he was diagnosed with non-Hodgkin's lymphoma and admitted to the in-patient unit. He was an intelligent, outgoing, athletic teen who was determined to go back to school and recover from his disease.

His family was comprised of his father, mother, and two siblings, Barbara aged fourteen, and George aged seven. Together they presented as a close and supportive family. His parents both visited

James in the hospital and took turns driving him to clinic visits once he was discharged.

During his many visits to the out-patient clinic for treatment, James tended to pace or stand restlessly until it was necessary for him to have his chemotherapy. The staff believed that his constant movement reflected both his anxiety and his attempt to control it. After his treatments, James was always in a hurry to leave the clinic to return to school and sports. He wanted to get on with his life and openly voiced his dislike of clinic visits. As his treatments continued, he would try to negotiate with the physicians to avoid being hospitalized at all costs. On two occasions hospitalization could not be avoided as James had developed pneumonia. This was especially relevant because of the size and location of his tumor which was large enough to impede his breathing.

In the hospital when he was acutely ill, James welcomed the company of the CLS as a companion in playing cards and engaging in other diversional activities. During these interactions, he would vacillate between hope for future health, denial of any major concerns, and fleeting moments of sadness and fear. When he felt better, he participated in the teen group activities, acting as if he was completely healthy.

Over the ensuing months, James struggled with keeping up with his school work and became increasingly distressed by his respiratory problems. Eventually he could not play sports and soon school and interacting with friends became almost impossible.

As James' physical condition deteriorated, he was admitted to the hospital and quickly moved to the Intensive Care Unit (ICU). There, it was arranged that a familiar CLS would prepare James for a difficult but necessary treatment. She helped him to relax his body and mind in a rehearsal of what was ahead. He was to be given a drug called Pavulon, a paralysing agent that would help him relax so that he could be intubated. This was frightening for James as he would be able to feel and hear, but would not be able to move or talk. During the preparation, he requested that, if his condition deteriorated and death was imminent, the dosage of Pavulon be reduced so that he could say goodbye to his family. The presence of the CLS helped James to accept his treatment.

His parents stayed with James in the hospital, helping to care for him and providing comfort and reassurance. Each day the CLS visited James, giving his parents time away from his bedside. They commented that they found this hospitalization was especially stressful and they had little energy left for their other two children. They were concerned that Barbara and George were both very anxious about the changes in their brother. Consequently, they asked the CLS to spend time on a daily basis with both children. She provided diversional activities and assisted them in the difficult task of saying goodbye to their brother.

As James deteriorated and death was imminent, his parents, with tremendous courage, faith, and wisdom, gave James permission to say good-bye. They held his hands and said:

> James, do you still want to fight? Are you ready to go and if you are, we will let you go. We will hold your hand until Jesus meets you, he will then take your hand and take over your care.

These words were spoken in privacy and several hours later, James died in peace.

CONCLUSION

Play for healthy children and children with acute, chronic, or terminal health problems is therapeutic and essential for their overall development. Diversional or medical play for hospitalized children has the unique power to assist them in gaining mastery over their environment and encourages recovery.

Family support and understanding in the preparation for procedures and therapeutic interventions creates a bond between the child life specialist and the parent(s). Together they observe the strengths and abilities of children who, through the activities of play, learn to understand and come to terms with their illness.

ACKNOWLEDGMENT

Appreciation is extended to Ruth Timney for her assistance and contribution to the art work.

REFERENCES

1. K. McCue, Medical Play: An Expanded Perspective, *Children's Health Care,* *16*:3, pp. 157-161, 1988.
2. R. H. Thompson, *Research on Pediatric Hospitalization*, Charles C. Thomas, Springfield, Illinois, 1985.
3. R. H. Schaffer and W. M. Callender, Psychologic Effects of Hospitalization in Infancy, *Pediatrics, 24*, pp. 528-539, 1959.
4. J. Bowlby, Separation Anxiety, *The International Journal of Psycho-Analysis, 61*, pp. 89-113, 1960.

5. N. Petrillo and S. Sanger, *Emotional Care of Hospitalized Children*, J.B. Lippincott Co., Philadelphia, Pennsylvania, 1972.
6. R. Thompson and G. Stanford, *Child Life in Hospitals: Theory and Practice*, Charles C. Thomas, Springfield, Illinois, 1981.
7. W. A. Rae, Hospitalized Latency-Age Children: Implications for Psychosocial Care, *Children's Health Care, 9*:3, pp. 59-63, 1981.
8. E. Plank, *Working With Children in Hospitals*, Year Book Medical Publishers, Inc., Chicago, Illinois, 1971.

BIBLIOGRAPHY

Adams, D. W., *Childhood Malignancy: The Psychosocial Care of the Child and his Family*, Charles C. Thomas, Springfield, Illinois, 1979.
Adams, D. W. and E. J. Deveau, *Coping With Childhood Cancer: Where do We Go From Here?* New Revised edition, Kinbridge Publications, Hamilton, Ontario, 1993.
Barr, R. D. (ed.), *Childhood Cancer, Information for the Patient and Family*, Vol.1, Canadian Cancer Society, Ontario Division, Toronto, 1989.
Bolig, R., Play in Health Care Settings: A Challenge for the 1990's, *Children's Health Care, 4*, pp. 229-233, 1990.
Bruner, J. S., A. Jolly, and K. Sylva (eds.), *Play: Its Role in Development*, Basic Books, Inc., New York, 1976.
Caplan, F. and T. Caplan, *The Power of Play*, Anchor Press, Doubleday, New York, 1974.
Erikson, E. H., *Childhood and Society*, W. W. Norton and Co., Inc., New York, 1963.
Fraiberg, S. M., *The Magic Years*, Charles Scribners' Sons, New York, 1959.
Gaynard, L., J. Wolfer, J. Goldberger, R. Thompson, L. Redburn, and L. Laidley, *Psychosocial Care of Children in Hospitals: A Clinical Practice Manual*, Association for the Care of Children's Health, Bethesda, Maryland, 1990.
Grollman, E. A., *Talking About Death: A Dialogue Between Parent and Child*, Beacon Press, Boston, Massachusetts, 1970.
Hughes, F. P. and L. D. Noppe, *Human Development Across the Life Span*, Collier MacMillan, Canada, Inc., Toronto, Ontario, 1991.
Kleinberg, S. B., *Educating the Chronically Ill Child*, Aspen Systems Inc., Maryland, 1982.
Linquist, I., *Therapy Through Play*, Arlington Books, London, 1977.
Oremland, E. K., Mastering Developmental and Critical Experiences Through Play and Other Expressive Behaviors in Childhood, *Children's Health Care, 3*, pp. 150-156, 1988.
Shaffer, D. R., *Developmental Psychology: Theory, Research and Application*, Brooks/Cole, Belmont, California, 1985.
Stone, L. J. and J. Church, *Childhood and Adolescence* (5th Edition), Random House, Inc., New York, 1984.

CHAPTER 5

The Use of Humor and Laughter in Helping Children Cope with Life-Threatening Illness

Gerry R. Cox, Eleanor J. Deveau, and David W. Adams

But let me laugh awhile, I've mickle time to grieve.
— John Keats

Storytelling, art, music, and play are approaches that provide forums of expression for all children, but especially for those whose lives are threatened with serious illness. Humor and laughter can offer another therapeutic approach that provides seriously ill children with relief from hospital routine and boredom, diversion during difficult treatments and procedures, respite from stress and anxiety, and opportunities to share special moments with family members, peers, and caregivers. For children facing life-threatening illness, laughter may be a very special, spontaneous, and welcome relief in a world filled with upset, confusion, pain, and suffering.

The therapeutic use of humor and laughter can engage children almost spontaneously. Children find it hard to remain passive observers when humor and laughter are present. Though a child may be determined to be angry and non-responsive, the antics of a clown or a funny scene in a movie make it difficult to maintain a sad face. Sometimes just seeing someone laugh, makes others laugh. In other words, laughter and humor have the unique ability to be infectious or contagious in a non-threatening and safe manner.

Humor is associated with laughter but the terms are not synonymous. Humor, which involves a cognitive, intellectual process, is developed as we grow up in society. Humor is not universal; what may be humorous to one person may not be humorous to someone in another culture. On the other hand, laughter is an instinctive, physiological process. We are born with a natural ability to laugh. In contrast to humor, laughter is universal; it is not culture-specific and can be shared with anyone regardless of language. Laughter may provide such a release of emotions that it can lead to crying, "I laughed so hard I cried!" Sometimes, we cannot distinguish where the laughter actually stopped and the crying began.

In this chapter, we will consider humor as an academic subject, address three different types of humor, identify the purposes of humor and laughter and their application to the lives of children, and discuss the use of humor and laughter as therapeutic approaches with seriously ill children.

HUMOR AS AN ACADEMIC SUBJECT

The intellectual treatment of humor is sobering. Criticism of humor is often defined by highly personal tastes, biases, and gut reactions, rather than evaluative or analytical standards. What is hilarious to one can bore or disgust another [1]. Humor is part of the North American tradition and is evidence of our societal resilience and capacity for self-criticism [2]. But we are not unique, as humor is a part of every society. Humor may consist of stories, cartoons, paradoxes, debunkers, superstition, sadism, masochism, nonsense, satire, and so forth. Levine suggests that the adult's sense of humor appears to develop out of the playful teasing behavior which is characteristic of children [3]. Responses to humor include facial expressions, amusing noises, and out-right laughter. Humor can be healing, or it can be cruel. Humor can be used to show love, loyalty, or faithfulness. It can also be used to show hatred, sickness, and prejudice.

Humor appears in many forums as an integral part of human interaction. It is included in ordinary conversations, speeches, lectures, and all types of human communication. Yet the study of humor has been sporadic [4-15].

Psychology recognizes the value of humor as a coping mechanism. In the early 1900s, Freud described humor as a liberating experience that signified the triumph of the ego in accomplishing the pleasure principle [16]. Freud suggested that humor and laughter were among the few socially acceptable means of releasing pent up frustrations and anger. Humor and laughter also provided a cathartic mechanism for preserving the psychic or emotional energy that would otherwise be released through negative emotional responses [17]. From Freud's perspective, the human being is directed by unconscious drives rather than by conscious thought. Infants laugh very early in life before complex cognitive processes develop. Laughter is also universal which suggests that it has some utilitarian purpose [18]. Freud's theory could serve as an explanation for the humor that dispels anger and aggression in some people. His theory might also explain the role of lust and violence in some humor, but it does not explain puns, riddles, epitaphs, and countless other forms of humor.

TYPOLOGY OF HUMOR

Although many typologies of humor exist, this chapter will focus on three major types of humor. These are constructive, philosophical, and destructive humor.

Constructive Humor

Constructive humor is essentially therapeutic in that it allows for a positive outcome. The intent is to laugh with one another or to laugh at oneself. Children, in families where humor and laughter enhance warmth and generate good feelings among family members, are more likely to develop positive attitudes toward the use of constructive humor.

One type of constructive humor is amusement. This humor comes from the perception of incongruity or illogical juxtapositions. Incongruity emerges in such jokes as, "There will be an eclipse of the moon tonight. Are you going to watch it? Sure, what channel?"

Nonsense jokes that are typically told by children are another type of constructive humor. For example, "What were Tarzan's last words? Who greased the vine?" or "Did you hear about the ghost who was so shy that he couldn't even spook for himself?"

Constructive humor can lead to a guilt-free release of tension. For example, death related jokes can act as a catalyst for the acceptance of an impending death [19]. One dying teen, in response to the hushed voices among family members gathered in her room asked, "Why are you all whispering? Are you afraid the ghosts will hear you and take me away?"

Tombstones can provide positive humor. In Schenectady, New York, a tombstone reads, "He got a fish-bone in his throat and then he sang an angel's note." An example that might appeal to teens is a tombstone found in Dodge City, Kansas, that reads, "Here lays Butch, we planted him raw. He was quick on the trigger, but slow on the draw."

Superstition can also be a form of positive humor. The ability to laugh at one's own superstitions can provide healthy release. Folk sayings may demonstrate an attitude toward life. For example, traditional Volga German proverbs demonstrate both superstition and an attitude toward life, "When someone dies, close his eyes immediately, or he will see who he should come and take next." Or, "An apple a day keeps the doctor away; a rosary a day keeps the devil away; an onion a day keeps everybody away" [20, pp. 165-166].

Philosophical Humor

Philosophical humor generally imparts wisdom, is not always funny, but can be thought-provoking. Some examples are as follows: "There was a man of our town, and he was wondrous wise—He moved away." "Jack be nimble, Jack be quick; Snap the blade, and give it a flick. Grab the purse, it's easily done. Then just for kicks, just for fun; plunge the knife, and cut, and run" [21, p. 26]. "Death is nature's way of telling us to slow down." "It's hard to view one's own death objectively and still carry a tune" [22, p. 92]. Such sayings may provide individuals with a different or unique perspective on their own troubling situations.

Destructive Humor

Destructive humor, on the other hand, is engaged in at the expense of someone else. Cruel and disrespectful humor, whether it be sarcasm, mockery, ethnic cuts, or sadistic comments, can be decidedly negative when intended to be harmful to others. Children, from families where members ridicule or poke fun at each other for faults and shortcomings, are more apt to use different forms of destructive humor.

There are many types of destructive humor. Hostile humor facilitates the expression of anger and frustration toward the objects of the jokes. It may be created by prejudice, fear, illness, impending death, or many other causes. Hostility can be expressed in the attacks of a comedian on the audience or in the ethnic jokes of a bigoted person. Such hostility may also appear in sex jokes that are designed to attack women or men rather than to laugh at oneself.

Sexist and racist jokes by students provide a great source of concern for educators. The greatest problems with such jokes probably exist in the high school system. The dean of boys was the object of hostility and jokes in one particular school experience. He was the person who disciplined students and because of his appearance, was criticized through the use of derogatory nicknames and outrageous imagery in the form of words and sometimes pictures.

Degrading jokes are another form of hostile humor. With this type of humor, one attempts to show the ignorance or foolishness of other people. Political cartoonists often illustrate the lack of wisdom of political leaders. Some ethnic humor is destructive in nature. Degradation also includes sick jokes that focus upon handicaps, disfigurement, personal failings, death, and so forth. Often these are hurtful and in poor taste. Occasionally, this type of humor may be innocuous or even healthy. For example, one tombstone inscription reads, "Here lies . . . , who finally held her tongue." In some instances, this type of humor may provide comic relief or aid in coping with anxiety and stress. It may provide a welcome escape from oppressing reality or help people to cope with crises. However, to debase people or to humiliate them because of their failings is seldom funny.

In another example of degradation, those who commit social blunders are the objects of ridicule and humor. A student who trips when crossing the stage at high school graduation may be readily degraded and seldom finds the embarrassment and ridicule truly funny.

It would seem that those who consciously attempt to be funny may provide a healthy form of humor, while those who accidentally or spontaneously do something that others find humorous may provide considerably less therapeutic value. What is healthy or constructive humor and what is destructive or harmful humor depends upon the perspective of the beholder.

THE PURPOSES OF HUMOR

Humor and laughter create both physiological and psychological effects that engage and exercise the systems of the body in a constructive manner. The therapeutic effects of laughter include:

- stimulating the cardiovascular system thus providing more oxygen for the blood
- exercising the respiratory system by causing deeper breathing
- moving the diaphragm thus stimulating nearby internal organs
- exercising the muscular system by toning and relaxing most of the body's muscles, including the facial muscles
- promoting more synchronization between the two hemispheres of the brain thus improving relaxation
- helping to possibly rebalance the body's endocrine system thereby activating natural painkillers and increasing the level of alertness
- generating feelings of sharing, togetherness, and intimacy [18, 23].

Recent research in humor and laughter indicates that not only do psychological and physiological benefits emerge, but that humor and laughter may provide spiritual and social value as well [12]. Besides coping with anger and aggression as Freud indicated, humor may function as a coping mechanism when people encounter a crisis by allowing them to avoid or deny feelings that are too frightening to face.

Thorson and Powell suggest that humor provides a means of seeking control over the uncontrollable [24]. For example, humor allows children to approach a topic that is both personal and serious with a degree of liberation that does not trivialize their losses. Thoughts and feelings associated with serious illness, the threat of death, and even death itself can be temporarily avoided or more readily dealt with through the use of humor. People enduring a crisis may humor one another in order to boost morale, even when they are not in a playful state of mind. After the tragic death of President John F. Kennedy, children told jokes similar to this one, "What did Caroline get for her birthday? She got a Jack-in-the-box" [25, p. 75]. Such humor provides individuals with an avenue to deal with suffering whether it is their own or someone else's. This type of morbid humor is known as "gallows humor." It also occurs among inmates in concentration or prisoner of war camps, and others who face impending doom. Often, from a self-preservation point of view, finding some humor in overwhelmingly painful or depressing situations can not only make such situations seem less intense, but can also help to preserve the positive energy needed to cope with the crisis.

DeSpelder and Strickland see humor as a means of reducing the anxiety that comes with an awareness of one's own mortality, although they worry that poking fun at death may not be genuinely facing it [26]. While children are not awaiting the gallows, they are still facing their own crises. For example, the topic of dying and death may induces fear in children. Humor encourages openness and communication. Dying children who were previously happy and had mutually supportive relationships may develop impaired relationships when normal communication is avoided in an attempt to conceal the truth from them or to pretend that death will not happen [27].

Pritchard and Epling suggest that open communication between dying children and their parents is not only beneficial to dying children, but also associated with greater optimism and adjustment in surviving siblings [28]. In such circumstances, one may cope with the fearfulness of the situation by the use of humor [29].

Sometimes it is helpful for adults to play games with children in order to promote their understanding of death through humor. For instance, marshmallow charades involves children acting out some common phrases that relate to the theme of death. If no one guesses the phrase, the children suffer the "torture" of being pelted by marshmallows. What is essential to the success of this game is to have an adult explain to the children the meaning of the phrases and the feelings suffered by the "losers."

Writing one's epitaph or planning one's funeral may also provide a potentially humorous way to introduce a difficult topic. As an educator, Cox has found this technique to be effective. Developing commercials for funeral homes, casket makers, or cemeteries can be a fun-filled learning experience. A life after death or a reincarnation party may be of similar value. The options chosen should be planned carefully, consistent with the leader's beliefs, and developed under adult supervision. It is difficult to teach with humor if one does not agree with the tenets of the humor. The leader must be able to laugh with the participants.

In some cultures, humor may also be introduced in special ways to help children deal with dying and death. Levine suggests that clowning or ritual joking was used by Native Americans to allay death related fears and anxieties [30]. Clowning provides a catharsis for the deepest antisocial feelings. It allows people to express their feelings of love, hate, and fear without guilt. Though clowning may be considered self-humiliating and self-punishing by some, it allows the expression of even the most repressed feelings that would not be tolerated in everyday life.

On the Day of the Dead (El Dia de los Muertos) in Mexico, for example, the souls of the dead are honored, and some would suggest that they actually return to earth. Children and adults enjoy this festive occasion including the candies and toys in the shapes of skeletons, skulls, caskets, and other symbols of death. Adults and children joke and exhibit humor surrounding the "return" of the dead. In this context, there is no fear or rejection of death. The humorous approach to the dead allows for a greater acceptance of death and a reduction of fear. Humor encourages the retention and expression of the fun-loving essence of childhood [31].

THE USE OF HUMOR WITH CHILDREN AND ADOLESCENTS WHOSE LIVES ARE THREATENED

Humor and laughter promote a feeling of wellness and good health. A humorous outlook has the potential to prevent, manage, and possibly cure diseases [32]. Humor and laughter are cathartic processes which release repressed emotions that cause anxiety and stress. Emotional stresses such as fear, anxiety, sadness, and anger have degenerative and debilitating effects on the body. These effects, which are evident and must be medically treated, can also be inhibited by humor [22]. Laughter and humor stabilize blood pressure, oxygenate the blood, massage the vital organs, stimulate circulation, facilitate digestion, relax the body, and produce a feeling of well-being [18]. How much pain people experience as part of illness is also influenced by their state of mind. The more people concentrate on the associated pain, the greater their discomfort. On the other hand, as many athletes have discovered, if the contest is close or one team is winning, minor injuries are quickly overlooked for the sake of the game.

When children's lives are threatened, they must face a complex array of changes and feelings. In a disease such as cancer or cystic fibrosis, children may encounter months or years of treatment and episodes of acute illness and hospitalization [33]. For these children, it is imperative to recognize that they may endure a complete range of intense emotions and be confronted by physical crises which bring them face to face with death. Their responses will be governed by their level of cognitive development and the reactions of their parents, other family members, peers, and caregivers. Zigler, Levine, and Gould suggest that while a child usually needs sufficient cognitive congruences to fully understand the humor stimulus, the child may still find reasons to view the stimulus as funny at times when the anticipated response would be the opposite [34].

The process of coping with illness and treatment includes many points where humor and laughter may be welcomed by children and their families. Children, who generally take themselves less seriously, often provide humor that uplifts their families and visitors. Perhaps this occurs through performing as if on stage, diverting everyone from the anxiety and sadness created by hospitalization, illness, and treatment.

The Candlelighters Childhood Cancer Foundation publishes separate newsletters for families and for teens. Humor is regularly presented as a feature in both publications. Russem cites the example of Missy, a nine-year-old girl with cancer, who had a reputation for being an endless source of humor on the pediatric ward. Missy explained why she liked telling jokes:

> It gets people laughing and I get attention for being funny, not for being sick. Now everyone always asks me to tell jokes and then they tell other people. It really lights up the day for . . . the staff. For some of the kids it's the first time they've laughed since they've been in the hospital. Their parents laugh too [31, p. 4].

Humor also provides an expression of individualism which may enhance children's feelings of self-control in the face of situations where they have little or no control. Michael, an Australian teen who lost his hair due to cancer treatment, wrote:

Q. Why did the chemo patient paint rabbits on his head?
A. From a distance it looked like hares. Ha! Ha! [35, p. 3].

Adams and Deveau note that children with cancer who lose their hair due to chemotherapy or gain excessive weight as a result of steroid medication, may become objects of degradation [33]. Taking their cues from comics who often perform comedy by deliberately committing social blunders, adolescents, in particular, may make themselves the objects of ridicule. One teen simply pulled off his wig and invited everyone to "laugh it out and get it over with" [33, p. 63].

Russem, in discussing children with cancer, points out how well children respond to jokes and riddles as part of communication. She suggests that:

The role of humor does not negate the child's pain and anger but encourages retention and expression of the fun loving essence of childhood [31, p. 3].

Without communication and humor, children who are unable to find anyone who is willing and able to listen and to understand their fears and feelings may die feeling lonely [27].

Clearly humor may be a non-threatening way to include death, mutilation, or injury as the subject of children's jokes. Their humor can become a safety-valve for releasing hostility, discontent, and otherwise unacceptable feelings [6]. Humor also tends to temporarily neutralize emotionally painful situations. Destructive humor may, at least for a time, ease the pain of an uncontrollable situation such as an impending death or painful illness.

Adams and Deveau discuss the behavior of a young boy seven years of age who, after many months of intensive chemotherapy and medical procedures, was playing with syringes as part of therapeutic play. He sprayed water in the face of all of the medical dolls, and when asked if he was giving them needles, he said, "No, I'm peeing all over them" [33, p. 31].

Humor may also help children and teens divert aggression or manage "touchy situations" at times when they feel threatened by illness, treatment, or the possibility of death. Eleven-year-old Tom's drawing of a gigantic syringe and needle chasing an ant-like figure, or twelve-year-old Scott's portrayal of the resident physician as a monstrous gorilla, both reflected their inner concerns about their illness, intensive treatment, and control by hospital personnel, particularly physicians. They had been defiant and angry with staff and their parents. But both also laughed at their drawings and displayed them on the bulletin boards in their rooms.

In other situations, for example, at summer camps for children with illnesses or disabilities such as cancer, cystic fibrosis, and muscular dystrophy, humor helps children to feel empowered to act and feel like their peers. Humor facilitates positive communication and social relationships, producing a feeling of solidarity and cohesion between children and counselors and between the children themselves. Humor is part of the bonds of friendship that bring happy memories after children return to their families and the consequences of having been labeled in their schools or neighborhoods as sick children.

In situations where children and teens are suffering from physical pain, the initial analogy about athletes holds true for children whose lives are threatened. Diversion and respite can be facilitated through laughter and fun which provide time out for at least brief periods. Even when children are extremely ill, they may enjoy watching their favorite type of humor such as "TV Bloopers" or age-appropriate videos. Humor may provide diversion and help them get through the day.

Lastly, humor can allow the seriously ill or dying child to deal with the paradox of life and death. One seventeen-year-old who recently died, illustrated this point. He responded to the long, sad faces of his family and caregivers by asking, "Did someone die around here?" He also planned his own funeral and requested that it be a happy occasion with much singing and laughter so that people might remember him with a smile.

CONCLUSION

In a comedy, laughs don't hurt.
— David Picker

Humor and laughter allow children and their families to escape, if only for a very short time, to a world where illness, pain, suffering, and impending loss do not exist. Yet, professionals and caregivers sometimes hesitate to use humor and laughter as a therapeutic approach because it is associated with happiness and a feeling of lightness [23]. When humor and laughter are integrated appropriately and sensitively in the right place and at the right time, bearing in mind the individual child's cognitive abilities, developmental level, and cultural and religious beliefs, the effects can be very positive and cathartic.

Humor and laughter, in conjunction with other therapeutic approaches, can help to dissipate difficult feelings of anger, fear, frustration, and helplessness. There is enough hurt, sadness, and gloom in the lives of these children and their families. As professionals we can encourage the use of humor and laughter, thus providing them with some lightness and happiness in their world of uncertainty.

REFERENCES

1. A. P. Dudden, *American Humor*, Oxford University Press, New York, 1987.
2. N. Walker, *A Very Serious Thing: Women's Humor and American Culture*, University of Minnesota, Minneapolis, 1988.
3. J. Levine, Approaches to Humor Appreciation, in *Motivation in Humor*, J. Levine (ed.), Atherton Press, New York, 1969.
4. M. L. Baron, A Content Analysis of Intergroup Humor, *American Sociological Review, 15*, pp. 88-94, 1950.
5. J. Burma, Humor as a Technique in Race Conflict, *American Sociological Review, 11*, pp. 710-715, 1946.
6. J. Coser, Some Social Functions of Laughter: A Study of Humor in a Hospital Setting, *Human Relations, 12*, pp. 171-182, 1959.
7. M. Davis, Sociology Through Humor, *Symbolic Interaction, 2*, pp. 105-110, 1979.
8. G. Fine, Humorous Interaction and the Social Construction of Meaning: Making Sense in a Jocular Vein, *Studies in Symbolic Interaction, 5*, pp. 83-101, 1984.
9. M. Flaherty, A Formal Approach to The Study of Amusement in Social Interaction, *Studies in Symbolic Interaction, 5*, pp. 71-82, 1984.
10. J. Flugel, Humor and Laughter, in *Handbook of Social Psychology*, G. Lindsay (ed.), Addison-Wesley, Cambridge, Massachusetts, 1954.
11. E. Gross, Laughter and Symbolic Interaction, *Symbolic Interaction, 2*, pp. 111-112, 1979.
12. P. McGee, *Humor: Its Origin and Development*, W. H. Freeman, San Francisco, 1979.
13. P. McGee and J. Goldstein (eds.), *Handbook of Humor Research*, Vols. I and II, Springer-Verlag, New York, 1983.
14. R. Stebbins, Comic Relief in Everyday Life: Dramaturgic Observations in a Function of Humor, *Symbolic Interaction, 2*, pp. 95-104, 1979.
15. M. Leming and G. Dickinson, *Understanding Dying, Death, and Bereavement*, Holt, Rinehart, and Winston, Fort Worth, Texas, 1990.
16. S. Freud, Jokes and Their Relation to the Unconscious, in *The Standard Edition of the Complete Psychological Works of Sigmond Freud*, Vol. 21, J. Strachey (ed.), Norton, New York, pp. 159-166, 1960.
17. D. Black, Laughter, *Journal of American Medical Association, 252*:21, pp. 2995-2998, December 7, 1984.
18. J. Goldstein and P. McGee, *The Psychology of Humor*, American Press, New York, 1972.

19. V. Robinson, Humor and Health, in *Handbook of Humor Research*, P. McGee and J. Goldstein (eds.), Springer-Verlag, New York, 1983.
20. T. Koberdanz, *The Volga German Catholic Life Cycle: An Ethnographic Reconstruction*, unpublished thesis, Colorado State University, Fort Collins, Colorado, 1974.
21. E. Merriam, *The Inner City Mother Goose*, Simon and Schuster, New York, 1969.
22. L. Peter, *The Laughter Prescription*, Ballentine Books, New York, 1982.
23. B. J. Jaffee, *Using Laughter as a Cathartic Process in Grief Counselling*, paper presentation, King's College Conference on Death and Bereavement, London, Ontario, 1993.
24. J. Thorson and F. Powell, To Laugh in the Face of Death: The Games that Lethal People Play, *Omega, 21*:3, pp. 224-239, 1990.
25. M. Wolfenstein and G. Kilman, (eds.), *Children and the Death of a President*, Doubleday, Garden City, New York, 1990.
26. L. DeSpelder and D. Strickland, *The Last Dance*, Mayfield, Compton, California, 1992.
27. P. Jeffrey and R. Lansdown, The Role of the Special School in the Care of the Dying Child, *Bereavement Care, 12*:2, pp. 14-16, 1993.
28. S. Pritchard and F. Epling, Children and Death: New Horizons in Theory and Measurement, *Omega, 24*:4, pp. 271-288, 1991.
29. H. Fitzgerald, *The Grieving Child: A Parent's Guide*, Simon and Schuster, New York, 1992.
30. J. Levine, Regression in Primitive Clowning, in *Motivation in Humor*, J. Levine (ed.), Atherton Press, New York, 1969.
31. J. Russem, Humor: Holistic Care for Children with Cancer, *The Candlelighters Childhood Cancer Foundation Quarterly, XXI*, pp. 3-4, Winter 1988.
32. G. Cox, *Sociology of Dying and Death: Theory and Research*, Fort Hays State University, Hays, Kansas, 1990.
33. D. W. Adams and E. Deveau, Coping with Childhood Cancer: Where Do We Go From Here?, Kinbridge Publications, Hamilton, Ontario, 1993.
34. E. Zigler, J. Levine, and L. Gould, Cognitive Challenges as a Factor in Children's Humor Appreciation, in *Motivation in Humor*, J. Levine (ed.), Atherton Press, New York, 1969.
35. M. McWilliam, riddle, *The Candlelighters Childhood Cancer Foundation Youth Newsletter, XII*, p. 3, 1990.

CHAPTER 6

Pets: A Source of Hope for Children with Life-Threatening Illness

Sharon M. McMahon

HISTORICAL HIGHLIGHTS

The relationship with and utilization of animals in humans' lives is not new [1]. Across many cultures, wild and domesticated animals have been associated with myths and legends for centuries. Ancient mythology and archeological evidence reveal that a great variety of selected non-human species shared the most intimate space and time with humans. Some animals were viewed as objects, accessories, and companions, as well as sources of security, transportation, hunting, sport, and diversion [2, 3]. Other animals had selected places of honor as totem figures, dream images, and class symbols. Reflection upon multicultural and spiritual traditions may reveal the significance of animals in an individual's spiritual and mental journey through history to this day [4]. Today, personal beliefs and needs blend with cultural norms and values to guide the definition and selection of species for domestication as a pet [5].

In our contemporary North American culture, pets usually meet eight expectations. They are non-utilitarian, aesthetically pleasing, singular, sociable, affectionate, and submissive as well as being a cohabitant and possession [6]. Today, pets are acquired or adopted for other roles because they possess qualities such as protectiveness, strength, agility, and "teachability." Some domesticated animals become therapeutic aides in animal-assisted therapy (A.A.T.) or animal-activity participation (A.A.P.) lifestyle enhancement programs which are available in many countries [7, 8].

For children with life-threatening illness, a therapeutic animal companion needs no label or definition. The endearing features of pets are noted consistently by children who enthusiastically and coherently talk about, paint, and draw their animal companions [9-12].

PEOPLE + PETS = POTENTIAL

The benefits of interspecies contact have been increasingly documented in the literature by many professions over the last ten years. They recognize that contact with pets can alleviate the negative outcomes of loneliness and separation. Domestic animals are reported to be comforting, gratifying, liberating, inclusive, educational, fun, and accepting. They can empower people, help create "eustress" (positive stress), and may be essential for holistic health [13, 14].

Bergler reports that dog owners when compared with non-dog owners have more frequent everyday happiness, less stress, more comfort, less depression and resignation, and a higher quality of life. They also engage in more normative, healthy, active behavior and communicate more about their problems. He also reports that cats satisfy human needs in individualized ways. Some are elegant, easy to care for, and offer lap-sized, huggable companionship. Others play spontaneously and provide a sense of calmness and security [15].

Together, pets and children have the potential for mutually beneficial relationships [16]. For all children, especially those with health challenges, animal companions can enhance socialization and acceptance by others [17]. Maggitti writes:

> Why shouldn't a pet mean as much and perhaps more to children who have not been blessed with sturdy good health or a loving, supportive environment. . . . (T)he child with special needs has a need for the special nurturing that only pets can provide [14, p. 7].

Pet affiliation encourages role modeling and teaching opportunities for children to learn how to assume responsibility, practice accountability, provide nurturance and empathy, show compassion, and be self-controlled.

Children do not have to own a pet to learn about animals and experience the benefits of pet affiliation. Regular visits with other owners' pets encourage activities such as touching (patting), grooming, walking, feeding, cleaning, conversation, and casual play. Such experiences can be enjoyable and beneficial especially when children view such visits as positive stress-reducing experiences [15].

Calming and centering activities help children feel good about themselves and their world. The warm, soft, supple quality of most animal coats encourages the pleasing sensation of gentle touch. Children learn to be gentle and calm in order to prevent the growls, scratches, and nips that may come from upset, mistreated pets, particularly dogs and cats. The immediate positive and negative responses from animals help children learn appropriate, consistent, interactive behavior. Through studying and interacting with pets, children can learn to trust, be caring, experience consistent relationships, feel good about themselves, achieve and complete goals, strengthen their relationship with others, and receive praise and unconditional love from the pet.

Children can experience first-hand the positive results of kindness, practice, interest, and attention given to pets. Animals give immediate feedback and will work toward long-term goal attainment with pleasure. Most children will feel proud and happy when their pet (usually a dog) can follow simple commands or comply with requests, and perform tricks that have consumed many hours of gentle teaching and positive reinforcement.

Pets can act as catalysts that hold a family together. They can encourage diversional or cooling-off activities in times of conflict [18]. Pearce states that, "The human-animal bond is more important than ever in these days of family break-ups" [19, p. 25].

DuVall reports that Levinson explains the child-pet bond in another way stating, "Probably the reason that most children take so readily and easily to animal pets as close companions stems from the need of the child to be close to a parent substitute that he can control and direct at will" [20, p. 20]. Levinson further theorizes that children's beliefs and emotions are perceived to be the same as the pet's. Therefore, if children and adolescents become angry with their parents, they believe that their pets must also feel the same. They see their pets as stalwart, truthful, and constant friends that never disappoint or confuse them [20]. As children nurture pets and begin to think for themselves, they can learn to actively problem-solve. They can share and take responsibility for optimal consistent care, protection, recreation, stress-reduction, and life enrichment activities for their dependent companion.

Pets have also proven to be a "bridge to maturity," especially for many children in crisis [21]. They can be safe sources of emotional projection when children have unresolved feelings or questions about family changes. Pets can be safe outlets for crying, hugging, pretending, role-rehearsal, and asking rhetorically about certain events that might have occurred or are about to happen. Safe expressions of anger such as talking-out-loud to a pet and going for a walk to "cool-off" can be much more effective than keeping feelings hidden inside or exploding in rage at familiar caregivers.

Professionals and caregivers must respect the decision of some families to avoid pet ownership. Personal beliefs regarding the value of pets should not be forced upon these families in spite of the positive outcomes that may be anticipated.

PETS AS PSYCHOTHERAPEUTIC AIDES

Advocacy for the use of pets as psychotherapeutic aides in various institutions, agencies, and programs has been summarized by numerous authors [10, 22-29]. The late psychologist, Boris Levinson, incorporated and prescribed companion animals in his work with families and children as follows:

> Early in the 1960's, my first insight into the use of a dog as an "accessory" in the treatment of disturbed children came about inadvertently. And it was my own dog, Jingles, who played the leading role in what proved to be a most startling drama [24, p. 41].

Before an A.A.T. or A.A.P. program can be initiated, professionals must determine the feasibility of such an arrangement for a particular child by taking into account any health risks, the family's cultural beliefs and practices, and the consequences of the presence of an animal pet in a shared space with other children. For some, pets are not desired or recommended due to allergies or risk of infection. For others, religious and cultural taboos clearly define certain animals as "unclean" (such as the dog and pig), and therefore, would not be suitable as a pet or an animal aide. In the shared space of a school, hospital, or clinic, the presence of an animal aide may make other children and families anxious or fearful. Desensitization to the fear of animals is not usually a priority in current oncology treatment programs, and hospice or palliative care settings. Consequently, though an A.A.T. or A.A.P. program may be recommended, it may not be feasible for some children.

PET SELECTION AND CARE
CONSIDERATIONS

For children living with long-term medical conditions, pet care and association with pets require planning and consideration of the important principles of epidemiology, zoonosis, and environmental hygiene, as some organisms exist that can cause sickness in both animals and humans. For example, organisms causing salmonellosis, toxoplasmosis, cryptocystis, mycobacteriosis, or cat scratch disease must be considered when humans and animals share a common environment.

In a medically fragile pediatric situation, guidance in the choice of a pet and ongoing health supervision for that animal is mandatory. Expert guidance can be sought from veterinary clinics, universities, and other organizations concerned with the health of animals. Prevention of illness for all participants is a common goal [30, 31]. Simple precautions such as wearing protective gloves and masks to clean pet excrement from litter boxes, cages, and yards can be maintained within any household or setting where immunocompromised children may live. Mandatory animal immunizations, regular stool checks for parasites, optional purchase of special medicated (antibiotic-coated) feed, and regular grooming to insure flea and tick prevention, are included in health promotion protocols for mammals and birds. Clean food, bedding, and housing are essential to quality care and health for all pets. Even fish and reptiles require regular bacterial swabs to monitor their health and living conditions.

While the total health of a pet is an important consideration, its suitability also depends upon many other factors such as: 1) the location and size of the family home; 2) legalities such as bylaws or tenant agreements; 3) lifestyle; 4) activity levels of parents and children; 5) monetary commitment; 6) interests and affinity for certain species; 7) special health concerns (such as allergies or immunosuppression); 8) other support resources; and 9) time available to assure life-long quality care for the selected animal companion [32]. An assessment of the needs and desires of potential owners must be conducted before a pet is selected.

Certain animals may be chosen for the specific qualities they bring to the interaction. Careful study of physical and personality traits is recommended to blend human, environmental, and animal qualities so that the likelihood of a healthy match is enhanced [27]. Horses, in particular, have breed characteristics that make the choice of one breed possible for selected functions. When matching dogs and cats, animal protection organizations, national dog and cat clubs, and veterinarians can help.

Pets should be chosen with care. It is important to plan ahead, to wait for the "right animal persona," and to consider the appropriate developmental stage of the child [33]. In an all-too-common scenario, a casual spontaneous "pick-a-pet" visit to a shelter, pet store, breeder, or a response to a media advertisement does not usually develop into a positive bonding experience [34]. Heart and mind must work together in the selection process as it often becomes the "choice of a lifetime" (the pet's at least).

Special training can prepare other species such as monkeys to provide practical and functional assistance and to be physical extensions of the person, thereby enhancing independence in self-care. Service dogs have proven to be reliable and cost-effective sources of mobility, exercise, physical care, self-esteem, protection, fun, communication, and sensory adjuncts especially for children during lengthy, confining periods of isolation or home care [18].

The author, in a similar manner to others, has witnessed the same calming and beneficial effects of goldfish and aquaria on the milieu of pediatric, psychiatric, intensive care units, and other office and clinic settings [35]. Birds and fish are frequently chosen for pet-keeping in institutional settings. Both species are fun to watch, relaxing, and content to be confined. However, some may require special equipment, safety devices, feed and cleaning protocols, and prevention of drafts, overfeeding, overheating, and crowding. Safety devices are available at reliable pet stores to secure cages and tanks to prevent accidents. The prevention of accidents and illness not only avoids grief from the death of a pet, but also avoids or defers replacement costs.

Small rodents such as rabbits, guinea pigs, gerbils, and hamsters are often chosen by teachers as classroom mascots. They are also frequent choices as family pets because they are "so cute" and make good "lap-sitters" on a towel. Rabbits can be litter trained, but other rodents are more difficult. Some breeds may bite if handled roughly by children. Pet owners must learn how to handle and feed rodents and determine if they can adapt to their sleep cycles and living patterns before making a selection. For instance, gerbils sleep in the daytime and are very busy at night. Therefore, they may be a good choice for children with insomnia, but would be inappropriate for children without sleep deficiencies. Chewing logs may help gerbils and other rodents keep their teeth short enough for comfort and proper eating. However, problems with overgrown teeth, ear mites, broken bones, and the tendency to be susceptible to human colds may make smaller rodents less practical as long-term pets than other mammals such as dogs or cats.

ANIMALS AS RESTORATIVE AGENTS AND MILIEU ENHANCERS

How can we deny children the opportunity to experience the richness of life with a pet? Their desire to be with and to share their world with a pet may be so strong that many children create make-believe creatures, walk mechanical pet substitutes, watch computer screen facsimiles, or sleep with silent stuffed animals.

Schaufl and Bergler support the importance of animals in children's imaginative play with puppets, drawings, cut and paste activities, and the reading, telling, and writing of stories [36]. Adults can engage children in storytelling, playing make-believe using animal costumes, manipulating animal models in zoos or farm scenes, visiting or watching videotapes of animal habitats, and walking in natural settings with time included for observation, listening, touching, and smelling.

Ongoing discussions and storytelling about one's own pet, favorite animals, and wishes associated with animals and nature, can provide valuable insights into children's relationships with the world. Pets can provide opportunities for children to demonstrate their compassion and respect for living things. Pets may serve as comfortable topics for social communication and provide motivation for goal setting.

Setting up and maintaining bird feeders, aquaria, butterfly gardens, insect farms, or other mini-habitats can: 1) keep children linked with the seasonal changes; 2) help prevent boredom; 3) stimulate inquiry and learning; 4) provide a purpose or create a passionate interest that can help children establish social linkages and communicate with others; 5) promote outreach beyond themselves; 6) foster experiences for self-growth; and 7) enhance recognition of their contribution to the world.

No age limit needs to be applied to the decision to incorporate pets as a topic in daily routines, diversions, treatments, or comfort. From the stylized animal creatures of juvenile television programs and classical tales of baby animals and forest species, to the sagas of undersea, jungle, intergalactic, or other adventure stories, fantasy creatures and talking animals can be inexpensive sources of relaxation, adventure, recreation, imagination, communication, learning, and self-validation.

RELATIONSHIPS: THE CHILD-PET BOND

Children raised with dogs, cats, and other "in-house" pets consider them to be "family." Many children even give animals the roles of brothers and sisters [37]. For many children, pets become part of their identity. When asked about the roles pets play, children described them as: a playmate; "my secret-keeper" and confidant; "my snuggle buddy;" "the only one who likes me just the way I am;" "my wet-nosed alarm clock;" "our team's best outfielder;" "my bodyguard;" and "my best friend." Pets always listen to everything. At all times, pets take children seriously and are discreetly silent! Many children consider dogs to be their best friends as they are so supportive.

For children experiencing life-threatening illness, constant long-term relationships with animal companions have even more significance because they help to validate the normalcy and viability of day-to-day activities. Child and pet relationships are treasured rather than taken for granted. Pets often provide a buffer to the stresses of life and help generate the perception of inclusion. Mood swings and anger are rare. When children are ill, dogs make ideal nursemaids because they remain close at hand. Their unconditional love and presence decrease feelings of isolation, provides comfort, and may improve compliance during necessary treatment [21, 40].

SOCIALIZATION OF PET AND CHILD

In order to enhance the positive attributes of pets, special socialization and education must be provided, especially for dogs and horses. Obedience schools can be excellent experiences for the pet dog and the family members, especially children. Puppy classes enhance acceptance of diverse experiences and provide pets with a sense of belonging, identity, and loyalty. As the pet grows in competence and learns to socialize appropriately, so does the child. Guidance from animal management books, veterinarians, kennel and cat clubs, magazines, canine or feline behaviorists (ethologists), and trainers may provide practical suggestions that can prevent traumatic accidents and unwanted behaviors such as biting, scratching, fearfulness, and conflicts caused by human ignorance of appropriate ways to interact with animals.

Parenting in the home must also extend to the pet. Parenting styles that are positive, informed, mature, respectful, nurturing, and focused on mentoring the child are often transferred positively to facilitate optimal socialization and care of the pet. Adult involvement in daily, routine pet care helps set a rhythm in daily living that is shared by all. Creative inclusion of the animal-care routines in family life takes planning but the results are often worthwhile.

For youngsters in crisis who may be denied many normal activities, pet care routines become reasons for being. Self-esteem is enhanced when pets depend upon children. Children can sense the security of an inclusive parenting style where their own needs and those of their pet are met. Children can be encouraged and assisted toward mastery of their developmental tasks by helping to care for the pet.

For medically challenged children, large animals can add a sense of social acceptance, power, release, control, competence, and being directly in touch with life around them, especially if mobility and assistance devices are part of a child's self-image and lifestyle [39, 40].

Watching animals work, touching them, and sensing their life (warmth, breath, smell, bodily functions) may help lift children's spirits and prompt them to reach out. Imagine the exhilaration of speed, the freedom of movement, the wind-on-the-face, and the sound of pounding power while astride a horse, or the joy of sight-seeing while riding in a pony, dog, or llama cart. Imagine being pulled along in one's own wheelchair by a large, trained, well-conditioned "service" or "ability" dog. Children are able to look up, smile, and enjoy the outing rather than exhaust themselves by pushing equipment, straining to reach elevator controls, and being on guard to make sure that no object or person gets caught in the spokes. There is great contentment when another living creature responds willingly and spontaneously to commands and gestures. Children's ability to involve pets in their activities and control them as partners increases their feelings of satisfaction and accomplishment and enhances their self-esteem.

PETS EMPOWER

When life is difficult, children often feel compromised. Pets may help them become positively empowered. Often children with life-threatening illness and their pets blend "as one," sharing moods, space, and essentials such as food and water. Together, they become mutually respectful of feelings including excitement, frustration, and fear. It is suggested that this is due to the aptitude of animals' intuition or instinct and their strength in perceiving changes in non-verbal and physiological conditions of humans.

Pets help children reach out beyond themselves and stretch their egocentrism to the point of "other-inclusion" and care [41, pp. 24-27; 42]. Some studies demonstrate that these interactions have long-term implications. For example, adults who have had a positive relationship with pets during their childhood have been found to be much more empathetic [43].

PETS AND CHILDREN WITH CANCER

In Erma Bombeck's book, *I Want to Grow Hair, I Want to Grow Up, I Want to Go to Boise*, many of the expectations of a positive, loving bond with animals are expressed by children with cancer [44]. Bombeck discusses a group of children with cancer who are gathered around a social worker to talk about their imaginary animal named Hope. The children describe Hope as about two and one-half feet tall, soft and fluffy, with blue eyes, and a short bottle brush tail that wags. One ear stands up while the other flops down. They state that Hope smiles and is the color of happiness and sunshine. At times, Hope is shy, loud (so it can talk louder than fear), or giggly. "Sometimes you can coax it to you, but most of the time you have to be patient and wait. Then it will come to you" [44, p. 142]. The children decided that Hope had to sleep inside with them because it was "too fragile." They also said that if you did not "take good care of it, it could die," "you can't cage it or buy it," and "it will come only when you need it" [44, p. 143]. Then the children created "Hopelets," the offspring of Hope. They realized that they were not to keep them. "Hopelets" must be shared with others who need them (as pets).

Pets are vital "links-to-hope" for children who are in the hospital or away from their own environment in alternate settings for treatment, palliative care, or special services. Arranged pet visits from home, time with ward mascots, looking at photographs or watching videos of their pets, and participating in A.A.P. or A.A.T. programs can help prevent, moderate, or reduce daily stress, sadness, and destabilization of self-esteem. These experiences provide opportunities to share, have fun, play, and experience devotion. They may also help children develop coping strategies for separation, continued illness, pain, death, and grief. Whether at home, in hospital, or in hospice/palliative care settings, children, parents, and caregivers can come together through the catalytic capacity of pets.

PREPARATION FOR THE PURCHASE OF A PET

The following suggestions will help parents select a pet that is most suitable for their family and manage its care:

1. Ask each family member about their wishes or concerns associated with introducing a pet.
2. Consult with reputable breeders, veterinarians, and humane-protection staff about pet characteristics, special health needs, and practices.
3. Read about animals to gain insight into their needs, nonverbal communication signals, and signs of health and distress.
4. Deal with concerns expressed by family members and make plans for housing and caretaking duties.
5. Take time to select a pet. Perform simple socialization tests to select the most compatible animal. Veterinarians can help with these. An impulsive decision will often end up as a mistake and the pet will be "forfeited," ignored, cast aside, or "dropped off."

6. Consider the selection of a pet to be as important as adopting another family member. Remember the pet will become part of the family unit and will influence relationships forever. The choice of a name should be by consensus.
7. Do *not* get a pet just as a present for a birthday or other (holiday) event. This is very stressful for the animal and humans and often sets up unnecessary tension right at the start.

Once the pet has been selected, the following suggestions will help to promote safe and happy bonds:

1. Do *not* designate the ownership of the pet to one family member. This creates jealousies and ignores the pet's natural selection of a "favored" person. It also isolates and reduces the bonding or unifying qualities that pets help to foster.
2. Set time aside for the pet, remembering that:
   a) A young animal requires more time for educating and socializing due to the need for frequent repetition of cues, rewards, prompting, correction, and safety precautions/ supervision.
   b) Mature animals may come with a history that should be known in detail to facilitate a positive transfer to a new family.
3. Allocate a yearly health care budget for the pet. Owners usually find that the larger the animal, the higher the cost to maintain it. Allow for immunizations, neutering, and some accidental "rainy-day" funds.
4. Keep a written record of the animal's history, resource people, health certificates, photos, anecdotes, and plans for care.
5. If hygiene management is a real or potential health problem, recruit help from local humane or animal-companion organizations, or veterinary resources such as a community college. Provide proper first-aid and medical attention for scratches, nips, or other zoonotic concerns. Prevention is the best precaution.
6. Do not expose the pet to extremes of heat, wind, sun, or cold. If you will not stay somewhere, the pet should not either (for example, a pet should never be left in a parked car, especially with windows rolled up in hot weather).
7. Learn how to humanely and properly handle, move, lead, and restrain the pet to prevent injury.
8. Allow time for the pet and family members to be mutually observant, to reflect, relax, be meditative, and enjoy the quietness and warmth of just being together.

9. Include the pet as part of family plans in activities such as vacations and outings. Kennel accommodation is possible but may have some drawbacks such as exposure to fleas, other animals, or contaminants.

10. Plan an escape route for the family and pet in case of an emergency.

11. Have a documented alternate plan in place in case the family situation changes.

12. Discuss and document what the family's wishes are if a pet dies or a family member predeceases the pet.

13. Make connections with organizations that share interests and have stories to tell, events to go to, and other pets and people to meet. Pets can help humans around the world reach out through magazines, clubs, obedience classes, computer bulletin boards, videotape exchanges, and other mass media.

REHEARSING COMPASSION

In the book, *To Live Until We Say Good-bye* by Kübler-Ross, the chapter about an adult woman, Louise, depicts through photographs the central and vital role played by her two faithful Labrador retrievers during her days with cancer [45]. Upon her return home after a period of care in a nursing home, Louise writes, "My two dogs welcomed me with a great display of emotion and very slurpy love, and it was the best medicine for me" [45, p. 97]. Kübler-Ross notes that, "Her home and her two dogs were her last attachments, and her great concern when she had to face the ultimate reality of her death" [45, p. 77]. She points out that they were at Louise's side as she became weaker and spent more time in bed. [45, p.89]. In concluding, Kübler-Ross says:

> Her two dogs stayed faithfully by her side and, she would spend more mornings looking at them and remembering the promise she made to herself that the dogs would be put to sleep when she died. They would be buried at the same time so they would not have to adjust to another owner, and they would follow her in death [45, p. 92].

When death is approaching, sometimes children may feel as Louise did. At other times, they may deny feelings or worries about death or the aftercare of a pet. Children may become angry, act out, regress, or become possessive, panicked, and fearful. Some may pretend that all is satisfactory in front of parents [46, p. 9]. Others may wish to "will" their pet to a special person. Parents, siblings, and others may find these feelings and actions difficult to acknowledge. Some family members may see a pet as a vital living link or bridge to their special loved one, especially a child who has died. Later on, the death of this pet may trigger a delayed grief reaction necessitating counseling and emotional support for surviving family members many years after the child's death.

The Death of a Family Pet

In their work, Iliff and Albright note that the loss or death of a pet "can be very traumatic to a child, depending upon what role the pet played in the child's life" [47, p. 125]. Children may express their grief differently than adults [37, 48]. "Children and adults often find that the death or loss of a pet among society at large is an event unworthy of much grief" [37, p. 69]. This means that the disruptions and emotional transitions following the death of a pet are generally ignored or insensitively dismissed [37, 42]. The social rituals, interpersonal outreach, and social cohesion that are available and practiced during bereavement *are not* traditionally present with the death of a pet, even when the emotional bonds, ties, and links with animals may be as strong as those with significant humans.

Family, friends, and significant others can provide the rituals to reduce the feelings of disenfranchised grief and to validate the transition from life to death [37]. Adults can permit bedside care and touching of the dying or deceased pet. They can accept children's tears and facilitate their input into and control of certain decisions. These may include the timing of events, the fulfilling of special wishes pertaining to the animal's comfort and manner of death (natural or by euthanasia), and the burial [37, 48].

In his writings about children and death, Grollman describes examples of age-appropriate dialogue that may be helpful for children and parents in discussions of death, both in respect to nature and interpersonal relationships [49]. A calm, authentic, respectful, dignified handling of "small deaths," such as a pet's death, can be reassuring and comforting for children who are facing this loss as a personal crisis. Papadatou and Papadatos write:

> . . . why not keep goldfish, gerbils, or other small animals as pets? What better way to help a child learn, firsthand, about the facts of life than with pets (especially a small pet with a short lifespan)? What better opportunity to teach the child to love, tend, and grieve for another creature? [50, p. 16].

A pet's illness and death can help children rehearse burial traditions, decide upon the pet's burial site or cremation, and plan aftercare visits. Children, with the help of their families, can create positive, tangible personalized memories through stories, photographs, videos, and drawings that can reinforce the fact that they have: 1) experienced dying and death; 2) been left with valuable memories; 3) contributed to their pet's life; 4) cherished it and experienced reciprocal feelings; and 5) loved a pet that will not be forgotten.

Opportunities also arise to explore the true meaning and universality of death and to clarify children's confusion, misconceptions, fears, and worries about illness, sleep, and death. These can be compared with the feelings of other family members and clarified within the child's level of comprehension.

Questions about death, attention to burial, and aftercare requests may help children to express their grief before and after the pet's death. Children should know that everything was done to ensure the pet's comfort and to prevent suffering. Everyone should be prepared for the normal changes in physiological responses after the pet's death including involuntary urination and defecation and the final expiratory sighing. Personal "closure" activities that are not rushed are vital to the fostering of recovery and compassionate grief work. Doka writes:

> If society is to recognize human grief reactions to the loss of a pet animal as legitimate and nonpathological phenomena, illustrative of the fact that human-pet bonds reflect more than property management, the enfranchisement of grief in caring communities becomes increasingly necessary [51, p. 157].

CONCLUSION

All children, but especially children with life-threatening illness, should not be denied the possible opportunity to LIVE life with a healthy, responsive pet. Caregivers who support these children should consider: 1) including real pets as companions; 2) studying the issues associated with the relationships between pets and children; 3) observing children with pets, while paying attention specifically to their faces and behaviors; 4) discussing personal concerns about pets with animal experts; 5) reaching out to other interested professionals and volunteers; and 6) trying new people-pet partnerships.

Everyone may find a richer world with the songs, barks, mews, splashes, and whinnies of sociable and healthy animal companions. Pets can be the agents of trust, acceptance, promise, activity, and comfort. They help to shape the world of children and facilitate the development of "active hope" as described by Hutschnecker [52, pp. 29-31]. Children with life-threatening illness benefit from the support that pets can provide. As Lebeck says, "Animals can help heal without words" [28, p. 1].

REFERENCES

1. S. B. Barker and R. T. Barker, The Human-Canine Bond: Closer Than Family Ties, *Journal of Mental Health Counselling*, *10*:1, pp. 46-56, 1988.
2. N. P. Alexandrovich, Animals As Totems at an Ancient Buelorussian Population, *Abstracts and Proceedings, The 6th International Conference on Human-Animal Interactions, Animals and Us*, Montreal, Quebec, July 21-25, 1992.
3. C. D. Bryant and W. E. Snizek, On the Trail of the Centaur, *Society*, *30*:3, pp. 22-35, 1993.
4. S. Ven Katraman, Animals and Tribals: A Case of Different Harmony, *Abstracts and Proceedings, The 6th International Conference on Human-Animal Interactions, Animals and Us*, Montreal, Quebec, July 21-25, 1992.
5. J. Meer, Pet Theories, *Psychology Today*, *18*:8, pp. 60-77, 1984.
6. J. Veevers, What is a Pet? Defining the Concept of Companion Animal, *Abstracts and Proceedings, The 6th International Conference on Human-Animal Interactions, Animals and Us*, Montreal, Quebec, Presentation #409 ABV, July 22, 1992.
7. L. Hart, A. M. Benfatto, P. Kass, and J. Serpell, The Lifestyles of People Who Live With Companion Animals, *Abstracts and Proceedings, The 6th International Conference on Human-Animal Interactions, Animals and Us*, Montreal, Quebec, Presentation #408 C, July 24, 1992.
8. G. Mallon, Some of Our Best Therapists Are Dogs, *Abstracts and Proceeding, The 6th International Conference on Human-Animal Interactions, Animals and Us*, Montreal, Quebec, Presentation #407 B, July 22, 1992.
9. S. Lowe, A Special Bond, *Equus*, *183*, pp. 24-28 and 30, January 1993.
10. M. Kale, What You Already "Knew", Fido and Fluffy are Good For You, *Interactions*, *10*:2, pp. 13-17, 1992.
11. L. Lloyd Nebbee, *Nature As A Guide: Using Nature in Counseling, Therapy, and Education*, Educational Media Corporation, Minneapolis, Minnesota, 1991.
12. A. Salomon, Animals and Children, *Canada's Mental Health*, pp. 9-13, June 1981.
13. S. Robb, Health Status Correlates of Pet-Human Association in a Health-impaired Population, in *New Perspectives in Our Interrelations with Companion Animals*, A. Katcher and A. Beck (eds.), University of Pennsylvania Press, Philadelphia, 1983.
14. P. Maggitti, Can Animals Help Us Heal? *Animals*, *120*:1, pp. 5-9, 1987.
15. R. Bergler, The Significance of Pet Animals for Human Well-being and Quality of Life, *Abstracts and Proceedings, The 6th International*

Conference on Human-Animal Interactions, Animals and Us, Montreal, Quebec, July 21-25, 1992.

16. M. E. Siegel and H. M. Koplin, *More Than Just A Friend: Dogs With A Purpose*, Walker and Co., New York, 1985.

17. M. Roberts, Unleashing Friendship, *Psychology Today*, *22*:8, p. 16, 1988.

18. D. C. Anderson, *The Interactions Bibliography*, Rockydell Resources, Penryn, California, 1991-1994.

19. S. Pearce, Animals and Us Conference, an International Success, *Dogs in Canada*, pp. 23-29, December 1992.

20. D. DuVall, Pets and People: Keeping A Pet Could Keep You Alive, *Single Parent*, pp. 18-21, May/June 1986.

21. G. Guttman, Animal Companionship and Cognitive Development. *Abstract and Proceedings, The 6th International Conference on Human-Animal Interactions, Animals and Us*, Montreal, Quebec, Plenary Session, July 25, 1992.

22. A. Siegel, Reaching The Severely Withdrawn Through A Pet Therapy, *American Journal of Psychiatry*, *118*, pp. 1045-1046, 1962.

23. A. Quaytman, Animals as Aids in Child Therapy, *Journal of the Long Island Consultations Center*, pp. 29-35, Spring 1963.

24. B. Levinson, *Pet-oriented Child Psychotherapy*, C.C. Thomas Publishing, Springfield, Ilinois, 1969.

25. A. M. Beck and A. H. Katcher, *Between Pets and People*, Putnam Publishing, New York, 1983.

26. A. M. Beck and A. H. Katcher, A New Look at Pet-facilitated Therapy, *Journal of the American Veterinary Medical Association*, pp. 414-421, 1984.

27. E. K. Kalfour, Pets Make a Difference in Long-term Care, *Journal of the Gerontological Nursing Association*, *15*:4, pp. 3-7, 1991.

28. S. Lebeck, Healing Without Words: The Effects of Animals on Depressed Populations in Psychiatric Hospitals, *The Latham Letter*, *13*:2, reprint, 1992.

29. R. Ruth, Animals are Helping Children Overcome Physical and Emotional Challenges, *Interactions*, *10*:1, pp. 16-18, 1992.

30. J. Harris, The Importance of Pets and the Prevention of Zoonotic Disease in Immunocompromised Individuals, *Abstracts and Proceedings, The 6th International Conference on Human-Animal Interactions, Animals and Us*, Montreal, Quebec, Presentation #409 B, July 25, 1992.

31. D. Waltner-Towes, Zoonosis Concerns in Animal-Assisted Therapy, *Abstracts and Proceedings, The 6th International Conference on Human-Animal Interactions, Animals and Us*, Montreal, Quebec, Presentation #409 A, July 25, 1992.

32. J. Stewart, The Family Dog: The Ins and Outs of Choosing the Right Breed, *Family Life*, pp. 160-167, December/January 1993.

33. C. Dobbs, Little Pets For Little People, *Harrowsmith*, *28*:112, pp. 20, 24, 1993.

34. A. H. Kidd, R. M. Kidd, and C. C. George, The Effects of Owner's Expectations on Successful Pet Adoption, *Abstracts and Proceedings, The 6th International Conference on Human-Animal Interactions, Animals and Us*, Montreal, Quebec, Presentation #408 C, July 24, 1992.

35. L. Hart, Aquarium Fish for Recovery of Coronary Patients in Intensive Care, *Abstracts and Proceeding, The 6th International Conference on Human-Animal Interactions, Animals and Us*, Montreal, Quebec, Presentation #408 C, July 24, 1992.

36. A. Schaufl and R. Bergler, Children and Dogs, *Abstracts and Proceedings, The 6th International Conference on Human-Animal Interactions, Animals and Us*, Montreal, Quebec, Presentation #407 B, July 22, 1992.

37. L. Lee and M. Lee, *Absent Friend: Coping With the Loss of a Treasured Pet*, Henston Ltd., Bucks, England, 1992.

38. B. J. Carmack, (ed.), The Human and Animal Bond: Implications for Professional Nursing, *Holistic Nursing Practice*, 5:2, 1991.

39. J. Eddy, L. A. Hart, and R. P. Boltz, Service Dogs and Social Acknowledgement of People in Wheelchairs: An Observational Study, *People—Animals—Environment: The Delta Journal*, p. 28, Winter 1986.

40. B. Mader, L. Hart and B. Bergin, Socializing Effects of Service Dogs for Children with Disabilities, *People—Animals—Environment: The Delta Journal*, p. 28, Winter 1986.

41. J. Pekar, Unconditional Love in the Person Pet Relationship, *Abstracts and Proceedings, The 6th International Conference on Human-Animal Interactions, Animals and Us*, Montreal, Quebec, Presentation #409 ABC, July 22, 1992.

42. C. Sanders, People in Disguise: Key Features of the Social Relationship Between Companion Animals and Their Caretakers, *Abstracts and Proceedings, The 6th International Conference on Human-Animal Interactions, Animals and Us*, Montreal, Quebec, Presentation #406 A, July 23, 1992.

43. B. Levinson, *Pets and Human Development*, C. C. Thomas, Springfield, Ilinois, 1972.

44. E. Bombeck, *I Want to Grow Hair, I Want to Grow Up, I Want to Go to Boise*, Harper and Row, New York, 1989.

45. E. Kübler-Ross, *To Live Until We Say Goodbye*, Prentice-Hall Inc., Englewood Cliffs, New Jersey, 1978.

46. A. Wolfelt, *A Child's View of Grief*, Centre for Loss and Life Transition, Fort Collins, Ohio, 1991.

47. S. A. Iliff and J. L. Albright, Grief and Mourning Following Human and Animal Death, in *Euthanasia of the Companion Animal*, W. J. Kay, S. P. Cohen, C. E. Fudin, A. H. Kutscher, H. A. Neiburg, R. E. Grey, and M. M. Osman (eds.), The Charles Press Publishers, Philadelphia, 1988.

48. J. Quackenbush and D. Graveline, *When Your Pet Dies: How to Cope With Your Feelings*, Simon and Schuster, New York, 1985.

49. E. Grollman, *Talking About Death: A Dialogue Between Parent and Child*, Beacon Press, Boston, 1976.
50. D. Papadatou and C. Papadatos, (eds.), *Children and Death*, Hemisphere Publishing Corporation, New York, 1991.
51. E. Doka, (ed.) *Disenfranchised Grief: Recognizing Hidden Sorrow*, D. C. Heath & Co., Lexington, Massachusetts, 1989.
52. A. A. Hutschnecker, *Hope: The Dynamic of Self-fulfilment*, G. P. Putnam's Sons, New York, 1981.

CHAPTER 7

Camps: A Therapeutic Adjunct for Children with Cancer or HIV/AIDS

John T. Maher

Disease-specific or disability-specific camp programs have operated throughout North America for decades. For example, there are camps for children with diabetes, and there are camps that are specifically designed and equipped to accommodate children with physical limitations. Some of these specialty camps have children attending who may experience sudden death (asthma); others serve children who will probably die in their twenties (cystic fibrosis); some are for children where 30 percent of them are likely to die of their disease (cancer); and still others are offered to children who are all expected to die (AIDS).

This chapter will focus on camps designed for the last two populations because they are both growing: the former in absolute numbers and the latter in incidence. Most of this chapter focuses on camps for children with cancer because we have accumulated a wealth of experience in their operation. Programs for children living with HIV or AIDS are relatively new. However, much of the discussion is applicable, *mutatis mutandis*, to them as well. Major differences for these camps will be considered following the information and discussion on camps for children with cancer.

CHILDREN LIVING WITH CANCER

It is expected that by the year 2000 one out of every thousand children in North America will be a survivor of some form of childhood cancer. Yet, even with two decades of remarkable treatment success, childhood cancer still remains the number one disease threat to children's lives.

Children with cancer have been denied access to regular camps because of fear or ignorance, disabilities, special medical needs which simply could not be met, or the increased risk of infections. We now know that an alternative is available that works effectively. In fact, any drawbacks of a cancer camp are outweighed by the benefits.

Camps for children whose lives have been affected by cancer are certainly not new. These specialty camps have operated for approximately twenty years in the United States and ten years in Canada. Over seventy camps now cater to different geographical and psychosocial populations. A national volunteer organization, Children's Oncology Camps of America, has been established in North America to organize national and regional workshops, and to help new groups form their own programs.

Although these camps are in a broad sense "normal" or "regular," there are special needs that staff members must be aware of and understand. Indeed, there is good reason to assert that the goals of these camps are therapeutic. Therefore, we have an obligation to seriously consider the philosophy which underlies cancer camps and establish both broad and narrow policy guidelines and operating standards (see Appendix). Camp experiences should never harm children, and we should take advantage of the camp environment to help as much as possible. For these reasons, I will present my thoughts about camp philosophies, goals, and operations which are the products of both personal experiences and communications with many directors of similar programs, hospital staff, camp staff, and, most important, the children and their families.

Hospital personnel are not always enthusiastic about the possibility of a child attending camp, but they are increasingly more aware of the benefits for these children. It is essential to have the active support of health care providers, and it should be clear from the outset that they have the final say in camp matters. A camp project should not be undertaken without a spirit of cooperation and trust. Camps take on serious obligations to the children, their families, and the children's health care teams.

Parents

Encourage parents to take an active role in camp planning and preparations. Specifically, ask them to help with publicity and fundraising, secretarial jobs, advisory board meetings, transportation, and supply pick-up.

Parents may hesitate to endorse a camp project for some of the following reasons:

- they do not believe that their children are sick enough to need a special camp (most children, in fact, do not),
- they do not believe their children can help and be helped by other children (they can),
- they are afraid that their children will find out something about their disease or treatment process that has not yet been revealed (children might, but this can be a very positive experience in a camp setting),
- their need to overprotect their children may make it difficult for them to admit that someone else can provide adequate care for their children,
- they are afraid that their children will be susceptible to disease-related injury,
- they want to spend as much time with their "dying" children as possible (what do the children want and need?).

These anxieties and fears must be acknowledged and addressed. Camps must realize that children may be coming to camp carrying a burden of guilt or fear as a result of parental worries.

Siblings

Siblings worry about their sick brother or sister, and may be under considerable pressure to care for the sick child at home. They may feel sad, guilty, jealous, left out, angry, and fearful. They may be afraid of what goes on in the hospital, afraid of what is happening to parental and family stability, and afraid that they will also get cancer.

Siblings have much to gain from, as well as to offer to, a camp experience. They may better understand and appreciate the complexities of cancer after going to camp [1]. Some children with cancer will not come to camp without the security of a sibling's presence. Only once did a child with cancer ask me not to permit her sibling to attend camp. This request stemmed from the healthy sibling's poor treatment of the sick child in the parents' absence. Such home conflicts have surfaced on several occasions, but with both parties at camp we were able to intervene appropriately. Hopefully, such interventions have led to improved home relations.

For bereaved siblings, grief that is shared may become easier to bear and survivors' guilt may be diminished. Children will often share with each other what they cannot share with parents.

CAMP: PHILOSOPHY, GOALS, ORGANIZATION, AND STAFF NEEDS

This section addresses five areas of concern: 1) the philosophy behind, and justification for, cancer camps; 2) camp goals; 3) the psychosocial care of the campers; 4) the practical organization of camps; and 5) staffing and staff needs. I will not attempt to cover these topics extensively because novel, camp-specific problems will always emerge. Nor will I address the serious problems which running any camp may engender. These matters are adequately treated elsewhere and experienced directors and counselors already know how to respond. However, I do hope the suggestions below may temper or nurture those responses.

1. WHY HAVE A SPECIAL CAMP?

Your response to this question may be rooted in some beliefs about compensatory justice. You may think that a camp experience should be offered to seriously ill children to make up for past, present, or future suffering. Or, you may believe that it is nice for dying children to have such an opportunity. While this motivation may play a role in establishing a camp, it should not be the primary justification. Starting a camp is a humanitarian venture, but its goals and benefits are therapeutic. Compassion and understanding are appropriate responses to suffering and disrupted lives, but pity is not. Pity is simply defeatist and ultimately counterproductive because it labels camps as "a last-chance-for-fun." We should not forget that some children will not come back, but this fact should provide the motivation for the extra effort that it takes to risk sharing ourselves and to work hard at making the program a success for these children.

Two developments in the field of pediatric oncology over the last twenty years have led to the feasibility and desirability of special camps. First, it is medically possible to both establish and maintain stable remissions and to permanently cure many patients. Second, as a consequence of increasing survival rates, the psychosocial and developmental needs of young cancer patients are being given much greater attention. Camps meet some of these needs very effectively [2, 3].

The shift in focus from medical cure alone, to both cure and psychological well-being, reflects the natural progression of a successful treatment program. A newly diagnosed child is suddenly thrown into a strange world where the cure often seems worse than the disease. Family life is dramatically disrupted and relationships are suddenly redefined. The child may fall behind in school or become a victim of the social stigma of cancer. Schoolmates may make fun of his or her physical appearance, they may make uninformed remarks, or they may ask disturbing questions such as, "When are you going to die?"

Children with cancer may have a fearful preoccupation with thoughts of death, suffering, and relapse. Psychological transformations wrought by the disease and treatment process may reduce the efficacy of future treatments. Being different isolates children from their peers, significant others, and even their former self. When considering a total cure, we cannot overlook the damage that cancer's fallout inflicts on children's minds and spirits. We need to help them see themselves as normal children again, or as children who can do normal things. Part of leading a normal life is going to camp. For many children it is a wonderful feeling to be able to go back to school in the fall bursting with reports of their own camp exploits. A camp for children with cancer sends a clear message to the community that these children just want to be "normal."

Given the frequent traumatic demands of living with cancer, I find it surprising that some camp philosophies insist that these children be treated as "normal" all of the time. Certainly, for the majority of children, being treated as "normal" is essential. Any other course would tragically reinforce a mentality of sickness. It would seem better, however, to view them as normal children with special needs. They generally do not want to be treated differently; yet, at the same time, some will want you to understand the hard times that they are having without feeling sorry for them.

Some campers should be seen as special children with special needs. Among these are the children who are dying. For them normal childhood development is impossible. The few children who fit into this last category are likely to define their own needs, and they will probably want you to treat them just like everyone else. The ultimate goal is to make all campers feel more than normal. They should feel precious and special, not because cancer has changed their lives, but because that is every child's birthright.

Children who have overly restrictive, highly structured environments, or who perceive themselves as having to do the "right thing" all the time may experience considerable anxiety when they need to express or act upon their basic instinctual needs. In psychodynamic terms, the ego may fear punishment from the external environment (e.g., parents, teachers, doctors, society). Or, it may be that the superego, which is an internalization of the moral attitudes of the external environment, compromises psychological and interpersonal health by being overly critical of self. This would lead to decreased self-esteem, less natural risk-taking behavior, and non-productive or excessive defences to id expression. This suppression of instincts means that children are less playful, less experimental, or less creative.

Camps, by design, permit gratification of selected instinctual needs through the provision of forums for their guided expression (play, arts and crafts, food fights, singing, campfires, openness to tears, and laughter). The balancing of superego development plus the modeling by adults who are permitted to be more expressive may help children feel more safe when acting out their natural developmental urges. It is hoped that reinforcement of positive experiences by so many people in many different ways may allow children to be more resistant to becoming overly self-critical. After all, risk-taking behavior is natural to human development and personal self-expression.

From a cognitive behavioral perspective, camps may challenge certain beliefs of children, i.e., "I could never play that sport," "I am too fragile . . . I couldn't possibly do anything without my mother." Such beliefs may restrict their actions and subsequently lead to negative feelings toward themselves. A new external environment presents different challenges and can stimulate new behaviors. Camps provide children with opportunities to expand their self-concept through doing; this is the most direct way to refute irrational beliefs and increase positive feelings toward self. As the behavior repertoire is evolving, self-validating thoughts and feelings foster progression through the natural stages of development.

There is a considerable amount of anecdotal evidence that for some children, anticipation of the next camp may play a significant role in their struggle to survive and live well.

2. CAMP GOALS

In addition to the obvious advantages that a camp experience may have for children, a cancer camp makes independence and personal growth possible for children who might otherwise be stifled by medical considerations, overprotective parents, or a sense of isolation. This evolution is accomplished both with the assistance of camp staff and through mutual self-help. The goals of camp should be:

1. To help children make new friends and improve, or catch up on, their social interaction skills. This means experiencing relationships that their disease may have denied them. For younger children, it includes just playing with other children in a normal way. For teenagers, it might mean experiencing the joy and

confusion of a budding romance. When you are no longer the only bald or disfigured person, the doors of possibility open.

2. To help children learn new skills, develop new hobbies, and generally be more adventuresome, both during and after camp.
3. To help children learn love and respect for nature.
4. To help children become more independent and confident; improve their self-image and sense of control; and develop a better sense of responsibility in their lives. A greater sense of self-worth should translate into better coping skills and less dependence on parents and health care providers. Children may become more active participants in their own medical management. Perhaps they will be more inclined to attend a regular camp in the future.
5. To help children learn to respect others, to work together, and to develop a sense of group identity. By providing a milieu where friendships are established and nurtured, a child's support network evolves and will be beneficial for future clinic visits and hospital stays, and for in-home contact such as letter writing or phone calls.
6. To enable children to share fun experiences with treatment staff in a non-medical and non-threatening environment. This contact helps to foster better relations during future formal exchanges. Medical staff also benefit from seeing these children outside of a sterile environment.
7. To help children grow emotionally and spiritually. Children will discover abilities and strengths which, because of cancer and dependency, they did not know existed or were afraid to exercise.
8. To give children with cancer the chance to meet, play, and share with children who have struggled or are struggling through similar life experiences.
9. To keep siblings from feeling left out of family experiences. Their presence adds to a more balanced camp atmosphere. Sick children also discover that they can do many of the same things as healthy children.
10. To give siblings the chance to meet children who are going through what their afflicted brother or sister is going through, and to meet others who share their own experiences of disease in the family.
11. To enable siblings of children who have died to help siblings whose brother or sister is going to die realize that life goes on even after death; and that it is alright to have fun again. They

may also provide support for one another through sharing their own experiences of death.

12. To enable counselors, especially former cancer patients, to share, learn, and grow with children who are often wise beyond their years.

13. To give parents the chance to rest, have time alone together, and reassess their relationships with their children and each other. Separation from their children can be very difficult for parents. The natural tendency is to be protective. By letting go and encouraging a positive attitude toward camp, parents can help their children learn, play, and discover on their own. If they attend a family camp with their children they can see first hand the benefits of independence and at least a modicum of separation.

14. Health education, research, professional development, and individual or group counseling may be additional goals of some programs.

The above goals are best accomplished through fun, laughter, play, and the joy and support of friendship. Mutual self-help does work. By meeting other children who have had similar experiences, children discover mutual feelings of anger, frustration, fear, loneliness, or guilt. They also discover that it is normal to have those feelings.

Prior to the beginning of camp children may be asked to fill out personal information sheets that ask non-medical questions. Information concerning children's hobbies and interests are useful in getting to know the campers and in planning suitable and interesting activities. Parents should fill out medical history and liability waiver forms on behalf of their children. Primary care physicians are asked to provide recent blood counts and specific medical information. Information on medical history forms and that provided by physicians is clearly confidential. A note in the registration package should inform parents that some confidential information may be passed on to counselors at the director's discretion.

3. PSYCHOSOCIAL ISSUES AND CONCERNS

It is unlikely that letting children, whose lives have been disrupted by cancer, live together will generate harmful and negative experiences. There will always be the usual "catastrophes" that children must deal with at any camp, and these may be exacerbated by the heightened emotional vulnerability of some children. However, past suffering often builds reserves of emotional strength. Children become much more sensitive to each other's feelings, are less likely to make hurtful fun of each other, and are quick to come to each other's aid. Unnecessary complaining, on the other hand, is seldom tolerated. This is not surprising since the standards against which discomfort are measured are often not those of normal childhood. There will be some very poignant and emotionally charged encounters and exchanges, but usually these will be both positive and rewarding for those involved. Appropriate safeguards and sensitive and experienced personnel will help to diffuse any difficult situations.

Camp Staff

Camp counselors must take their roles and obligations seriously because they have a profound influence on children and are responsible for their day-to-day psychosocial well-being. I suggest a 2:1 or 3:1 camper-staff ratio which is certainly higher than necessary (up to 5:1 would be reasonable), but this decreases the likelihood of important incidents going unnoticed or unreported. A high ratio also ensures that children receive adequate attention and supervision.

Counselors who do not have professional medical or psychological training should not initiate discussions about cancer related matters, nor should they offer advice. Their role as friend and counselor is to offer a sympathetic ear. They should be mature and competent enough to deal with the usual worries of campers, but in their training they should be advised that a camper's apparently innocuous remarks and concerns may reflect a more serious problem. For this reason, there should be two options open to counselors. First, they must know where to go for assistance (i.e., doctor, nurse, social worker, therapist, pastoral worker, or director). Second, they must be encouraged to report incidents at the daily staff meeting. When in doubt, tell someone. Incident reports may also serve as the basis for a follow-up camp report to hospital personnel not in attendance. Professional staff should not be too quick to usurp the fiduciary role which counselors have established. Everyone needs to work together.

If possible, someone with professional counseling experience or psychological training should attend camps for children older than seven years. Even for younger children it is desirable to have a professional attend, however, this is not necessary if camp staff are sensitive and phone consultation is available. Professionals who attend camp should understand the psychosocial concerns of young cancer patients and their families and be familiar with effective intervention strategies. Additionally and ideally, professionals should be familiar to the children and should be aware of their current family situations.

Though a professional with counseling skills may be present this does not mean that there must be either individual or group counseling sessions. Camp should give children an opportunity to escape the burden and threat of assessment and treatment. Camp is a child's time to just be a child.

On the other hand, there are no other situations that compare with camp which offer children unique possibilities to support and help one another. Sometimes formal counseling may directly conflict with camp goals. Yet some children find camp the best possible environment to explore their feelings. The challenge is to find a balance.

There are two ways to proceed: The first option is to let fun be its own therapy and let the talking that children inevitably do among themselves do its work. This sharing can be facilitated by: encouraging children with the same forms of cancer or siblings of similar backgrounds to share the same cabins or tents; by giving children unstructured free time; by teaming old and new campers; and by assigning specific counsellors (i.e., those who have had cancer themselves, who have a sibling with cancer, or who have lost a sibling to cancer) to appropriate campers.

Interpersonal dynamics and emotional developments during camp can be monitored through shrewd observation and acute sensitivity. Perhaps a play therapist can design activities which reveal feelings or an art therapist can develop an art program where sentiments are exposed. There must, however, be respect for privacy. It would be a serious mistake to deny children the freedom that camp promises.

The second option would be to offer special discussion sessions as a natural part of the camp program, but children should know that these sessions are optional. Sessions must be guided or monitored by a professional and should make use of the children's natural desire to help each other. Offerings may include: individual artwork or play under the direction of an appropriate therapist; children in the same cabin or tent discussing why they are at a special camp; posting "cabin hours" that indicate when and where children can find professional help on their own; separate campfires or meetings with associated discussion themes (i.e., "What having cancer means," "What it means for your brother or sister to have cancer," "What it feels like to have a brother or sister die," or "What cancer does to your family"); and health education sessions where sick children and/or siblings can have their questions answered and doubts resolved. Health education might be especially important toward the end of camp to clear up misinformation that surfaced during the camp. Self-help sessions will be most effective after the children have learned to know and trust each other through spontaneous and structured play activities.

The second option requires prior assessment of the needs of the particular camp population. Questionnaires for the children and parents and discussions with parents may be the most accurate way to assess particular needs. It is unreasonable to dismiss counseling options out of hand with a "recreation first, communication later" slogan.

Specific Issues and Concerns

Self-image

It is crucial that a positive self-image be reinforced. Children with no hair, amputations, or disfigurements should be made as comfortable as possible, especially when swimming. Provide adequate privacy for taking off wigs and limbs and for getting changed.

Young Love

Flowering romances will always be a highlight of any adolescent's camp stay. They can also be the source of great anguish. Many love triangles have been laid bare during our closing camp dances. Offer consolation and reinforce a positive self-image.

Feeling Homesick

There are bound to be times when children long for home. There will be occasional unpleasant experiences which only a mother can make better. Some of these moments can be overcome with fun diversions. If you let children call home it should be to say hello and to report on how camp is going. They should not call while they are upset.

Parents should never send children to camp against their will. Nor should they tell their children that if they do not like camp they can come home. They should not send letters or make calls which induce homesickness; nor should they visit camp. Some parents look for an excuse to bring their child home because they need the child, not vice versa.

Discipline

Discipline should always be gentle, but do not let campers get away with transgressions just because they are sick.

Disclosure of New Information

It is sometimes difficult to determine what information means to a particular child. For example, a child may be told that when you die you go to heaven. Suppose he is told that Uncle Fred is already in heaven. What if Uncle Fred was a scary figure for him when he was younger? Heaven may be seen as a dangerous place. Similarly, it is hard to know how children will interpret the comments of other children. Misinformation should be corrected on the spot (if other children have not already done so), and you must keep your ears open to expressions of concern. Make yourself available for discussion.

Sibling Jealousy and Rivalry

Healthy siblings who are ignored at home may be very frustrated and angry, especially because they know that they should not get angry at sick people. If healthy siblings have been forced to assume responsibility for the care of the sick child at home, they need a rest and the chance to just be children for a while. Follow-up by the social worker with the parents to discuss siblings' needs and concerns may be important. Counselors must be careful not to favor one sibling over the other.

Campers' Participation

The camp program should offer meaningful roles and challenges for every child, regardless of health. Routines and structure give children a secure place from which to venture forth. Help children to succeed in a non-threatening and non-competitive environment.

What to Say and Do about Those Who Have Died Since the Last Year

If and when deceased children or counselors are discussed, be comfortable in talking about them. Let children know that you miss them. By your example, show them that life goes on. You might want to look at pictures or videotapes from last year's camp and reminisce together. Or, you may wish to have a more formal ritual or ceremony. A word of caution in relation to this last option: do not open the door on feelings or issues that you are not equipped to handle at that moment and follow up on later.

Animals

A camp dog lets some of the more withdrawn children find a canine cure for loneliness.

Reintegration

Children and counselors off treatment can be an inspiration to those who are on treatment. However, if cured children are not involved in a counselor-in-training program, you might consider encouraging them to attend a regular camp in the future. Having said that, one cannot deny the benefits of returning to a familiar place, and to friends with whom one shares a common bond. A loyalty and identification develops that can be a tremendous source of future security. When one considers the uncertainty of cure in many cases, it is difficult to determine just when a camper would benefit from moving on to a new, and potentially less supportive, environment.

Siblings of Children Who Have Died

These children should not be refused admission to camp just because their brother or sister has died. A reasonable alternative to a joint camp might be to offer a transition camp just for surviving siblings. Such a camp permits them to be once removed from the reminders of sickness without ignoring their great loss. It also opens up the possibility of running bereavement counseling sessions.

Pastoral Support

If children want to discuss matters of life and death from a religious perspective, it is helpful to have a member of the clergy available. However, such a formal presence is not necessary beyond days of religious observance.

Should Dying Children be Treated Differently?

Dying children will define their own roles. We should not automatically treat them differently, but must respect and meet their special needs. Outwardly, dying children may look as healthy as many of the other campers. They may even be more active if chemotherapy has been withdrawn. Staff may not know that a child is terminally ill unless the child has informed them. It is quite natural to give dying children extra attention, but they must not be overwhelmed or robbed of their desire or capacity to control their own lives. Nor should they be segregated. Dying children still want to have fun, perhaps even more than other children.

4. PRACTICAL ORGANIZATIONAL MATTERS

Every camp will be different. Novel circumstances will demand novel responses. If your priorities are the health, safety, and well-being of campers and staff, the fun will surely follow. Start with the goal of giving children the most wonderful time of their lives and you cannot go wrong, as long as you operate within responsible limits. In what follows, I will make some brief comments concerning those limits, and offer other practical suggestions.

The Name of the Camp

Children may want to be able to talk about going to camp without necessarily revealing their diagnosis, therefore, do not use disease-related terms for the camp name. Likewise, do not use names that suggest special problems or disability.

Should Children with Cancer Attend a Camp which is Open to Children with Other Chronic Diseases?

Yes. In fact, one camp accepts campers with over twenty different diseases. However, from a practical perspective, it is much more difficult to organize a camp requiring such diverse medical and psychological needs. Such a program should likely exclude siblings. An all-encompassing camp may not reinforce children's personal feelings about being normal or cured. On the other hand, exposure to children with serious debilitating diseases may help children with cancer see themselves as better off than they thought they were. It might also arouse suspicions about their own status.

Without denying the reciprocal benefits, children with cancer can be very active. The program potential with respect to activity level is likely greater for cancer camps because cancer is not chronic in the same sense as other diseases. With cancer, chronic usually means uncertainty of cure. This uncertainty and the much shorter dying process when cancer is uncontrolled, distinguish the psychological support needs of pediatric oncology patients from children with other diseases.

How Much Should Campers Pay to Attend Camp?

The answer to this question will depend on your operating costs and revenue. Children should not be charged more than a regular camp and I would encourage charging less. Families may have already incurred a great many treatment-related expenses (e.g., drugs, supplies, travel, accommodation, baby-sitting). The community of donors is often very generous and therefore, you may not have to charge a fee. While this latter course will arrest the exclusion of some children for financial reasons, a small token fee can still be charged so that parents see camp as a service, not a charity. Always be willing to waive fees, and let parents make contributions if they desire.

What Should the Medical Criteria Be for Accepting Campers?

Medical staff will set certain criteria (i.e., a high enough blood count) but beyond specific medical restrictions, accept any child who is not too sick to benefit. A child may only be able to visit camp for a couple of hours, but these visits can be very special if specific activities or opportunities to interact are in place.

If Possible, Do Not Perform Invasive Medical Procedures at Camp

Usually, treatments can be scheduled before or after camp.

Medical Staff Have the Primary Responsibility for Children's Health

When children are at camp, non-medical staff should never diagnose and should be quick to report suspicions. Staff training must include familiarization with significant symptoms. If a child needs to be sent home or taken to the health center or hospital, this should be done without delay. If a communicable disease is suspected, the sick staff member or child should be isolated immediately and seen by medical personnel.

Medical Staff Must Supervise Medication Schedules

Encourage children who show initiative to assume greater responsibility for their own care. However, do not make announcements in front of a group that will take children away from activities in order to take their medications. Ease children in and out of activities with discretion. A formal sick parade or sick call is not necessary.

The Influence of Medical Personnel

Medical personnel should be aware that they have both a conscious and unconscious influence on children and non-medical staff. They must maintain a positive stance and actively support camp activities. Silence can be misinterpreted as disapproval.

All Staff Must Be Well Informed

Staff must be aware of specific medical restrictions and problems for specific campers, for example, prolonged exposure to sunlight, getting wet, weakness, fatigue, seizures, allergies, etc., especially when these may effect swimming ability. Children who have Hickman Catheters are able to participate in waterfront programs by using waterproof tape over the catheters.

Activities Should be Designed So That Everyone Has a Meaningful Role

Competitive activities where a child is sure to fail because of his or her disease should be avoided. However, challenging undertakings serve to build self-confidence. Do not separate sick children from healthy children. If a sick child wants to drop out of an activity, make sure it is not a programming fault. Even very weak children can be referees or participate in games where players team up (and carry each other, for example). Do not offer contact sports. Establish the rules for a game well before the activity starts. Proceeding in an ad hoc manner may make children fearful and self-conscious. If necessary, provide alternate activities for scared, worried, tired, or sick children. Make sure that everyone is comfortable and has fun.

Give Children a Sense of Control Over Their Day by Letting Them Choose Some of Their Own Activities

Schedule unstructured time so that children can talk, share, and do things together that they enjoy. Arrange opportunities for them to improve at certain activities (e.g., archery) that are challenging for them. Also, provide progressive challenges both during camp and from year to year. Schedule sufficiently long, appropriately spaced, and enforced rest periods.

Smoking

Given the nature of these camps, smoking should be banned for both children and staff.

Children are Naturally Divided by Age and Sex for Sleeping

If you wish to have children who have the same disease sleep in the same cabin or have healthy siblings together, be careful the divisions are natural. Some siblings from the same family may be more comfortable sleeping together. If you intentionally put oncology patients together, make sure you mix children on treatment with children that are cured.

Leader-in-Training and Counselor-in-Training Programs

These programs offer the best potential to guarantee a future camp staff who have special insight into children's feelings and problems.

Full Attendance

If spaces are limited and expansion is absolutely impossible, I suggest the following order be used to select children: first, dying children; then, children still on treatment; next, children off treatment; then, siblings of the first three groups in corresponding order of priority; and finally, siblings of children who have died.

Camp Memorabilia

Awards, medals, certificates, tee-shirts, and camp newspapers are important souvenirs and remind children of camp accomplishments. Group photographs should be distributed to everyone. A camp "yearbook" or a camp photo album can be compiled and created to be left in the treatment center so that children can look at it. This will give newly diagnosed children some idea of what camp is like. If children work on a video presentation and/or a mural, these should be made available and displayed at the hospital.

A Closing Ceremony

A family picnic or awards banquet provides an opportunity for parents to witness their children's accomplishments. Consider allowing the whole family to stay for the last weekend of camp. Camps for both parents and children give them an opportunity to get away from the reminders of the disease and provide relief, if only temporary, from their sadness.

Children's Privacy

Do not allow indiscriminate visiting by the curious. Publicity (e.g., newspaper articles, radio and television interviews, video or slide presentations) may be necessary for fund-raising, but once you have funds it should be stopped. Parents' permission must be obtained prior to including names or pictures in any public literature or display. The fact that some children have cancer is confidential information which must be protected.

New Programs

New programs may evolve out of, or build upon, residential camp experiences. Theme weekends designed to help children cope, adolescent programs, winter camps, and camp reunions can strengthen and reaffirm summer friendships. Other options include volunteer visiting or home assistance offered by camp counselors, youth groups, special adolescent programs, support group meetings, or educational seminars. Special seasonal events like a sugar bush outing, an autumn colors nature walk, or cross-country skiing always seem to work well. Or, consider combinations of the above for parents and children together. For parents, there might be support or bereavement group meetings, short respite periods or retreats, or special event weekends. Do not let the benefits of camp wither.

Evaluation

Evaluations are a good way to improve your program, assess efficacy, and compile data. If you intend to document the results of your program, establish a professional research advisory committee to ensure that research is properly conducted. There is nothing wrong with doing research, provided it does not threaten the goals of the camp. The problems that camp relationships and environments engender, the various ways campers satisfy their needs, and the efficacy of interventionist strategies should all be subject to review. Psychosocial research done at camp will lead to better camps and may be used in providing service to children outside of the camp environment.

Insurance

Each camp must have a liability policy that covers the actions of the camp counselors. It is also beneficial if they have their own personal insurance. Note that certain activities (i.e., windsurfing) may require special inclusion in a general policy. Your lifeguards must be certified members of an association. Medical staff must have their own malpractice insurance.

5. STAFF AND THEIR NEEDS

A camp program can be run by paid or volunteer counselors, or a combination of both. Staff are usually easy to find through employment ads and word-of-mouth. Running an all volunteer program is less expensive. Though most volunteers will not accept remuneration, you may choose to give honorariums. People usually offer their services for personal reasons: some simply and genuinely care, others want career-related experience, some personally know the ravages of cancer and want to help others by sharing their experiences, and others are looking for personal help with matters related to cancer or death. Those who fit into the last category should not be offered staff positions but referred to other sources for help. Camp is not the place for staff to be working through their own serious problems. Parents of children with cancer may be very effective counselors, however, they should be excluded from consideration if their children are campers. The separation of children from parents may be more beneficial for both in the long run.

Applicants must be screened carefully using individual and group interviews. Consider the following questions when judging a candidate's suitability:

- Does the person have a good personal support network of family and friends?
- Is the person mature, emotionally stable, patient, and caring? Or, is the person anxious, pushy, or out to prove something to others?
- Has the person experienced cancer's effects on the life of someone close? How were those experiences handled?
- Is the person comfortable working with sick, disfigured, or dying children? Can the person treat these children normally?
- Does the person have camp experience and/or special skills?
- Why is the person applying for this position?
- Does the person have good references?
- Will the person be available in future years? Staff continuity is very helpful for the smooth functioning of the camp, for consistency, and for renewed relationships with children and parents.
- Does the person function well in a group?

- Does the person demonstrate initiative, an independent spirit, and a generally fun-loving and happy disposition?
- Does the person have training in first-aid and CPR?

Staff Orientation and Training

An orientation for volunteers and paid staff members should include the following:

1. A resource library which is available on site and readily accessible. This library should include the following: a) comprehensive books on childhood cancer (for a practical guide, I recommend *Coping with Childhood Cancer: Where Do We Go From Here? ***); b) a specialized cancer camp counselor's manual (available from the larger established camps); c) films or video presentations on childhood cancer (a list of learning resource materials and sources is available from the Candlelighters Childhood Cancer Foundation*).
2. An orientation program which includes five sessions that provide adequate opportunities for new staff members to ask questions and have their concerns addressed by the following people: a) A pediatric hematologist/oncologist who explains the medical aspects of childhood cancer, cancer treatment, physical symptoms, and restrictions to watch out for at camp; b) A social worker who describes the psychosocial aspects of childhood cancer and what to be alert and sensitive to at camp; c) A parent or panel of parents who explains the effects of cancer on children and their families; d) An adolescent or young adult who describes what it is like to have cancer; e) A sibling who shares his or her feelings and the difficulties associated with living with a brother or sister who has cancer; and f) a counselor who discusses feelings, experiences, and camp concerns.
3. Provide training for first-aid and CPR.

Staff Requirements

For efficient camp operation, roles, responsibilities, and avenues of communication must be clearly defined. If camp is viewed as an alternative health-care setting, then clear policy guidelines should be established that further therapeutic goals. Staff must be trained adequately and must operate within certain defined limits.

---

* See Bibliography.

The training program outlined above is designed to give camp staff who have no prior hospital experience a sense of the suffering and burdens that families of children with cancer must carry. Camp staff should have an appreciation of the contrast between the world of sickness and the world of camp. Staff members who understand the effects of cancer tend to be more caring and patient, more effective as counselors, and more dedicated to furthering the goals of the camp. Staff may serve as ambassadors for the camp long after camp is over and may, in turn, educate others in positive ways.

An adequate understanding of the emotional impact of childhood cancer enables staff members to be more effective and to feel more secure in their dealings with these children. Non-professional staff members should not initiate cancer-related discussions with children in any formal way. However, if a child initiates a cancer-related conversation staff must have adequate knowledge and information. Children who share the fact that they are dying, need staff members who possess the strength of character to both cry with (not for) them, and continue to have genuine fun with them.

Staff Concerns

Many staff members are concerned about how they will behave around sick, disfigured, or dying children. This apprehension is less likely to lead to problems for staff members during a short camp. However, over a full summer program, the consequences can be very unfortunate for campers and staff alike. Medical, nursing, and other professional staff or students usually have achieved a functional balance prior to their camp experience. One possible way to increase staff comfort is not to reveal the prognosis of their charges. Some staff members claim that if they do not know that a child is dying, they can function normally as counselors. Unfortunately, ignorance has its pitfalls. For example, staff may respond inappropriately to the attention-seeking behavior of a dying child. Or, they may jump to false conclusions when a child's health status is unclear. Sometimes, staff cannot tell who is sick, especially if siblings are present.

The Issue of Disclosure of Information

The issue of disclosure must be rooted in more than concerns regarding staff comfort. The confidentiality of medical information and the effectiveness of intervention strategies are also at stake. A balance must be established concerning how much staff should be told because, ultimately, they must have enough information to respond appropriately to existing circumstances.

Should Staff Members Be Told More than the Child Already Knows?

Staff members should always be honest but should they open wounds with the sword of truth? At one summer camp we had a child who was not told that he was dying. It is not possible to determine how this knowledge may have colored his camp experience, however, staff must respect the wishes of parents in matters related to information disclosure.

On the other hand, parents may not be able to predict the content of interactions that may be generated by camp experiences, nor how much information a staff person will need in order to respond most effectively. What if a dying child already has an intuitive sense that she is dying and seeks confirmation from her counselor? One important role that a staff member can fulfil is to be a good listener rather than someone who offers advice. In this case, it would be appropriate to suggest that the child speak with a professional counselor. Sometimes disclosing the child's concerns may lead him or her to believe that secrets are being betrayed. However, staff members must be aware that a loss of trust may be ultimately less important than finding proper help for a particular child.

What Information is Appropriate to Pass On, and How Should it Be Done?

These questions must be answered on an individual basis. For most campers, personal information sheets filled out prior to camp will suffice if staff are well informed about the general problems which might emerge.

Doctors, nurses, social workers, therapists, and the director require free access to a child's medical information. Some medical information will need to be divulged to all staff members to ensure the child's safety and emotional well-being. Examples include information about seizures, allergies, psychological problems such as acute depression, and learning disabilities. Some medical information may be shared in confidence with a staff member responsible for a particular child. Examples include information about drug reactions, fatigue, bed-wetting, and psychosocial adjustment problems. These latter disclosures may, or may not, include additional information about a child's cancer or prognosis.

Students, in professional programs who provide their services in part because of professional development goals, should have controlled access to medical information provided they clearly understand their obligation to protect the confidentiality of these children and their families.

Should Non-Professional Staff Know which Children
Have Cancer and Who has had a Brother or
Sister Die of Cancer?

You may answer that they do, in order that they can be sensitive to subtle hints from children who want to discuss things that bother them. However, if staff are well-informed concerning the general signs to watch for, specific knowledge may not be necessary. Additionally, if staff members do not know who has had what life experiences, children may more likely receive similar amounts and types of attention.

In the end, the issue of disclosure should be settled on two grounds: 1) the proper role and responsibilities of a staff member, and 2) the desires of the children. Staff members do not always need confidential information to safeguard their campers well-being, to be their friend in fun, or even to be sensitive to psychological idiosyncrasies. Some camp staff actually function better not knowing more than is necessary. Some children appreciate having the option to tell "special" staff only as much as they want them to know. Controlling information flow is quite a change for these children from their usual hospital world. Since more information is readily available from the director, non-essential disclosure should be an option, not an automatic given.

Avoiding Staff Burnout

It is important that staff members be properly supported. When staff live and share with children as they do in a camp setting, there are always emotional involvements. While a certain amount of detachment is desirable, risking oneself in an intimate friendship produces many mutual benefits. Staff must be careful, however, not to foster dependency or stifle initiative.

Working with sick, dying, or troubled children can be exhausting and emotionally draining. It can also be the most rewarding experience in one's life. To ensure staff effectiveness, staff members should be given ample time off and time to share with and support each other. Periodic, formal, guided sessions can relieve some of the tension and allow staff members to share their collective concerns and needs. Informal gatherings, after children are asleep, also provide opportunities to share and develop coping strategies. Professional counseling staff should be available to individuals as needed. Staff conflicts and worries should be dealt with accordingly. Emotions will surface during an extended camp program because sharing in suffering can really hurt.

In some cases it may be beneficial for staff members and campers to maintain contact after camp. Exchanging letters, making hospital or home visits, or sending condolences may all be appropriate. A word of caution: staff members may not be welcome at difficult times or they may create expectations that they cannot live up to outside of the camp environment. Having said that, it is important to recognize that some staff members become a source of primary support for a particular child and family [4].

CHILDREN LIVING WITH HIV OR AIDS

The number of children with HIV or AIDS in North America increases as the number of infected women increases; this is because 70 percent of all pediatric HIV infections are the result of transplacental transmission [5]. The estimates on how many women are actually infected vary, but they all point to terrible increases. Half of the remaining 30 percent currently infected with HIV are children with hemophilia; fortunately, the sterilization of blood products has eliminated this group as a vulnerable population. The balance have been infected through intravenous drug use, transfusions, and sexual contact.

Camps for Children with HIV/AIDS

As previously mentioned, much of the information on camps for children with cancer can be adapted to camps for children with HIV/AIDS. Because most of the children infected with HIV are under the age of five, and will probably not live much beyond the age of ten, the best camp models are a day camp, residential family camp, or residential mother/child camp. These last two models open the door to providing support for infected parents, or for infected mothers in particular.

The Issue of Confidentiality

The great fear of discovery means that it takes real courage for some people to get involved with support programs. They need to be reassured that their diagnoses will be safeguarded, and that there will be no violations of their rights to privacy.

This protection extends to limitations on publicity that uses the camp name or location, even for fund-raising purposes. Of sad note is the fact that in a few places local community members have organized protests against the presence of people with HIV at camps in their area.

Universal Precautions with Body Fluids

This topic is broached because people are very fearful of or exaggerate the risk of contagion. The reality is that the normal precautions that must be in place at any camp, for any group of children, are completely adequate.

Truthtelling

In the past decade there has been a major shift toward truthtelling in the domain of pediatric oncology. Parents of children with HIV are likewise encouraged to develop and maintain open and honest relationships with their children. However, the reality is that many children are not told about their diagnoses because there is such a long and potentially symptom free (or limited symptom) period between diagnosis and the development of AIDS.

Children who do not know their diagnoses will probably go to a regular camp. However, if you are running a family camp or a mother/child camp, you will have to deal with the disclosure issue head on. While one of the strengths and remarkable things about cancer camps is the freedom to talk openly about the disease, HIV camps may operate with strict discussion limitations for both campers who know why they are there, and for counselors. The risks of discovery or verbal slips are great. Unfortunately, until the stigma and social persecution that attend a diagnosis of HIV are eliminated, these webs of secrecy and complicity will be necessary. The alternative is to only run programs for families who have already handled this very difficult problem prior to camp.

Hope

The need for hope is universal, whatever the sorrow or challenge. At present, people living with HIV expect to die prematurely because of their infection. This disease is more brutal than other afflictions because of the burden of secrecy that it forces on so many, the number of orphans that it is producing, and the isolation and guilt that it engenders. Camps can foster a sense of community while waiting for an ignorant society to learn to love without condition.

CONCLUSION

Summer camp is a cultural icon. It is part of the nostalgic myth of childhood innocence and freedom; a symbol of how the world should really be; and a challenge to the way the world really is.

In the face of suffering we attempt a response. From fun, friendship: from friendship, support: from support, hope . . .

APPENDIX

The following provides an example of operating standards for oncology camps:

Accreditation

1. The camp must comply with the standards of the state or provincial camping association in whose jurisdiction it falls. Formal accreditation of the camp by the appropriate camping association will constitute evidence of having met this requirement. A camp so accredited must remain a member in good standing of the camping association.
2. In those cases where an oncology camp hires the services of another established camp to develop and deliver a specialized cancer program, the camp so engaged must be accredited by the appropriate camping association, and must comply with any additional operating requirements set forth in this document.

Affiliation

3. The camp must operate in formal association with a recognized pediatric oncology clinic. Evidence of such association must be available in writing in the form of a letter from the medical director of the recognized clinic.

    Formal association means that the camp can publicly declare its association with the clinic on its literature and during public addresses, and/or that the medical director or his/her delegate is a member of the management board or body that governs operations of the camp.
4. A camp may also have formal association with the Cancer Society or a recognized parent association.

Funding

5. A camp must not accept any funds from manufacturers or distributors of tobacco products.

Finances

6. An independent annual audit should be carried out by certified accountants. Annual financial statements must be available for review by donors.

Governing Body

7. The membership of the board which governs camp operations must include at least one parent, and should include at least one survivor of childhood cancer.

Campsite

8. The campsite must not be more than one hour from a tertiary care center using any mode of transportation (including helicopter). This time limit must include the time required for any non-resident vehicle to travel to the campsite.

   Written emergency evacuation procedures must be in place in advance of all camp sessions.

Staff

9. Each day or residential camp must maintain a ratio of at least one staff person for every seven campers. Each family camp must maintain a ratio of at least one staff person for every ten campers, where "campers" is understood to include parents.
10. The camp must provide a compulsory training session for camp personnel in advance of the arrival of any campers. The duration of the training session may vary in relation to the qualifications of the personnel, but it must be thorough, structured, and serve to adequately prepare the staff for all of their anticipated responsibilities. At a minimum this session must include formal instruction and opportunities for discussion related to the following topics:
    a) Handling of body fluids.
    b) Confidentiality of personal/medical information.
    c) Physical and sexual abuse patterns in society.
    d) Talking about difficult or sensitive subjects.
    e) Respecting cultural and personal values.
    f) Reporting on the psychological well-being of campers.
    g) Identifying and reporting important physical symptoms.
    h) Personal support options for staff.

Confidentiality

11. All medical forms, medical information, and psychosocial information about both campers and staff must be safeguarded and treated
as strictly confidential. The camp must have disclosure policies
governing what information may be revealed to what staff,
by whom, and for what purposes. Each staff person (including
Counselors-in-Training) must understand these policies, and as a
condition of working at the camp must agree to abide by them
during the camp and in perpetuity thereafter.

    Each parent should sign a consent form authorizing the discre-
tionary release of information to staff by the camp director or
medical director.

Psychosocial Support

12. The social worker(s), psychologist(s), child-life worker(s), or
nurse(s) with formal responsibility for ongoing psychosocial support of each camper must: i) be present at the camp, or; ii) be "on
call" and readily available for consultation by telephone with the
camp directors or medical staff, or; iii) identify in writing another
professional who is competent to assume these responsibilities on
their behalf.

Medical Care

13. The pediatric hematologist/oncologist(s) with formal responsibility
for ongoing medical care of each camper must: i) be present at the
camp, or; ii) be "on call" and readily available for consultation by
telephone with the camp directors or medical staff, or; iii) identify
in writing another doctor who is competent to assume these
responsibilities on their behalf.
14. At least two health professionals (nurse or doctor) must be in camp
and on-call. There should be a ratio of at least one health professional to every thirty campers.
15. The head nurse must have a minimum of three years experience in pediatric oncology, or five years in general pediatrics.
All other camp nurses must have a minimum of one year of
pediatric experience, or two years of active nursing care in any
other area.
16. A complete first-aid kit and a nurse or doctor must accompany
campers on "out-trips" which will take campers more than twenty
minutes walk from the base camp.

17. The camp health center must be equipped to handle common medical problems arising in a camp setting, and in addition should contain supplies and equipment consistent with the level of care that the camp is providing (e.g., intravenous versus oral chemotherapy).
18. Each camp health center must have a locked storage space for drugs and medicine, and must have a written policy governing access and supply tracking.

Siblings

19. The camp should have a camping option for siblings. A separate sibling's program may be offered, however, participation in the same program as the children with cancer, or in a family camp, is preferred.

Warnings

20. An advisory notice must be sent to all parents in advance of camp reminding them of the dangers of contagion, and advising them to report any suspected or real contacts to camp medical staff in advance of letting their children come to camp.

REFERENCES

1. O. J. Z. Sahler and P. J. Carpenter, Evaluation of a Camp Program for Siblings of Children with Cancer, *American Journal of Diseases in Children,* *143,* pp. 690-696, 1989.
2. R. A. Seeler, Disease-Specific Camping for Children, *The Journal of Pediatrics, 116*:2, pp. 271-272, 1990.
3. M. Bluebond-Langner et al., Children's Knowledge of Cancer and its Treatment: Impact of an Oncology Camp Experience, *The Journal of Pediatrics, 116*:2, pp. 207-213, 1990.
4. D. Adams, *Parents of Children with Cancer Speak Out: Problems, Needs and Sources of Help,* Candlelighters Childhood Cancer Foundation Canada, Toronto, Ontario, 1992.
5. J. Sherr, *HIV and AIDS in Mothers and Babies,* Blackwell Scientific Publications, Oxford, England, 1991.

BIBLIOGRAPHY

Adams, D. W. and Deveau, E. J., *Coping with Childhood Cancer: Where Do We Go From Here?* (revised edition), Kinbridge Publications, Hamilton, Ontario, 1993.

Candlelighters Childhood Cancer Foundation Canada, 10 Alcorn Ave., Suite 200, Toronto, Ontario, M4V 3B1.

The Candlelighters Childhood Cancer Foundation, Suite 460, 7910 Woodmont Ave., Bethesda, Maryland 20814.

CHAPTER 8

Helping Lethal Suicidal Adolescents

Antoon A. Leenaars and Susanne Wenckstern

During the last few decades, one of the greatest misconceptions in helping suicidal adolescents is the underestimation of the pain of these young people. Often that pain was unbearable. The hurt, anguish, depression, and especially hopelessness and helplessness was too much to bear. Such individuals are in need of treatment, often long-term psychotherapy with possible milieu therapy, medication, and in some cases hospitalization. The oversimplification has been our error.

Suicide is not uncommon in adolescents [1, 2]. There is an even higher number of suicide attempts in teenagers. Smith and Crawford reported that 8.4 percent of adolescents have attempted to kill themselves [3]. An even greater number think about suicide. The study by Smith and Crawford reported that 62.6 percent of high school students had experienced some degree of suicidal ideation (i.e., thoughts of suicide) [3]. Although it is not unusual for people to think about suicide, the current prevalence [1, 4] warrants considerable concern. Yet, the allocation of resources has been minimal according to the American government's own report [5]. In part, this is reflective of the lack of understanding of suicide itself and the high demand for long-term services that these young people need.

A MISCONCEPTION

A current popular formulation regarding suicide is that it is simply due to an external event or "stress"; for example, the rejection of a friend or the influence of the music of a pop singer. Although precipitating events (e.g., deprivation of love, sexual abuse, death of parent, divorce, a rejection) do occur in the suicides of adolescents, there is much more. Here we are reminded of a clinical example, which is quite similar to one reported by Menninger [6]:

> A sixteen-year-old was found dead in a car, having died of carbon monoxide poisoning. People were perplexed, "Why did this young person, from an upper middle class family, kill himself?" The parents learned that his girlfriend rejected him the day of his suicide. That was the reason: When a young person gets rejected and is so in love, he may kill himself. A few friends and his teachers knew that he had been having problems in school. That was the reason. A few others knew that his father was an alcoholic and abusive. That was the reason. His physician knew that he had been adopted and had been recently upset about that. She knew the real reason. And others knew . . . .

Often, the adolescent is equally blinded by a single event. Here we are speaking about moderately to highly lethal suicidal adolescents. The teenager who is about to put a bullet through his head with his father's gun or the teenager who is about to take her mother's prescription pills, at the moment of decision, may be the least aware of the essence of the reasons for doing so. The adolescent's conscious perception is a critical aspect. Yet, to simply accept that perspective is not only simplistic but may well be suicidogenic. The pain simply makes it impossible for the adolescent to give a complete and accurate recitation of the event. Suicide is complex, more complicated than the adolescent's conscious mind is aware [7]. For example:

> Dennis, a sixteen-year-old male, was referred for psychotherapy, following a suicide attempt. The attempt had resulted in a month-long stay in hospital. When asked about his perception, i.e., what caused the pain in the suicidal scenario, he said, "a break-up with a girl." He reported that the loss of that relationship was unbearable. Yet, much later he revealed that the relationship was only a fantasy. He had been in love with the girl for six months, since the beginning of the school year. He had never spoken to her. He simply could not stop looking at her. One day one of her friends said, "She wants you to get lost." He simply caved in. That was a reason. It was also known that his parents had been divorced and the relationship with his father was strained. His relationship with his mother, on the other hand, was overly dependent; he was his mother's only friend. And it was also known . . . Our point is that Dennis' state of mind is prototypical, not unique. As a further example:

Robert, a fifteen-year-old male, was referred for crisis intervention after engaging in a great deal of overt verbalizations at school about wanting to kill himself and appearing very agitated and upset. It became quickly apparent that from Robert's perspective, there were two "blinding" events leading to his suicidal behavior, i.e., within the space of several weeks, he had, not once but twice, been involved in serious car accidents in his father's car which resulted in extensive damage to the car. He presented as being quite agitated and made many self-depreciating comments, focusing almost entirely on the feeling that he was letting his parents down. Over the course of several months, Robert began to paint a picture of long-term personal problems and family dysfunction, e.g., he reported that he took more than 50 pills at age nine, requiring hospital admission. It then became known through Robert's self reports, as well as those of his mother and father, that he had a history of behavior adjustment difficulties since grade 2, including acting out problems, low grades, and school truancy. Later, alcohol and substance abuse became prevalent in this boy's attempts to halt his pain. His mother reported that his father also had a "drinking problem." Robert was aware that his parents were on the verge of separation and were staying together "for my sake." In addition to Robert's and his parents' reports, a public health nurse informed the therapist that he was being tested for HIV. And it was also known . . .

Shneidman has noted that the common consistency in suicide is not the precipitating event but life-long coping patterns [8]. Even in youth, one can see a continuity despite developmental changes. Adolescents who kill themselves experience a steady toll of threat, stress, failure, challenge, and loss that gradually undermines their adjustment process. They are unable to cope. One merely has to reflect on the frequent statement that Sally killed herself because her boyfriend rejected her. Most of us would not, why Sally?

The suicidal adolescent is unable to cope with the demands of life. The pain is unbearable and suicide becomes functional. The ego has been weakened. A mere focus, therefore, on suicide as "stress" grossly underestimates the problem that these young people face and is instrumental in the subsequent lack of help that they receive.

LETHALITY AND PERTURBATION

In understanding suicide in adolescents, one needs to be aware of behaviors that are potentially predictive of suicide. However, there is no *one* definitive behavior. Suicide is a multi-dimensional malaise [8]. Two concepts that are extraordinarily useful and helpful are *lethality* and *perturbation*. Lethality, a psychological state of mind, refers to the probability of a person's killing him/herself and on a quantification scale ranges from low to moderate to high. Perturbation refers to subjective distress (disturbed, agitated, sane-insane, discomposed) and can also be rated from low to moderate to high. Both concepts are needed in order to understand the depth of pain of suicidal adolescents. Lethality kills, not perturbation. All sorts of adolescents are highly perturbed but not suicidal. Perturbation is often relatively easy to observe; lethality is not. When we are discussing suicidal adolescents in this chapter, we are referring to individuals who exhibit at least moderate risk in lethality. Of course, a suicidal act (deed, occurrence, event, threat, attempt) of whatever lethality is always genuine in its own light and merits serious consideration.

PREVENTION/INTERVENTION/POSTVENTION

The classical approach to the prevention of mental health and public health problems is that of Caplan [9], who distinguished among primary, secondary, and tertiary prevention. The more commonly used concepts for these three modes of prevention are prevention, intervention, and postvention, respectively. All have a place in helping the suicidal adolescent in a reasonably prudent fashion.

Prevention relates to the principle of good mental hygiene in general. It consists of strategies to ameliorate the conditions that lead to suicide: "to do"—venire—something before the event occurs. Preventing suicide is best accomplished through primary prevention. Prevention is education. Young people (and their gatekeepers) must be educated about suicide. Such education—given that suicide is a multi-dimensional malaise—is enormously complicated, almost tantamount to preventing human misery.

Intervention relates to the treatment and care of a suicidal crisis or suicidal problem. Secondary prevention is doing something during the event. Obviously, suicide is not solely a medical problem and many persons can serve as lifesaving agents. Nonetheless, professionally trained people, psychologists, psychiatrists, social workers, and psychiatric nurses continue to play the primary roles in intervention. A great deal has been learned about how to intervene—in crisis intervention and therapy with suicidal young people.

Postvention, a term introduced by Shneidman in 1971, refers to those things done after the event has occurred. Postvention deals with the traumatic aftereffects in the survivors of a person who has committed suicide (or in those close to someone who has attempted suicide). It involves offering psychological services to the bereaved survivors. It includes working with all survivors who are in need: children, parents, teachers, friends, and so on. School systems are an especially critical force in these endeavors.

Each of these modes of prevention is needed to address suicide in adolescents. Here we will focus on intervention. Intervention was chosen because it is generally agreed that teenagers who are at moderate or high risk are in need of treatment [10-12]. A recent analysis of the treatment of suicidal people [13] warrants that conclusion. Even the research by Shaffer, Vieland, Garland, Rojas, Underwood and Busner, despite its obvious limitations in its application to prevention in schools, suggests that young attempters are in need of intervention [14]. Intervention is not prevention. Prevention has enormous value in the overall approach to adolescent suicide [15]; however, it does not address the needs of a moderate to highly lethal individual.

An example of the error in the treatment of suicidal young people is the growing trend toward peer counseling. We are not suggesting that peers have no utility, only that it does not address the need of truly suicidal young people [16]. Peer counseling is not psychotherapy. There is no research to suggest that peer counselors can provide the therapeutic care that suicidal youths need. On the other hand, a peer, teacher, guidance counselor, minister, etc., may assist in the identification and provide support in the process; yet, they must refer the adolescent to a professional. The fact that teenagers prefer to talk to teenagers is no justification to follow their wishes, often defensive ones. The defense is an expression of the magnitude of the pain and the inability to cope with it.

We wish to point out, despite the central role of the professional mental health worker, others have an equally valuable role. Parents have a critical contribution [17]. Often the family, once evaluated to be on the side of life, is in need of treatment [18]. Frequently the suicide risk in an adolescent signals a system dysfunction. Robert's suicide risk, for example, signaled his family's long-standing dysfunction. One should, in fact, use all resources with suicidal adolescents. These include support, behavioral techniques, hospitalization, medication, etc., and especially the involvement of others, not only parents, friends and siblings but also "social" individuals—teachers, priests, elders, the Chief, doctors, anyone—all of whom serve, directly or indirectly, to mollify the pain.

Although an outline of the strategies of intervention warrants a book by itself [e.g., 19, 20], we would like to provide a few comments about intervention with some guidelines for assessment and prediction. As a word of caution, however, it is worth noting that the search for a singular universal response to suicide in adolescents is a chimera, an imaginary and non-existent conceptual fabrication. The search for a simplistic response is a foolish and unrealistic fancy. There is no one method for helping suicidal adolescents.

ASSESSMENT AND PREDICTION

Assessment and prediction of suicide risk in adolescents is abstruse [19, 21-23]. Elsewhere, we [21, 24] and others [e.g., 8, 25, 26] have outlined a digest for such assessment. In the 1960s and 1970s, there was a focus on the *prediction* of suicide, and suicidologists believed that eventually it would be possible to predict which individuals out of a population would eventually complete suicide [27]. However, it was soon realized that the statistical rarity of suicide and the imperfection of the prediction instruments led to an enormously large number of false positives, so many in fact, that the prediction instruments were of little use to clinicians or to those planning suicide prevention services.

In the 1980s and 1990s the focus shifted to assessment [22]. That is, rather than predicting the future occurrence of suicide in people, the focus became assessing potentially suicidal people in a more general sense, taking into account all of their characteristics, life experiences, and psychological factors, which are relevant to future suicidal behavior. Indeed, it is our belief that prediction and assessment are mutual processes and any separation is an artificial one. They are not separate categories.

Are there any avenues that could help us predict that a teenager is a suicide risk? Recently, due to awareness of the phenomenon of suicide in youth, the National Institute of Mental Health (NIMH) organized a think tank in the assessment of suicidal behavior in adolescents to answer this question [28]. This group found that there were inherent difficulties in the assessment of suicidal behavior. Suicide is not a psychopathological entity in the DSM-III-R [29]. Within this frame, they reviewed all available assessment instruments used to study suicidal behavior in adolescents. The conclusion: *Few, if any, are useful.* The NIMH group found numerous problems in the way professionals evaluated suicide; for example, ambiguity of the purpose of the instrument, insufficient attention to validity, the lack of discrimination between suicide risk and other forms of self-destructive behavior, and the lack of theoretical models. Our own impression agrees to date, each of these single tests or measures, *by themselves,* has little utility. They are like a sign of a "bump on the head," making us regress back to the days of phrenology. However, it was also concluded that within the context of the clinician's skill, suicide can often be evaluated.

Suicide can be defined as an event with biological (including biochemical), psychological, interpersonal, situational, sociological, cultural, and philosophical/existential components [8]. Each of these components can be an avenue to assessment. Here are a few behavioral observations that may be seen in some—not all—suicidal adolescents.

1. PREVIOUS ATTEMPTS

Although it is obvious that one has to "attempt" suicide in order to commit it, it is equally clear that the event of "attempting suicide" need not have death as its objective. It is useful to think of the "attempter" (now often referred to as a parasuicide) and the "completer" as two sets of overlapping populations: 1) a group of those who attempt suicide, a few of whom go on to commit it; and 2) a group of those who commit suicide, a few of whom previously attempted it. A good deal has to do with the lethality of the event. The ratio between suicide attempts and completions in the general population is about 8 to 1—one committed suicide for every eight attempts; however, some studies on teenagers report a rate of 50 to 1, even 100 to 1.

A previous attempt is a good clue to future attempts, especially if no assistance is obtained after the first attempt. *However*, not all previous attempters go on to attempt again (or kill themselves); about 15 percent do so, versus 1.5 percent for the general population. Unfortunately, all too frequently, such behavior is not taken seriously.

2. VERBAL STATEMENTS

As with behavior, the attitude toward individuals making verbal threats is often too negative. Such statements are seen as being made *just for attention*. This attitude results in writing off or ignoring the behavior of a person who is genuinely perturbed and potentially suicidal. Examples of verbal statements from young people are the following: "I'm going to kill myself" or "I want to die," both being very direct. Other more indirect examples are the following: "I am going to see my (deceased) mother" or "I know that I'll die at an early age."

3. COGNITIVE CLUES

The single most frequent state of mind of the suicidal person is *constriction*. There is a tunnel vision, a narrowing of the mind's eye. There is a narrowing of the range of perception, opinions, or options that occur to the mind. Frequently the person uses words like "only," "always," "never," and "forever." Examples from young people are the following: "No one will ever love me. Only mom loved me"; "John was the only one who loved me"; "Dad will always be that way"; and "Either I'll kill my brother or myself."

4. SUDDEN BEHAVIORAL CHANGES

Changes in behavior are also suspect. Both the outgoing individual, who suddenly becomes withdrawn and isolated, and the normally reserved individual, who starts to become outgoing and seeking thrills, may be at risk. Such changes are of particular concern when a precipitating painful event is apparent. Changes in school performance, such as sudden failure, may be an important clue. Making final arrangements, such as giving away a record collection, a favorite watch, or other possessions, may be ominous and often not responded to by the receiver; the receiver is simply too pleased to get the "gift." A sudden preoccupation with death, such as reading and talking about death, may also be a clue.

5. EMOTIONAL CLUES

The single most frequent emotional state in a suicidal adolescent is depression. However, it must be understood that not all suicidal youth are depressed and that not all depressed youth are suicidal. Depression and suicide are *not* equivalent. Yet, Pfeffer has noted that depression distinguishes many suicidal adolescents from non-suicidal groups [30]. As many as 40 to 60 percent of suicidal adolescents show some signs of depression [23]. Depression can be noted in mood and behavior (ranging from feeling dejected and some hesitancy in social contacts, to difficult to contact, isolation, serious disturbance of appetite and sleep), verbal expression (ranging from talk about being disappointed, excluded, blamed, etc., to talk of suicide, being killed, abandoned, helpless), and fantasy (ranging from disappointed, excluded, mistreated, etc., to suicide, mutilation, loss of a significant person). Behaviors such as excessive aggressiveness, sleep disturbance, change in school performance, decreased socialization, somatic complaints, loss of energy, and unusual change in appetite and weight have all been associated with depression [30]. However, not all depression is overt. Teenagers often exhibit what has been termed masked depression. Anorexia, promiscuity, and drug abuse, for example, have been associated with depression.

It is paramount to remember, however, that depression does not equal suicide in a simple one-to-one fashion. Most suicides experience *unbearable pain*, but not necessarily depression [8]. The unbearable emotion might be depression, hostility, despair, shame, guilt, dependency, hopelessness and/or helplessness. What is critical is that the emotion—pain—is unbearable. In teenagers, the pain is often expressed in anger. In fact, very angry and hostile adolescents may be more at risk for suicide than adolescents exhibiting more traditional signs of depression [19].

6. LIFE-THREATENING BEHAVIOR

We recall a seventeen-year-old teenager who died in a single car accident on an isolated road after having had several similar accidents following his mother's death. *Self-destructiveness is not rare.* Often alcoholism, drug addiction, mismanagement of medical treatment, and auto accidents can be seen in this light. Farberow [31] has referred to this as, "the many faces of suicide." Here are a number of questions:

- Why did a teenager play with the gun, knowing it was loaded?
- Why did a teenager drive so fast on a slippery wet road when he knew, for the last three months, how bad his brakes were?
- Why did a person, knowing how cocaine could affect her, get hooked?

We are not suggesting that these young people intentionally want to die; yet, their behavior made them "as good as dead."

The few ideas presented here for understanding suicide and, by implication, assessment and prediction of suicide risk, are only the beginning. Predicting suicide in adolescents is a complicated ongoing process [4, 19, 21] that warrants a text by itself.

INTERVENTION

Intervention with highly—and often moderately—suicidal adolescents differs from other human relationships [32-36]. The goal is simple: To keep a person alive. However, the procedures are often not simple. Working with such adolescents demands a different kind of involvement than usual psychotherapy.

1. Rapport

Intervention with suicidal adolescents begins in the first encounter. The encounter requires the development of an active, non-judgmental rapport. It requires a "strong interest in, affection for another person, a willingness to give up something for another person, a willingness to assume responsibility for another person" [37, p. 103]. In a sense, to establish rapport, love predominates over hate. If an interventionist has difficulties expressing attachment, he or she would do best not to try doing intervention (or therapy). From our view [7, 38], in fact, the key to working with suicidal adolescents is the relationship itself.

A thirteen-year-old female comes to mind, who was seen in individual therapy for over three years. She was initially referred for self-mutilating behaviors, i.e., Jennifer's school principal had noticed cuts, bruises, and what looked like scars from cigarette burns on her arms and legs. She had also made two moderate suicide attempts. Each attempt had occurred at a time of perceived total abandonment and rejection by her family. She was the youngest of ten children (of an unwanted, late in life pregnancy). Her parents divorced when she was quite young and for many years she had resided alone with her drug dependent mother. She related to the therapist that after many years with her mother and virtually no other familial contact, she was suddenly "snatched away" from the only home she had known to live with virtual strangers, i.e., her biological father and adult siblings. This followed a "messy" custody battle, wherein her mother was declared as unfit. Now, as a teenager, Jennifer was reliving (recapitulating) many of these experiences, thoughts, and feelings in her own tumultuous relationships with her peers and family. She described feelings, for example, of unbearable pain and of "being pulled in all directions." During this time, it was most remarkable and perhaps life-saving to this troubled and hurt adolescent that she was able to, not only form an attachment but, maintain a meaningful relationship with her therapist, which was for a time her only reported stable relationship. Our point here is that, aside from the therapist's theoretical framework or therapeutic technique(s), it is suspected that the important aspect of this therapy was the therapeutic alliance/relationship itself between Jennifer and the therapist.

2. The Goal

Response to an intensely suicidal person, like Jennifer, Dennis, or Robert, is a special task. The goal of treatment is quite simple. It consists almost by definition, of lowering the lethality; in practice, this amounts to decreasing or mollifying the level of perturbation. We defuse the source of the person's constricted focus on suicide. We create social interest around the person. We make that person's temporarily unbearable pain just bearable enough so that he or she can stop to think, reconsider and discern alternatives to suicide. The way to decrease lethality with the individual is by dramatically decreasing the felt perturbation—a process in which the relationship is the key. The therapist works to improve the situation related to pain and other aspects of the suicidal state, to achieve a J.N.D. (Just Noticeable Difference). This can be accomplished initially through ventilation, interpretation, instruction, and realistic manipulation in the outside world.

When fourteen-year-old Joey was first encountered in the therapist's office, it was readily evident that he was at moderate to high risk for suicide. Many of the signs were there; i.e., Joey had, in the past several weeks, increasingly distanced himself from family members and friends, spending hours brooding alone in his bedroom. His verbalizations included many references to wanting to give up, that there was no reason to live, and no point in talking to anyone because it could not help anyway. His current interests included reading horror books, watching horror films over and over, and writing about and ruminating on death. In response to many questions about school, his home life, friends, etc., he merely replied, "I don't care." He also reported previous suicide attempts, although the lethality of these attempts was not clear. In this case, especially in view of Joey's reluctance to talk, a timely (i.e., same day) realistic manipulation in the outside world was viewed as offering the best chance at a J.N.D. Help was procured from Joey's mother and from the school's gym teacher/coach. It was learned that Joey had a special interest in basketball. His mother and gym teacher quickly moved to enroll a reluctant, though compliant, ("I don't care") boy onto the school basketball team, with practice to commence that very evening. Activity was created around Joey. Moreover, in light of significant signs of agitated depression, Joey's mother followed a strong recommendation to immediately have Joey undergo in-depth physical/medical evaluation. With consultation, he was put on a medication regime that was closely monitored and adjusted as needed, and that reduced the level of perturbation, achieving a J.N.D. Medication and hospitalization are always complicating events with an adolescent, but in some cases are essential. The changes were enough to allow the therapist to engage Joey in a relationship. In addition, Joey's progress was closely monitored by the school, with daily contact arranged with significant school staff. Long-term treatment was then planned and subsequently followed with the therapist.

3. Crisis as a Perception

A crisis, as we have seen with Dennis, Robert, Jennifer, and Joey, is defined by a perception; i.e., the way an individual construes his or her circumstance. A "B" on an examination is acceptable to many students but to others it may be the occasion of unbearable pain. The belief that a crisis is defined by a subject's perception does not, however, mean that one accepts the person's view of the problem without questions, as illustrated in the case of Dennis. Given the person's view, suicide has adjustive value. It abolishes pain. One must translate the adolescent's perception into a wider adaptive view. One has to widen the blinders. One does not talk only about the low grade or the lost girlfriend or boyfriend. Despair over a low grade, for example, can be translated into a need for perfection. Dennis' "loss" of a girlfriend, for a specific example, can be translated into a need for attachment.

As one explores, one redefines to the individual the trauma as painful but tolerable. One develops the adaptive potential of the adolescent. If the intervener accepts the perspective, "I can't live with this" then we tacitly collude with the person's decision to die and the adolescent cannot survive. Yet, we cannot provide naive reassurance by simply saying, "You can too!" A better response to the teenager would be something like, "When you say I can't live with *this,* what is the *this?*" The interventionist can then redefine (reframe) the problem in terms of, say, a need for perfectionism, or another limiting, intolerable value (view).

It is imperative for the intervener, however, to understand how the suicidal teenager defines the trauma; i.e., what it is that cannot be endured. This is true for all the teenagers discussed so far. A crisis is a perception, not a thing-in-itself. These adolescents often cannot concentrate; they are too perturbed. Therefore, when one helps these youngsters, it is useful to bear in mind the question: "What is it that we are going to focus on?" Typical questions when focusing are: "What is the problem?" "What were you hoping to accomplish?" "What would be most helpful?" "We've talked about a lot, what do you want to discuss?"

4. Active Participation

Experience has shown that it is neither useful nor wise to respond to an individual in an acute suicidal crisis with punishment, moral suasion, confrontation, or the like. The most effective way to help a suicidal adolescent is to assuage the anguish of the trauma, reducing the perturbation. It is the elevated perturbation that drives and fuels the elevated lethality; therefore, one tries to reduce the person's trauma—his anguish, tension, and pain. The rule is: Reduce the elevated perturbation and the lethality will come down with it.

Suicide is, thus, an effort by the teenager to stop unbearable anguish and intolerable pain. The anguish and pain usually relates manifestly to only one thing—e.g., the loss of an imagined girlfriend, letting one's parents down—but latently to much more. They want action and need prompt relief. To save a person's life, we have to do something! This may include putting out information that the person is in trouble into the stream of communication, letting others know about it, breaking what could be a fatal secret, proffering help, and, always showing interest and deep concern. We do not agree with those individuals who argue for a "no rescue" stance in this field. One should have, at least a rescue approach with moderately lethal adolescents (although in adults such may be provisional in some moderately lethal individuals), and always an action plan with highly lethal adolescents.

Bear in mind three things when helping suicidal adolescents: First, a key to intermediate and long range effectiveness with the suicidal teenager is to increase the options of actions available, to increase awareness of adjustment processes, to widen the angle of the blinders, and to increase the number of people available to help. Second, when the adolescent is no longer highly suicidal then the usual methods of psychotherapy can be usefully employed. One does not leave the adolescent with his/her weakened, not adequately developed ego. He/she needs therapeutic assistance. Finally, given all that, we need to be reminded that work in suicide prevention is risky and dangerous, and there are casualties.

5. Blocking the Exit

The highly suicidal adolescent wants out. It follows that, when possible, the means of exit should be blocked. A practical application of this view is to "get the gun" in a suicidal situation where it is known that the individual intends to shoot himself or herself and has a weapon. The explosive situation needs to be defused until that person no longer has the need for a suicidal weapon [see 39]. Maltsberger's consultative words [39] on such cases may guide us here:

> I would consult as much to avoid charges of negligence as to deal with my own anxiety. I think that any time I get into a difficult case, where I am concerned that somebody is imminently suicidal . . . I would want to be careful. It is enormously helpful to ask a colleague to help to monitor one's own judgment when in a tense, anxiety-provoking situation [39, p. 118].

6. Desiderata

Clearly, consultation is needed in some cases. As we have learned, the focus in intervention with lethal adolescents should not be on "why" suicide has been chosen as the method of solving the problems. This is probably better addressed in more usual psychotherapy, once the lethality is lower. Instead, the focus should be on solving the problem(s), so that pain becomes mollified. The problems are discussed and addressed in terms of what can be done about them. The person needs to see some hope, although simultaneously we would agree with some (e.g., [12]) who point out how critical the hopelessness is for the therapeutic intervention. One talks about practical items—school grades, conflicts with parents, rejection by friends, whatever. The individual needs immediate partial reduction of the urgently felt suicidal impulses or wishes.

Here is a list of some further special desiderata that were derived from discussions with E. Shneidman (Personal communication, June 29-30, 1991):

1. Monitorship: A continuous, preferably daily, monitoring of the adolescent's lethality.
2. Consultation: There is almost no instance in a therapist's professional life when consultation with a peer is as important as when he is dealing with a highly suicidal adolescent. The items to be discussed might include the therapist's treatment of the case; his own feelings of frustration, helplessness or even anger; his countertransference reactions generally; the advisability of hospitalization for the adolescent, etc.
3. Hospitalization: Hospitalization is always a complicating event in the treatment of a suicidal adolescent but it should not, on those grounds, be eschewed. Obviously, the quality of care—from doctors, nurses and others—is crucial.
4. Confidentiality: Careful modification of the usual canons of confidentiality. Admittedly, this is a touchy and complicated point, but the therapist should not ally himself or herself with death. Statements given during the therapy session relating to the adolescent's overt suicidal (or homicidal) plans obviously cannot be treated as a "secret" between two collusive partners.

For further details please refer to E. Shneidman [e.g., 8, 25, 40]. As a note, one must limit one's case load to crisis intervention with only a very few highly lethal adolescents. It is impossible to deal effectively with many highly lethal individuals without risking therapist "burnout" or emotional withdrawal from the demands of such adolescents.

7. Referral for Psychotherapy

Early intervention with suicidal adolescents does not completely fix situations. Once the lethality is lowered, and the difficulties are more bearable, one moves toward more usual therapy—psychoanalytic, cognitive, existential, behavioral, whatever. This has been one of our greatest errors in helping suicidal adolescents; the underestimation of the pain and the level of their ability to adjust to life's demands. Their ego has been weakened and they need long-term assistance. In a professional psychotherapeutic exchange the focus is on feelings, emotional content, and unconscious meanings, rather than the immediate difficulties. This was true for Dennis, Robert, Jennifer, Joey and, if we can be constricted, all suicidal adolescents. The emphasis is on the latent significance of what is being said, more than on the manifest and obvious difficulties. However, these endeavors usually come after the lethality is lowered, although it is sometimes possible to embark on these efforts in one's earliest interventions [13].

A FEW NOTES ON TRANSFERENCE AND COUNTERTRANSFERENCE IN INTERVENTION

Although the issues of transference and countertransference are critical, they are so broad that space here only allows a brief note (for examples see [11, 41-43]). Yet, every crisis worker must be fully aware of these concerns.

Transference is a process arising in a therapeutic situation which involves reactivation of the person's previous experiences, recollections and unconscious wishes regarding (often early) significant people (objects). Such processes in object relations must be identified in treatment, even in crisis intervention.

Suicidal adolescents, for example, could feel angry, injured or rejected in the following situations:

• after premature termination or discharge
• with excessive waiting for help (even 1 hour, or 1 day!)
• when treatment time was short and they felt "cut off"
• if referred to others
• dealt with too directively
• given inadequate rapport, interest, etc.
• disappointed by a therapist who forgets important details
• confronted by a therapist about an issue too early
• presented with simplistic use of a written suicide contract
• contacted by a person other than the crisis interventionist.

Countertransference comprises all the therapist's unconscious reactions to the adolescent and the adolescent's transference. These reactions originate in the therapist's own conflicts and/or real objective interactions (object relations). They may not necessarily be negative; indeed, they can be most constructive in developing an understanding of our youths (and ourselves). It is, however, the negative ones that can be, not only problematic but, suicidogenic. The following reactions in the therapist may arise if confrontation with the suicidal teenager provokes feelings of guilt, incompetence, anxiety, fear, and anger, and when these feelings are not worked through:

- underestimation of the seriousness of the suicidal action
- absence of discussion of suicide thoughts, attempts, etc.
- allowing oneself to be lulled into a false sense of security by the teenager's promise not to repeat a suicide attempt (such as in the use of a simplistic written suicide contract)
- disregard of the cry for help aspect of the suicide attempt and exclusive concentration on its manipulative character
- exaggeration of the adolescent's provocative, infantile and aggressive sides
- denial of one's own importance to the young person
- failure to persuade the adolescent to undergo further treatment
- feeling of lacking the resources required by a particular teenager
- experiencing an exaggerated sense of hopelessness in response to the adolescent's troubled social situation and abuse of drugs or alcohol
- being pleased when the adolescent claims to have all problems solved after only a brief contact, without reflecting closely on the plausibility of this statement
- feeling upset when the youngster shows insufficient progress after a brief course of assistance, despite the therapist's initial profound commitment.

Obviously, issues of transference and countertransference are complex and the interventionist experiencing them can benefit from contact with a supervisor or consultation with a colleague, as well as consideration of the broader literature on such reactions written for psychotherapists.

CONCLUDING REMARKS

Ultimately, we must understand that there are no universal formulations regarding how to help a suicidal adolescent. We can speak of helping, but never with precision. When our subject matter is suicide intervention with teenagers, we can be no more accurate or scientific than the available ways of responding that our subject matter permits. Yet, the yearning for simplistic universal response persists. There is no one method to help. There is no cookbook!

To quote Berman and Jobes: "It is axiomatic that adolescents identified to be at risk for suicide or suicidal behavior need help" [10]. The goal of that help is simple: To keep a teenager alive. The procedures are often not simple, however. Our greatest error to date is underestimating the need for help. Many, if not all of these adolescents are in need of psychotherapy, usually long-term. First, we must address the trauma and then we must deal with the underlying inability to cope. We must recognize the risk in these young people and not act like ostriches with our heads in the sand, something that these youngsters are more than manifestly wanting us to do.

To help suicidal adolescents, prevention, intervention and postvention are needed. Intervention, including the assessment and prediction of risk, is only one aspect of the avenues that we need to address for suicidal adolescents [5]. Yet, intervention is an essential facet for those at risk. Help cannot be reduced to prevention or vice versa (and postvention adds another aspect when the event has occurred [44-47]). We should not underestimate the complexity of helping suicidal adolescents.

REFERENCES

1. D. Lester, A Cross-cultural Look at Suicide Rates of Children and Teenagers, in *Suicide Prevention in Schools*, A. Leenaars and S. Wenckstern (eds.), Hemisphere, Washington, D.C., pp. 17-25, 1990.
2. J. McIntosh, Epidemiology of Suicide in the United States, in *Life-span Perspectives of Suicide*, A. Leenaars (ed.), Plenum, New York, pp. 55-70, 1991.
3. K. Smith and S. Crawford, Suicidal Behavior Among "Normal" High School Students, *Suicide & Life-Threatening Behavior, 16*, pp. 313-325, 1986.
4. D. Lester, *The Cruelest Death: The Enigma of Adolescent Suicide*, The Charles Press, Philadelphia, 1993.
5. U.S. Department of Health and Human Services, *Report of the Secretary's Task Force on Youth Suicide*, U.S. Government Printing Office, Washington, D.C., 1989.
6. K. Menninger, *Man Against Himself*, Harcourt, New York, 1938.
7. A. Leenaars, Unconscious Processes, in *Suicidology: Essays in Honor of Edwin S. Shneidman*, A. Leenaars (ed.), Aronson, Northvale, New Jersey, pp. 125-147, 1993.
8. E. Shneidman, *Definition of Suicide*, Wiley, New York, 1985.

9. G. Caplan, *Principles of Preventive Psychiatry*, Basic Books, New York, 1964.
10. A.L. Berman and D. Jobes, Treatment of the Suicidal Adolescent, in *Treatment of Suicidal People*, A. Leenaars, J.T. Maltsberger and R. Neimeyer (eds.), Taylor and Francis, London, pp. 89-100, 1994.
11. J. Eyman, Countertransference when Counseling Suicidal School-aged Youth, in *Suicide Prevention in Schools*, A. Leenaars and S. Wenckstern (eds.), Hemisphere, Washington, D.C., pp. 147-158, 1990.
12. K. Smith, Therapeutic Care of the Suicidal Student, in *Suicide Prevention in Schools*, A. Leenaars and S. Wenckstern (eds.), Hemisphere, Washington, D.C., pp. 135-146, 1990.
13. A. Leenaars, J.T. Maltsberger, and R. Neimeyer, (eds.), *Treatment of Suicidal People*, Taylor and Francis, London, 1994.
14. D. Shaffer, V. Vieland, A. Garland, M. Rojas, M. Underwood, and C. Busner, Adolescent Suicide Attempters: Response to Suicide Prevention Programs, *Journal of the American Medical Association, 264*, pp. 3151-3155, 1990.
15. A. Leenaars and S. Wenckstern, Suicide Prevention in Schools: An Introduction, *Death Studies, 14*, pp. 297-302, 1990.
16. A. Leenaars, 1990: Suicidology in Schools, in *Suicide Prevention in Schools*, A. Leenaars and S. Wenckstern (eds.), Hemisphere, Washington, D.C., pp. 257-264, 1990.
17. A. Leenaars, Crisis Intervention with Highly Lethal People, *Death Studies, 18,* pp. 341-359, 1994.
18. J. Richman, Family Therapy with Suicidal Children, *Suicide Prevention in Schools*, A. Leenaars and S. Wenckstern (eds.), Hemisphere, Washington, D.C., pp. 159-170, 1990.
19. A.L. Berman and D. Jobes, *Adolescent Suicide: Assessment and Intervention*, American Psychological Association Press, Washington, D.C., 1991.
20. J. Zimmerman, D. Grosz, and G. Asnis (eds.), *Treatment Approaches with Suicidal Adolescents*, Wiley, New York, 1995.
21. A. Leenaars and D. Lester, Assessment and Prediction of Suicide Risk in Adolescents, in *Treatment Approaches with Suicidal Adolescents*, J. Zimmerman, D. Grosz and G. Asnis (eds.), Wiley, New York, pp. 47-70, 1995.
22. R. Maris, A.L. Berman, J.T. Maltsberger, and R. Yufit, *Assessment and Prediction of Suicide*, Guilford, New York, 1992.
23. R.J. Myatt and M. Greenblatt, Adolescent Suicidal Behavior, in *Suicidology: Essays in Honor of Edwin S. Shneidman*, A. Leenaars (ed.), Aronson, Northvale, New Jersey, pp. 186-206, 1993.
24. A. Leenaars and S. Wenckstern, Suicide in the School-age Child and Adolescent, in *Life-span Perspectives of Suicide,* A. Leenaars (ed.), Plenum, New York, pp. 95-108, 1991.
25. J.T. Maltsberger, *Suicide Risk*, New York Universities Press, New York, 1986.

26. E. Shneidman, *Suicide as Psychache*, Aronson, Northvale, New Jersey, 1993.
27. A.T. Beck, H. Resnik, and D. Lettieri, *The Prediction of Suicide*, Charles Press, Bowie, Maryland, 1974.
28. P. Lewinsohn, C. Garrison, J. Langhinrichsen, and F. Marsteller, *The Assessment of Suicidal Behavior in Adolescents: A Review of Scales Suitable for Epidemiological Clinical Research*, National Institute of Mental Health, Rockwell, Maryland, 1989.
29. American Psychiatric Association, *Diagnostic and Statistical Manual of Mental Disorders* (3rd Edition, revised) (DSM-111-R), Author, Washington, D.C., 1987.
30. C. Pfeffer, *The Suicidal Child*, Guilford, New York, 1986.
31. N. Farberow, (ed.), *The Many Faces of Suicide*, McGraw-Hill Book Co., New York, 1980.
32. L. A. Hoff, *People in Crisis*, Addison-Wesley, Menlo Park, California, 1984.
33. L.A. Hoff, Crisis Intervention in Schools, in *Suicide Prevention in Schools*, A. Leenaars and S. Wenckstern (eds.), Hemisphere, Washington, D.C., pp. 123-134, 1990.
34. A. Leenaars, Suicide Notes and their Implications for Intervention, *Crisis, 12*, pp. 1-20, 1991.
35. R.A. Mackinnon and R. Michels, *The Psychiatric Interview in Clinical Practice*, W.B. Saunders, Philadelphia, Pennsylvania, 1971.
36. H. Parad, *Crisis Intervention*, Family Service Association of America, New York, 1965.
37. S. Tarachow, *An Introduction to Psychotherapy*, International Universities Press, Inc., New York, 1963.
38. A. Leenaars, *Suicide Notes*, Human Sciences Press, New York, 1988.
39. A.L. Berman (ed.), *Suicide Prevention: Case Consultation*, Springer, New York, 1990.
40. E. Shneidman, Psychotherapy with Suicidal Patients, *Suicide & Life-Threatening Behavior, 11*, pp. 341-348, 1981.
41. S. Freud, The Future Prospects of Psycho-analytic Therapy, in *The Standard Edition of the Complete Psychological Work of Sigmund Freud, Vol. 11*, J. Strachey (ed. and trans.), Hogarth Press (original published in 1910), pp. 139-151, 1957.
42. P. Heimann, On Countertransference, *International Journal of Psychoanalysis, 14*, pp. 81-84, 1950.
43. J.T. Maltsberger and D. Buie, Counter-transference Hate in the Treatment of Suicidal Patients, *Archives of General Psychiatry, 30*, pp. 625-633, 1974.
44. B.F. Carter and A. Brooks, Clinical Opportunities in Suicide Postvention, in *Suicide Prevention in Schools*, A. Leenaars and S. Wenckstern (eds.), Hemisphere, Washington, D.C., pp. 197-212, 1990.
45. F. Lamb, K. Dunne-Maxim, M. Underwood, and C. Sutton, Postvention from the Viewpoint of Consultants, in *Suicide Prevention in Schools*,

A. Leenaars and S. Wenckstern (eds.), Hemisphere, Washington, D.C., pp. 213-227, 1990.

46. S. Wenckstern and A. Leenaars, Suicide Postvention: A Case Illustration in a Secondary School, in *Suicide Prevention in Schools*, A. Leenaars and S. Wenckstern (eds.), Hemisphere, Washington, D.C., pp. 181-195, 1990.

47. S. Wenckstern and A. Leenaars, Trauma and Suicide in our Schools, *Death Studies, 17*, pp. 151-172, 1993.

CHAPTER 9

The Suffering of Children and Adolescents with Life-Threatening Illness: Factors Involved and Ways Professionals Can Help

David W. Adams

> To look at her she is a picture of health;
> to look inside her, she is crying [1, p. 10].

As adults, we often have the life experiences and the cognitive capability to understand the nature of suffering, and recognize that it is an integral part of life that may be activated at any time. Children, on the other hand, frequently lack the life experiences and cognitive capability to understand suffering. They must rely on parents and other adults to interpret its meaning and help them to deal with it.

Suffering has been differentiated from pain as being more complex in origin, broader in scope, and longer in duration. Whereas pain has usually been viewed as a physically related and stressful phenomena associated with disease, injury, or bodily disorder, suffering has been attributed to intense emotional as well as physical distress. Cassell points out that:

> Suffering occurs when an impending destruction of the person is perceived and continues until the threat of disintegration is passed or until the integrity of the person is destroyed in some other manner [2, p. 640].

Copp suggests that suffering is a human state of anguish due to pain, injury, or loss [3].

Maes points out that there are a range of complex causes of suffering that include phenomena such as physical disability, depression, anxiety states, bereavement, and economic loss [4]. Suffering also conjures up thoughts of terror, horror, pain, agitation, anxiety, dread, and confusion [4]. It is an unwanted intrusion that lasts too long. It may rob the afflicted person of the opportunity for pleasure and enjoyment of actions and events that have been appreciated in the past or were anticipated in the future. The person who suffers responds to stimuli that others may see as being real or imagined, but, for the sufferer, are always real and hurtful. The degree to which we are prone to suffering and the array of changes and feelings that accompany it depends upon our perceptions—our personal feelings, beliefs, and reactions to trauma that prey upon us, demand more than we have to offer, and make us pay the price for exposure to whatever unearths and capitalizes on our vulnerability. Basically, suffering takes away the pleasures that we may take for granted and, through time, may erode our endurance.

As children, we were shaped by experiences that we encountered in each stage of our development. We evolved cognitively, behaviorally, socially, and spiritually. While our evolution into adulthood provided us with the tools to benefit from life experiences, it also taught us to respond negatively to what we perceived to be threatening or hurtful. As adults we are prone to reacting to what we think and feel, to what others think and feel, and to who we determine ourselves to be within the universe. In adulthood, it seems reasonable to expect us to be fully equipped to be sufferers depending upon what we encounter and how we approach what life offers. However, children are different. They are less prepared. Is it reasonable to expect that children will suffer? If so, when and under what circumstances?

CHILDREN AND ADOLESCENTS AS SUFFERERS

Society tends to see suffering as an undesirable phenomena of adult life that is to be avoided, controlled, or eliminated. However, in reality, suffering is very much a part of everyday living that extends beyond the adult world into the protected and potentially sacred ground of childhood. Suffering is even more unwanted and unwelcome in this domain as it is hoped that children will be healthy, happy, and energetic rather than being ill or in pain. Most adults would prefer a falsely optimistic view of childhood fueled by adult denial. In short, adults tend to be ethnocentric about suffering, willingly relegating suffering to the confines of adulthood.

Given these perceptions, some questions readily emerge. Can children really be threatened to the extent that Bradshaw suggests where suffering is seen as a "hole in the soul?" [5, p. 271]. Do children experience the entire range of feelings that are characteristic of suffering? We know that children may be easily frustrated and feel helpless, but do words like anguish, despair, apathy, and hopelessness fit into their repertoire?

In their progression toward adulthood, children and adolescents are extremely vulnerable and often ill equipped to cope with the impact of:

- physical pain that may vary in intensity and duration, and become chronic
- damage to or loss of a body part
- hurtful and damaging assaults on their ego
- change resulting in severe and lasting disruption of their family or social lives
- grief associated with personal tragedy, family illness, and loss
- afflictions that may range from coping with an abusive parent to living in a violent neighborhood.

In each situation, children and adolescents are prone to experiencing what Patricia McGrath refers to as "noxious stimuli" that may threaten the integrity of themselves and their families, and make them suffer [6, p. 13]. Children are the innocent victims of what Van Eys calls "undeserved adversity" [7, p. 124].

When we remember five-year-old Peter and his struggle with leukemia, ten-year-old Kevin with a tumor that eroded his intestinal tract, twelve-year-old Betsy whose skin was stretched tight with scleroderma, thirteen-year-old Billy who was afflicted with a severe head injury, or sixteen-year-old Emily whose joints were chronically inflamed and swollen with a progressive destructive arthritic disease, the word suffering takes on a meaning that transcends most human experiences.

In this chapter, I will concentrate on suffering that is associated with life-threatening illness, often referring to childhood cancer to illustrate what transpires when children and adolescents suffer. Throughout the process of diagnosis, relapse, use of experimental therapies, and terminal care, many children and adolescents experience the suffering incurred from the threat of disintegration described by Cassell [2]. Their lives may be destroyed, or the threat of destruction may be present in varying degrees of intensity throughout their illness and potentially their lives [8, 9]. The experience of living with childhood cancer also parallels Battenfield's description of the three phases of suffering [10]. These include: 1) initial impact; 2) turmoil without resolution; and 3) recovery involving coping, accepting, understanding, and finding meaning. The time of diagnosis and relapse is in tune with Battenfield's first phase and includes shock, disbelief, and various types of pain and discomfort. Phase two is readily associated with the period following diagnosis, times of intense treatment, the period after relapse, and terminal care. These times may be fraught with confusion, difficult emotions, and feelings of helplessness or hopelessness. Recovery, the third phase, occurs when children, adolescents, and their families learn to cope with the disease, accept temporary or long-term limitations, and find meaning through self-awareness and personal growth. In recent years, entering this phase of recovery is a reality for an increasing number of children with cancer who pass through the most difficult phases on the way to long-term survival and cure.

Despite the parallels with Battenfield's phases, it is imperative to recognize that there is no practical framework for understanding the dimensions of suffering for each individual child with cancer or any other disease. There will always be individual variation in respect to the causes, characteristics, and duration of suffering.

In the rest of this chapter, I will discuss:

- who influences the suffering child
- how parents and families affect the suffering of children and adolescents
- why children and adolescents suffer
- what happens when they suffer
- what they tell us about their suffering
- how parents, children, and adolescents can be helpful in coping with suffering
- how professionals can help.

WHO INFLUENCES THE SUFFERING CHILD: THE ROLE OF PARENTS AND LIFE BEYOND THE FAMILY

In examining the suffering of children and adolescents, it is imperative to recognize that their responses to noxious stimuli are influenced by their parents, family members, and people they encounter outside of the family.

The Role of Parents

From birth, children come under the intense and pervasive influence of parents or guardians who serve as nurturers, controllers, role models, and protectors so that children can thrive as physical, psychological, social, and spiritual beings. Parents are their anchor, and ideally should offer constancy and stability through time [10].

Nurturing implies that parents have a lasting commitment to feed, shelter, clothe, and promote the personal growth of children. Unfortunately, illness and other afflictions may impede parents' efforts to nurture their children in the way that they had anticipated. Adverse conditions created by pain and suffering may make parents feel frustrated to the point where they transmit their distress directly to their children. The process is self-defeating, makes them feel guilty, and directly opposes what they wish to achieve.

Controlling is associated with parents' need to provide direction and boundaries that enable their children to grow up in keeping with legal, moral, and ethical expectations of society. In most situations, parents try to be flexible as children approach adolescence and learn to reason as adults, but boundaries are still needed until children become totally independent from their parents. When children are suffering, it may become increasingly difficult to maintain control as both the effects of the illness and children's reactions to noxious stimuli may be beyond parental influence. Their difficulties may also be compounded by the distress of siblings who may be upset by the appearance of the child who is suffering, worried about what is happening, or be jealous of the attention given to the sick child. Relatives, too, may be upset and interfere with parents' ability to manage family life. At the extremes, parents under duress may become rigid in order to maintain control, or they may be so overwhelmed that they flounder or withdraw, leaving their children without the necessary reassurance and guidance.

Role modeling by parents provides a pattern for children to learn to manage their daily lives through observation and emulation as they pass through various developmental stages. As part of this process, many parents try to instill confidence in their children by being confident and positive themselves as they successfully manage a variety of situations. However, parents may find it difficult to be confident and positive when they realize that their children are suffering. In stressful situations, they may see their behavior as being less than ideal, especially when they lose control of their emotions. They worry about what they are role-modeling for their children, often believing that they should not show their true feelings as it may upset their children further or be seen by other adults as a sign of weakness.

Protecting involves parents' commitment to providing a safe, secure environment for their children. Parents place their children under an "umbrella" of parental protection that shields them from physical, cognitive, and spiritual harm [11, p. 17]. As protectors, parents are often vigilant, conscientious, and prepared to advocate on behalf of their children under any circumstances. When children are in distress due to illness, parents may have difficulty balancing their desire to be protective with their children's needs to play and be active like healthy children. If they are too protective, children may become less confident and less willing or able to control or overcome their suffering. When parents are effective protectors, the likelihood that children and teens will be subjected to additional, unnecessary pain and suffering is minimized.

By performing each of these roles, parents establish a framework for family life. Children are indoctrinated into family routines and rituals and, in ideal situations, benefit from family relationships that are encouraged, monitored, and heavily influenced by their parents. This experience lays the ground work for children's behavior outside of the home.

Becoming Independent: The World Beyond Parents and Family

As children proceed through the stages of childhood and adolescence, they gradually distance themselves from their parents and rely on them less for guidance and role modeling. They are increasingly exposed to the influences of schools and other organized systems that ensure that they are shaped and moulded to adult standards. These influences are augmented by a range of informal and spontaneous interactions that vary in intensity and frequency with peers, neighbors, and others at each stage of their development. Peers, in particular, become increasingly influential as children reach adolescence. Teens tend to spend more time with their peer group than with their families.

As a result of these experiences, it is hoped that children and adolescents will learn to accept themselves as worthwhile individuals who are acceptable to others, capable of functioning positively, and able to overcome obstacles as they arise. They are expected to be able to interact, understand, give love, and receive it from others. It is anticipated that they will be able to live by rules, judge their own abilities, and feel positive about themselves. Maes suggests that children become strong due to "acceptance, approval and interaction" that helps them hold "introjects of images, feeling and memories" and other reassurances that have been "filed away for future use" [4, p. 47].

Ideally, the world should be a safe place where children and adolescents are integrated into a supportive social structure where social isolation, loneliness, and feelings of inadequacy and incompetence are minimized.

When children are suffering, they may be removed from the umbrella of parental protection, making it more difficult to keep them free from harm. They may be subjected to repeated hospitalizations, a continuous barrage of treatments, and an endless array of caregivers. They may also be isolated from friends and family, rejected by peers, and unable to continue with regular activities. Their independence under such circumstances is premature, anxiety provoking, and exposes them to experiences that are suppose to be reserved for those who have passed beyond the innocence of childhood.

HOW PARENTS AND FAMILIES AFFECT THE SUFFERING OF CHILDREN AND ADOLESCENTS

Sadly, the expectations that society places on parents and that parents place on themselves are unreasonable. Parents may feel anxious about their ability to provide their children with emotional support and guidance in every situation, feel hurt and alienated when their children deviate from prescribed expectations, and feel guilty in circumstances affecting their children that are beyond parental control. Yet, parents are expected to be pinnacles of strength and wisdom, and to be the primary caregivers for their children, whatever the circumstances.

When their children are ill, parents often serve as a buffer between the health care system and the child. They continue to be role models, set the tone for the behavior of the rest of the family, and actively seek out what is best for their children. In fact, as I have always been quick to point out, "as the parents go, so goes the child" [12, p. 10]. I strongly believe that as Spinetta and his associates validated in their work with children with leukemia, children manage best when the communication pattern in the family is open and honest [13, 14]. However, we must also recognize that when children's lives are threatened and they are suffering, parents are severely taxed. They worry about their children's pain, the potential for lasting disability, physical deterioration, and death [6]. When they have difficulty understanding or accepting what is happening, they may convey their anxiety to their children, be in conflict with each other about how to cope, have difficulty disciplining their other children, or express adult attitudes and beliefs that may confuse the sick child. For example, parents may minimize or deny their children's suffering, or believe their children are being tested, punished, or subjected to the will of God [15]. Van Eys points out that we should be very concerned about the impact of such parental behavior when he says:

> They (the children) are at the mercy of adult values by which they are judged . . . Children are seen, at best, as wholly dependent and totally beholden to the adult in whose care they find themselves [7, p. 118].

Such a picture suggests that children and adolescents who are suffering from life-threatening illness are locked in and unable to help themselves. They are in the hands of parents who are often powerless, or are given over to medical personnel in hopes that they have the power to help them to control or escape from their suffering. When parental influence is weak or lacking, the vulnerability of children and teens often increases proportionately.

WHY CHILDREN AND ADOLESCENTS SUFFER

In the previous paragraphs, I pointed out how much children and adolescents are affected by the behavior of their parents. Coppolillo suggests that when parents react severely to a child's life-threatening illness, the child suffers "from the anguish of seeing the parents suffer and the uneasiness of being treated in an unfamiliar manner" [16, p. 57]. Children and adolescents may also have difficulty sorting out what is happening and may respond more to emotional messages than to the illness [16]. When they are suffering from a multiplicity of noxious stimuli, it is often difficult to define the specific source of their suffering or the stimuli that aggravate or intensify the process. Patricia McGrath in her monumental book on children and pain, supports this perspective. She notes that children's perceptions of pain are not necessarily linked to the extent of bodily injury or the severity of an illness [6]. Factors such as their cognitive development, previous experience with pain, the degree of importance allocated to the illness, their social situation, expectations that pain will be relieved, and children's ability to control the pain themselves all affect their perceptions and reactions [6].

WHAT HAPPENS WHEN CHILDREN AND ADOLESCENTS SUFFER

The author modified Chesler and Barbarin's categories of challenges faced by parents of children with cancer and applied these revised categories to the experiences of children themselves [17, 18]. These can readily be applied in examining the challenges faced by suffering children. These include: 1) intellectual; 2) practical or instrumental; 3) physical; 4) emotional; 5) social or interpersonal; and 6) existential challenges.

Intellectual Challenges

These challenges are associated with the need for suffering children to make sense out of what is happening to them in language they can understand. Medical terminology, the nature of communication or lack of it, and the paradoxes associated with illness and treatment are all complicating factors. For example, young children with cancer who are bombarded by chemotherapy may receive messages about how treatment will make them feel better while at the same time, it imposes severe side effects such as vomiting, hair loss, lethargy, and repeated infections that make them feel miserable. Children may also be confused and anxious because what they are facing may be beyond the control and understanding of their parents on whom they must rely to provide and interpret information. By pre-adolescence as children develop their capacity to think rationally, their ability to inquire, seek answers to their questions, and gain a satisfactory level of understanding may assist them to reach a level of comprehension of their suffering that is equal to or greater than that of their parents.

Practical or Instrumental Challenges

Practical challenges include the need to comply with treatment, hospital rules, and the dictums of professionals as well as coping with practical concerns such as scheduling treatments, doing rehabilitation exercises, and being immobilized. Practical demands are particularly intrusive and distressing for adolescents who wish to be in control, have the freedom to take action on their own, and be like their peers.

Physical Challenges

Physical challenges are often associated with major visible sources of suffering especially when the impact of a physical stressor is intense or prolonged. Physical pain may emanate from inflammation, distortion, destruction, and deterioration of body parts. Patrick McGrath and his associates in studying the pain of children with cancer, conclude that children suffered pain from the disease, the diagnostic and monitoring procedures, and the treatment. They suggest that a key concern is the control of pain from invasive medical procedures, chemotherapy, and active disease processes [19]. In a broader based approach to pain, Patricia McGrath pays special attention to the suffering from chronic pain which is different from acute pain because its persistence gradually changes a child's life [6]. She suggests that the suffering of children and adolescents in chronic pain may arise from a variety of serious and life-threatening illnesses including:

- arthritis accompanied by tissue changes, joint inflammation, and systemic reactions
- hemophilia involving repeated joint inflammation or disability from hemorrhage
- reflex sympathetic dystrophy with symptoms of vasomotor dysfunction
- childhood cancer that may involve cumulative, systemic pain from aggressive treatment programs, or pain resulting from impairment or destruction of body parts
- sickle cell anemia affecting only black children. The disease impedes the oxygen flow to body tissues with the potential for varying degrees of obstruction.

In most instances, it could be suggested that the greater the intensity, the longer the duration, and the more physical pain impedes functioning, the more children will suffer.

Emotional Challenges

Emotional challenges may be related to any type of major stress prevalent in the lives of children and adolescents who are suffering. These may include:

- anxiety generated by the uncertainty of others, the threat of medical or rehabilitative procedures, and the prolonged effects of a severe illness or treatment
- sadness associated with the changes in their lives or the lives of their families, the damaging effects of pain, or restrictions that prevent them from going to school or participating in their regular activities
- anger generated by the frustration of being subjected to frequent tests and procedures, having to comply with rules and regulations, and being forced to relate to a variety of caregivers
- loneliness due to prolonged isolation from their families, friends, and peers

- guilt associated with the emotional and financial demands that their illness makes on the family or their assumption of responsibility for causing their own illness.

When children and adolescents are suffering, their behavior may include:

- passive resistance to caregivers exhibited through non-compliance, tearful outbursts, body rigidity, or pulling away
- active resistance shown through acts of aggression such as lashing out verbally or physically, gesturing, using vile language, or running from situations where they feel threatened
- passive acceptance demonstrated by compliance accompanied by a complete lack of questioning or emotion
- active acceptance highlighted by their efforts to cope with and reduce their suffering by their own acts or by seeking the assistance of others.

I encountered a classic case of active acceptance when I met Gary. He was thirteen years old when he was left with weakness in his lower limbs and difficulty keeping his balance due to the removal of a brain tumor. His parents worried about him and were very protective. He pleaded with them to allow him to attend a teen weekend with other adolescents with cancer, and they reluctantly consented to let him participate. In the company of other teens, he became more talkative and willing to take part in most activities. The other teens were very supportive and helpful, and on the second day they encouraged Gary to fulfil his desire (under adult supervision) to swim again. This achievement was a surprise to his parents and changed their approach to their son. Swimming lessons became a source of respite for Gary in his struggle to recover and gave him renewed confidence.

In order to protect themselves and gain at least some degree of mastery, children and adolescents may also invoke a number of defense or coping mechanisms [20]. These may include:

1. *denial* in order to avoid blame, provide respite from the effects of noxious stimuli, and enable them to participate to some degree in regular or special activities. Adolescents, in particular, use denial to avoid receiving information that may threaten their physical or emotional well-being or restrict social activity,
2. *displacement* so that frustration with themselves or their caregivers is projected onto someone else such as a parent or sibling,

3. *regression* which provides relief from having to perform at the same level as their peers. By regressing, children and teens exhibit behavior associated with younger children. This may provide secondary gains through increased dependency on parents or give them the license to rebel against rules and regulations of the hospital,

4. *rationalization* which helps them to justify what is happening to them in order to make their situation more palatable,

5. *projection* that enables them to attribute their anger and other difficult feelings to others, essentially holding them accountable. This is particularly common in adolescence,

6. *sublimation* which helps them immerse themselves in activities that they deem to be constructive or helpful, thus diverting their attention from negative feelings associated with their illness,

7. *aggression or acting out* by expressing anger externally in ways that may release pent up feelings positively, or be destructive and hurtful to others.

These coping mechanisms may be activated at any time, especially when noxious stimuli are intolerable and children and adolescents are suffering intensely. However, these mechanisms can also be invoked at times when some children and teens see an opportunity for secondary gains by making parents feel guilty in order to obtain rewards such as special treats or compromises. Further, if children and adolescents are unable to activate sufficient coping mechanisms to maintain their ego integrity and self-esteem, the psychological consequences may be severe and lasting.

Social and Interpersonal Challenges

These challenges are also a major problem for children and teens who are suffering. They are associated with disruptions in relationships with family, peers, and community. When children and teens suffer, their roles in the family change. Instead of being active participants in the life of the family, they may become the focus of attention, the consumer of the family's emotional and physical energy, and the source of increased sibling rivalry and resentment. For example, after her brother was diagnosed with cancer, Tanya, age sixteen, said:

I have developed my own disease from my brother's. My side effects are: sympathy pains, a craving for affection that the family doesn't have time to give me any more, and jealousy [21, p. 6].

Tanya reflects the pathos, ambivalence, and frustration that many siblings in her situation experience. The companionship, alliances, rivalry, scheming, role modeling, and fun of sibling relationships may be undermined or lost when a brother or sister is suffering.

At the same time, when children and adolescents are unable to remain involved in school or community activities, they may become increasingly displaced and isolated. Often their peers do not understand why they are suffering and behaving differently. Some peers may become disillusioned and pull away due to their uncertainty and may be left wondering why their friend or playmate is so irritable and unwilling to participate in activities that used to be fun.

When suffering becomes restrictive, it is usually difficult for children and adolescents to attend school, concentrate, and keep up with academic work when their lives are continually taxed or interrupted by painful stimuli. In addition, they may become entrenched in behavior that bonds them to their parents and home so that they are reluctant to relinquish the attention and protection of the family. When suffering is prolonged, returning to the outside world can be anxiety provoking and may require more emotional and physical energy than they can muster [22].

Existential Challenges

Existential challenges become increasingly important with older children and adolescents, and are associated with how they view their existence, the nature and purpose of life, and their sense of what is fair and just [18]. These challenges are closely related to spirituality and religion, and children's ability to use abstract thought. Religious beliefs and practices of their families often influence what they think, feel, and believe. As children reach pre-adolescence, they may seek their own answers to spiritual questions and when suffering, may be more concerned about the existential question, "Why me?" Teens, in particular, may be anxious, ruminate about their futures, and increase their physical and emotional pain at times when it is difficult for them to deny what is happening. Issues pertaining to God may also surface due to their indecision about whether God exists, and whether or not God is benevolent or punitive. They may contemplate the meaning of fate and try to determine how what is happening relates to their need for freedom and justice. It is their ability to think as adults, link their thoughts with their experiences, and assimilate information about what is happening that helps children and adolescents to deal with existential concerns.

Any or all of these challenges may be part of either the noxious stimuli associated with their suffering, or the source of strength that enables them to cope with this distress. Their vulnerability to any or all of these challenges is most closely associated with their level of cognitive development. Coppolillo suggests that children need to develop a "cohesive and lasting sense of self" and determine how it matches the requirement of inner and outer worlds in a child's life [16, p. 55]. When children's lives are threatened, their internal sense of cohesion may be fragmented by the implosive experience of acute pain or the gnawing anguish of chronic pain and suffering. Their ability to perform complex functions may be replaced by more primitive functions as their lasting sense of self is compromised. This may result in regressive behavior, immaturity when compared with healthy peers, or an inability to move toward recovery.

The components by which children's reactions are governed emerge from the external world and their internal "physiological and psychological awareness" [16, p. 56]. By the time children reach pre-adolescence, they have an increasing ability to comprehend the external world more effectively and often assert their individuality in how they respond to illness and treatment. They become increasingly articulate about what they think and feel and may want to manage as much as possible on their own. In the following section, children and teens tell us about their suffering in their own words.

SUFFERING FROM THE PERSPECTIVE OF CHILDREN AND ADOLESCENTS

Children and teens are the best sources for increasing our understanding of what happens to them. Wesley, age five, vividly describes his perceptions of the physical impact of leukemia in his poem:

HOW MUCH I HATE COMING TO THE CLINIC
My toes turn green.
My face turns yellow.
My belly turns brown.
My arms turn red.
My smile turns black.
My fingers turn purple [23, p. 10].

It could be said that Wesley's reaction simply focuses on his concrete experiences and observations described in the language of a five-year-old. However, this would be understating Wesley's case. His poem is loaded with emotion associated with an experience he vehemently dislikes, and clearly reflects a sense of anguish that may be the result of months or years of suffering.

In his dramatic account of his battle with physical pain, Rajeev describes the extent of his suffering, anxiety, and fear of disintegration in a stanza of his poem:

CANCER
Pain, what is this
thing called pain.
Turns eternity into hell,
death comes to reality,
life becomes intolerable,
separates us from
our loved ones
who mean so much.
It gnaws at our insides,
tearing our outsides,
forever eroding our sanity [24, p. 9].

In a later stanza from the same poem, Rajeev describes his feelings of sadness and isolation, and continues the theme of disfiguration.

Fears of rejection,
tears of sorrow and
loneliness set in.
Are these all for nothing
remaining at the back
of my mind, poisoning it?
Slowly it deteriorates
letting all its
frustrations be known.

In the midst of her struggle with cancer, Debbie, age fifteen, likens her life to that of a rose as she describes the emotional impact of her suffering and alludes to the hole in her self created by her suffering:

I often feel helpless.
Each day that passes by, I bloom.
Yet, in another sense, I die
This feeling I can no longer hide [25, p. 1].

As she continues, she reflects on the physical and existential components of her suffering.

Now I am no longer beautiful.
I have become shrivelled and lifeless.
I long to be that beautiful bud I once was,
But that cannot be.
Now, I know all roses die,
But, please, will someone help me?
This naked rose wants to live.

Landi, a fourteen-year-old with Hodgkin's disease, emphasizes how difficult it is to see the emotional impact of her illness on her family and friends:

Right now is a rough time. Not only for me, but also for my family. It hurts me so much to see my parents cry, my brother is so quiet, and my whole family disrupted just for me. It's tough on my friends because they're all short on words, careful to say just the right thing, never knowing if something will upset or hurt me [26, p. 11].

After battling cancer for seven years, Patricia says that she still suffers from physical setbacks that are currently associated with periodic joint pains. These were previously linked to bouts of dizziness and fainting. Her article "My Life" contains a description of the haunting reality of her emotional as well as her physical suffering. She writes:

There is much pain involved with having cancer, both physical and emotional. Although the physical pain I've suffered has been substantial, the emotional pain has had more of an impact on me. Physical pain comes and goes, and with time, is practically nonexistent. The emotional suffering, however, is still present, and I assume will never go away completely [27, pp. 6-7].

Sloane, a teen who experienced the removal of a malignant brain tumor, highlights the cognitive, social, and physical sequelae of being left only with partial vision in one eye and weakness extending down one side of her body. She was fourteen when she wrote a letter to her teachers, saying:

Communicating with others is also troublesome for me now. Sometimes the words I want to say do not come out easily. My brain processes everything a bit slower than before; but I am learning to understand this and hope others do too. It takes me a little bit longer to get around and sometimes I get real tired. Having my classes close together will be a big help [28, p. 8].

In her commentary, "Now I See," Dawne, a long term survivor of childhood cancer, notes how her perspective on life changed, and even after all the treatment ended she felt defeated and sad. She describes the lasting influence on her sense of self as she wrote:

Dreams that were dreamed were gone, shattered, never to be achieved. Failure set in and I wondered why I ever came through cancer and why I didn't die [29, p. 11].

Jeanie, a sixteen-year-old with osteogenic sarcoma, reflects on the bittersweet nature of existence in the first stanza of her poem:

Life—a word with so much meaning—
Many take it for granted and don't look deep into it.
For those of us who do can see that it is full of pleasure, peace, conflict and pain.
We have been through much of this conflict and a lot of the pain.
Because of this we have suffered all throughout [30, p. 1].

COPING WITH SUFFERING

How Parents and Families Can Help

When we think about how children learn to cope, there are several factors to consider. Earlier, I briefly touched on how parents can be a positive influence in helping children to alleviate and adapt to suffering. In his work, Coppolillo suggests that when children's lives are threatened by illness, parents must mourn for the loss of the child that they had before the diagnosis and for the child they had anticipated having in future years. He stresses the need for parents to grieve and learn to manage their feelings. Only then can they address what he terms "the healthy components of the child's personality" [16, p. 59].

If parents relate to children and adolescents on the basis of their pathology, they tend to lose sight of the potential for children and teens to cope with their illness and potentially to enjoy life [16]. Parents' negative reactions may also have a profound impact on siblings and impede the ability of the family to function effectively [8, 9, 31].

Children and adolescents who are suffering cope best when nuclear families are involved in activities together, supported by extended family and friends, free of other emotional or social burdens, and led by parents who have a positive history of managing difficult life experiences. At the same time, parents manage best when they adopt specific techniques such as writing down questions for discussion with medical personnel, living one day at a time, and taking a positive approach to life that is characteristic of the martial art, Aikido. Bull suggests that the Aikido philosophy involves living with the illness and treatment, respecting a life-threatening disease as the enemy, and flowing with whatever transpires while maintaining one's own integrity and self-esteem without panicking and being swept away [32].

Sometimes children demonstrate this philosophy in their own special way. Susie was six years old when she developed leukemia and lost her hair due to the treatment of her disease. Her mother and grandmother were very concerned that Susie would feel self-conscious if she returned to school totally bald, so they bought her a wig. After her first day back at school, Susie came running home laughing and carrying her wig. In her mother's words, "She bounced in as bald as a billiard ball and told us she did not need the wig. She said that nobody laughed at her and she would never wear it again" [9]. Susie's spontaneity and freedom from adult anxieties truly reflects the spirit of Aikido. Susie was not about to be compromised by the thoughts and actions of others or by the consequences of her illness. She confronted life at school, and emerged with her self-esteem and integrity intact.

In the following section, children and teens demonstrate their resilience in managing the stress created by their illness.

How Children and Adolescents Help Themselves

Although the poetry and prose of these children and adolescents with cancer may seem to be filled with frustration and despair, it is important to recognize that they cannot be stereotyped. Many are creative, resourceful, determined to control and, if possible, to overcome their suffering. In another stanza of her poem, Jeanie poignantly tells us how much she values life:

> Since we have been cursed with this deadly being,
> life is more of a wish come true for us.
> Now we look forward to our future and our dreams,
> and most of all, the pleasures of life [30, p. 1].

Landi, too, now looks on the bright side although she continues to suffer emotionally, and she tells us:

> However, I do not view this (the illness experience) as a negative thing. I have learned to look out for myself, but at the same time be aware of other people and their feelings. I have been forced to develop my own theories on death and dying. And, when I want something badly enough, I don't let anything stand in my way of

getting it. I have fought the battle for my life—and won. After that kind of victory, nothing will hold me back [26, p. 11].

Many other examples can be cited including the words of Sloane who, despite her visual problems and communication difficulties, continues her story by telling us:

It is important for me to be open with you about myself as it helps me to take a big step toward accepting my life as it is to-day. I am handicapped and have certain limitations but I still want to laugh and be accepted by people around me [28, p. 8].

Michael, a teen who had one leg amputated due to bone cancer, points out how his illness helped him learn to confront death. He says, "My own encounter with death has permitted me to be more open about death because I was forced to face it and then grew to understand it" [33, p. 5].

It is often through their writing, poetry, and participation in camps or group programs that children and teens help each other. Richard, age nineteen, is a long-term survivor of a pelvic tumor. The suggestions he offers other young people with cancer include:

• Never give up on the belief that you WILL get better.
• Believe in what the doctors tell you, but also believe in YOUR ability to heal yourself.
• Never let others run your sickness.
• Take an active role in your recovery.
• . . . never despair. That is the worst thing you could do for yourself and your recovery. It tells your body that you are giving up . . .
• Don't feel sorry for yourself and start with the "Why Me?" questions. It doesn't matter why it happened to you. It happened, by accident, and there is NOTHING you can do to change it.
• I could feel sorry for myself, but I don't. Why? Because there are always people in the world who are worse off [34, p. 14].

He closes his article by telling his readers that there is:

. . . the hope that lies at the end of it all. This experience, the strength that you gain from having beaten one of the worst diseases known to us, can help you change your life, realize how precious each day is, and live life to the fullest [34, p. 14].

As Richard points out, if they remain preoccupied with their suffering, children and teens may lose sight of their potential to cope with or recover from their suffering. However, it is imperative to recognize that in order to cope or recover, children and adolescents must be allowed to grieve for their losses, experience their difficult feelings, and to the greatest extent possible, have their physical pain controlled.

When physical pain is managed effectively, their illness is in long-term remission, and they are without severe mental or physical handicaps, children and teens are likely to recover from childhood cancer and other life-threatening illness with little or no impairment.

As professionals, in our interactions with young people, it is important to examine what is most helpful to them. In the following section, I have used the categories of challenges cited earlier to note ways that we can be effective as caregivers.

HOW PROFESSIONALS CAN HELP CHILDREN AND ADOLESCENTS COPE WITH SUFFERING

Professionals are most effective when they tailor their assistance to the challenges that children and adolescents face intellectually, physically, emotionally, practically, and existentially [17, 18].

Intellectual Challenges

Professionals can be most helpful when they provide child and adolescents with:

1. concise, timely, age-appropriate information about their illness and treatment that is in keeping with the information given to their parents. Information should be conveyed in an honest, straight-forward but sensitive manner,
2. time to converse with staff so that their questions are answered and concerns discussed,
3. preparation for what lies ahead in respect to medical, nursing, and rehabilitative care,
4. assistance in making their needs and concerns known to parents and the health care team. Professionals may be a bridge for communication that promotes empathy, understanding, and cooperation.

Practical or Instrumental Challenges

Life in hospitals and rehabilitation centers includes practical challenges that are especially aggravating and frustrating for pediatric patients who are in distress. They are helped most when professionals:

1. advise them about what is negotiable in respect to rules, regulations, and requirements for compliance by the hospital and health care team. If rules are flexible and reasonable, children and teens are often very willing to comply,
2. offer choices that help them to gain control of their lives. These may include selecting the time of day for bathing, going to the playroom, having time alone, or choosing injection sites, diversionary activities, and foods to eat,
3. advocate on their behalf to counteract the rigidity of rules and restrictive practices that add to their feelings of isolation and detachment, and
4. help them to make their own decisions about how to reduce suffering. They may decide that specific measures of control are most helpful and should be administered in a certain manner. Professionals often provide them with tools and training to take action on their own behalf.

Physical Challenges

Professionals provide the greatest assistance to child and adolescent patients who are suffering from physical pain, loss of a body part, and disability when they:

1. accurately assess the nature, extent, and influence of physical symptoms on their suffering,
2. engage them in a dialogue about what they see, think, and feel in relation to their physical pain,
3. involve parents in observing, describing, and monitoring their children's reactions to noxious physical stimuli,
4. prepare patients for invasive medical procedures, anxiety provoking tests, painful treatments, and stressful rehabilitative routines,
5. maintain effective continuous pain control through the use of analgesics and other pharmacologic measures,
6. encourage parents to provide gentle back rubs, warm baths, ice packs, massages, and other comforting measures, and
7. offer patients choices regarding the timing and method of managing necessary body movements in order to minimize their pain and suffering.

Emotional Challenges

Professionals must help children and adolescents deal with the intensity of their emotional distress by providing:

1. a caring environment that meets the patient's needs for security by consistently relating to regular caregivers,
2. order, routine, and preparation so that upsetting surprises are avoided;
3. time for diversion and respite from treatment, rehabilitative, and physical maintenance programs,
4. periods when they can converse freely and informally about their feelings,
5. opportunities for them to achieve small successes in controlling or eliminating noxious stimuli using their own initiative. These successes may also help to enhance their self-image and to regain control of their feelings,
6. a goal-orientated approach that helps them face reality and use their strengths to overcome obstacles that prevent them from participating in regular activities,
7. assistance to defuse emotionally charged crises precipitated by factors such as physical changes, new treatments, relocation, distressing information, or parental anxiety,
8. opportunities for therapeutic play and self-expression through writing, art, and music,
9. training in the use of psychological techniques that help them to express and manage their feelings. These techniques may involve their parents as coaches [6, 35]. They include: 1) visual imagery; 2) relaxation and diversion; 3) biofeedback; 4) hypnosis; and 5) operant reinforcement,
10. an approach that at all times is empathic, non-judgemental, and positive. Professionals must believe in the abilities of their pediatric patients and help them to believe in themselves and maintain hope.

Social and Interpersonal Challenges

Professionals must be aware of children's needs to interact with others and remain involved in activities in the family, on the ward, and at the rehabilitation center. Professionals can help suffering children and adolescents most by providing:

1. opportunities for them to have siblings and friends visit, or have siblings join them in their activities,

2. access to play and group programs in keeping with their wishes, level of energy, and ability to tolerate interaction with other children,
3. support and encouragement for them to return to school or other social activities, even if their attendance is brief and their participation is limited,
4. assistance to parents to determine which athletic or other physical activities are suitable so that children and teens can participate to their maximum capacity without inflicting permanent damage or intolerable pain,
5. family focused intervention to use their family's strengths to cope with lifestyle changes or deal with dysfunctional behavior patterns such as enmeshment, rigidity, overprotectiveness, and inability to resolve interpersonal conflicts that may amplify their suffering [8, 36],
6. access to social support from other children facing similar difficulties e.g., through attendance at support group meetings, camps, conferences, and other gatherings.

Existential Challenges

Children and adolescents whose lives are threatened often struggle with existential questions about themselves, their families, illness, and their future. They may receive information and guidance from their families or if communication is lacking, closed, or poorly developed, may be left to arrive at their own conclusions. Unless they are able to reason like adults, their conclusions may be flawed and distorted by fantasy. Existential concerns associated with religion and spirituality require exploration and dialogue so that children can reach a level of understanding that matches their cognitive ability. Professionals help children and teens most when:

1. they talk with them about existential concerns,
2. they are willing to listen to what they think, feel, and believe,
3. they help them to reach realistic, age-appropriate conclusions on their own or with the help of their parents,
4. they are honest when they are unable to answer their questions,
5. they are prepared to consult with others who are knowledgeable regarding cultural, religious and spiritual matters, or engage them in assisting children and adolescents directly.

In closing, in each situation that I have encountered with children and adolescents who are suffering from physical or emotional pain, I have been touched by their tremendous desire to use their own strengths and the strengths of their parents, family members, peers, and other adults in order to cope with whatever transpires. Their warmth, sensitivity, energy, and resilience often help them temper Copp's "state of anguish," Cassell's "threat of disintegration," Battenfield's "turmoil," and Maes' picture of terror, horror, anxiety, dread, and confusion that all characterize suffering [2-4, 10]. As professionals, we must remember that they are also extremely perceptive and often see right through adults. For example, in her poem about her parents, Diane, age ten, a child with leukemia, shows her perceptiveness:

> WHAT I KNOW
> It seems as though I can see
> Right through you.
> When something's wrong,
> I see fear.
> When something goes wrong,
> I see anger.
> When you are scared,
> I see courage.
> When something goes right,
> I see pride in you.
> But throughout it all,
> I see you love me,
> And I love you [37, p. 7].

When we are working with young people like Diane, we are acutely aware of their need to have us work with the parents who love and care for them, to include them in learning to manage whatever they must face, and to understand how difficult it is for them to be confined or afflicted by an illness that stops them from being the same as their peers. We must recognize that they are individuals with capabilities that increase with each stage of development and each new experience that they encounter.

At the same time, we must never underestimate the healing power that parents impart to their children when they help them to deal with their suffering. It is when parents are able to cope with their children's life-threatening illness in the spirit of Aikido that children at any age manage best. By keeping the family together, being open and honest, and assisting children to the best of their ability, parents offer a valuable antidote to suffering.

From this beginning, I challenge you in your professional work to learn more about the conditions which make children and adolescents suffer, obtain a greater understanding of the noxious stimuli involved, and participate in helping them to work with their families to overcome whatever afflictions they face.

In closing, the hopeful message of Helen Keller reminds us of the rewards in taking a positive approach in our work.

Although the world is full of suffering, it is full also of the overcoming of it [38, p. 1].

REFERENCES

1. R. Beaumont, Eighteen More Months—Fingers Crossed, *The Candlelighters Childhood Cancer Foundation Youth Newsletter, X*:2, p. 10, 1988.
2. E. J. Cassell, The Nature of Suffering and the Goals of Medicine, *New England Journal of Medicine, 306*, pp. 639-645, 1982.
3. L. A. Copp, The Spectrum of Suffering, *American Journal of Nursing, 74*, pp. 491-494, 1974.
4. J. L. Maes, *Suffering: A Caregiver's Guide*, Abingdon Press, Nashville, Tennessee, 1990.
5. B. Justice, Suffering in Silence and the Fear of Social Stigma: Survivors of Violence, in *The Hidden Dimensions of Illness*, P. L. Starck and J. P. McGovern (eds.), National League for Nursing Press, New York, 1992.
6. P. A. McGrath, *Pain in Children: Nature, Assessment and Treatment*, Guilford Press, New York, 1990.
7. J. Van Eys, Therapeutic Interventions for Suffering: Professional and Institutional Perspectives, in *The Hidden Dimensions of Illness*, P. L. Starck and J. P. McGovern (eds.), National League for Nursing Press, New York, 1992.
8. D. W. Adams, *Childhood Malignancy: The Psychosocial Care of the Child and His Family*, Charles C. Thomas Publisher, Springfield, Illinois, 1979.
9. D. W. Adams and E. J. Deveau, *Coping with Childhood Cancer: Where Do We Go from Here?*, (New Revised Edition), Kinbridge Publications, Hamilton, Canada, 1993.
10. B. L. Battenfield, Suffering—A Conceptual Description and Content Analysis of Operational Schema, *Image: The Journal of Nursing Scholarship, XVI*, pp. 36-41, 1984.
11. A. K. Gordon, The Tattered Cloak of Immortality, in *Adolescence and Death*, C. A. Corr and J. N. McNeil (eds.), Springer Publishing Company, New York, 1986.
12. D. W. Adams, When a Child Dies of Cancer: Care of the Child and Family, in *The Dying and Bereaved Teenager*, J. D. Morgan (ed.), The Charles Press, Philadelphia, 1990.
13. J. J. Spinetta, D. Rigler, and M. Karon, Personal Space as a Measure of a Dying Child's Sense of Isolation, *Journal of Consulting and Clinical Psychology, 42*, pp. 751-756, 1974.
14. J. J. Spinetta, D. Rigler, and M. Karon, Anxiety in the Dying Child, *Pediatrics, 52*, pp. 841-845, 1973.

15. M. E. Duffy, A Theoretical and Empirical Review of the Concept of Suffering, in *The Hidden Dimension of Illness*, P. L. Starck and J. P. McGovern (eds.), National League for Nursing Press, New York, 1992.
16. H. P. Coppolillo, Disintegration Aspects of Childhood Illness, in *The Mind of the Child Who is Said to be Sick*, D. R. Copeland, B. Pfefferbaum, and A. J. Stovall (eds.), Charles C. Thomas Publisher, Springfield, Illinois, 1983.
17. D. W. Adams, *The Moment When Everything Changes: The Diagnosis of Life-Threatening Illness in Childhood*, Lecture, University of Quebec, Montreal, Canada, 1994.
18. M. A. Chesler and O. A. Barbarin, *Childhood Cancer and the Family*, Brunner/Mazel, New York, 1987.
19. P. J. McGrath, E. Hsu, M. Cappelli, B. Luke, J. T. Goodman, and J. Dunn-Geier, Pain from Pediatric Cancer: A Survey of an Outpatient Clinic, *Journal of Psychosocial Oncology, 8*:2/3, pp. 109-124, 1990.
20. F. F. Worchel, Adjusting to Childhood Cancer: A Model for Psychosocial Care, in *Teaching More Than Medicine*, J. Van Eys, D. R. Copeland, and E. R. Davidson (eds.), The University of Texas, M. D. Anderson Cancer Center, Houston, 1992.
21. T. Moran, My Brother Has Cancer, *The Candlelighters Childhood Cancer Foundation Youth Newsletter, XI*:1, p. 6, Winter 1989.
22. E. J. Deveau and D. W. Adams, We Can Help Ourselves: Family Relationships and Coping Skills, in *We Can Help Ourselves: Proceedings of the 1989 Childhood Cancer Conference*, University of Alberta, Edmonton, Canada, 1990.
23. W. Bunderson, How Much I Hate Coming to the Clinic, *The Candlelighters Childhood Cancer Foundation Youth Newsletter, X*:1, p. 10, Spring 1988.
24. R. Dalal, Cancer, *The Candlelighters Childhood Cancer Foundation Youth Newsletter, X*:2, p. 9, Summer 1988.
25. D. Buardo, I Often Feel Helpless, *The Candlelighters Childhood Cancer Foundation Youth Newsletter, XI*:1, p. 1, Winter 1989.
26. L. Lowell, I'm Going to Keep Walking the Same Path, *The Candlelighters Childhood Cancer Foundation Youth Newsletter, XI*:1, p. 11, Winter 1989.
27. P. Holmes, My Life, *The Candlelighters Childhood Cancer Foundation Youth Newsletter, X*:2, pp. 6-7, Summer 1988.
28. S. Caglia, Hi! Fellow Classmates, *The Candlelighters Childhood Cancer Foundation Youth Newsletter, X*:2. p. 8, Summer 1988.
29. D. Fowler, Now I See, *The Candlelighters Childhood Cancer Foundation Youth Newsletter, X*:2, p. 11, Summer 1988.
30. J. Lee, Life—A Word With So Much Meaning, *The Candlelighters Childhood Cancer Foundation Youth Newsletter, X*:2, p. 1, Summer 1988.
31. D. W. Adams and E. J. Deveau, When a Brother or Sister is Dying of Cancer: The Vulnerability of the Adolescent Sibling, *Death Studies, XI*, pp. 279-295, 1987.

32. M. Bull, Lifetime Losses, in *We Can Help Ourselves: Proceedings of the 1989 Childhood Cancer Conference*, University of Alberta, Edmonton, Canada, 1989.
33. M. Motyka, Personal Statement About Death, *The Candlelighters Childhood Cancer Foundation Youth Newsletter, X*:1, p. 14, Spring 1988.
34. R. Emond, My Story, *The Candlelighters Childhood Cancer Foundation Youth Newsletter, XI*:1, p. 14, Winter 1989.
35. L. Kuttner, Management of Young Children's Acute Pain and Anxiety During Invasive Medical Procedures, *Pediatrician, 16*, pp. 39-44, 1989.
36. S. Minuchin, L. Baker, B. L. Rosman, R. Liebman, L. Milman, and T. Todd, A Conceptual Model of Psychosomatic Illness in Children: Family Organization and Family Therapy, *Archives of General Psychiatry, 32*, pp. 1031-1038, 1975.
37. D. Wise, What I Know, *The Candlelighters Childhood Cancer Foundation Youth Newsletter, XI*:1, p. 7, Winter 1989.
38. H. Keller, Optimism, in *The International Thesaurus of Quotations*, R. T. Tripp (ed.), Harper and Row, New York, p. 620, 1970.

BIBLIOGRAPHY

Adams, D. W., Helping the Dying Child: Practical Approaches for Non-Physicians, *Childhood and Death*, H. Wass and C. A. Corr (eds.), Hemisphere Publishing, Washington, 1984.

Altman, A. J., N. L. Schechter, and S. J. Weisman, The Management of Pain, *Supportive Care of the Child with Cancer*, A. R. Ablin (ed.), The Johns Hopkins University Press, Baltimore, 1993.

Callaghan, D., *The Troubled Dream of Life: Living with Mortality*, Simon and Schuster, New York, 1993.

Drotar, D., Psychological Perspectives in Chronic Childhood Illness, *Journal of Pediatric Psychology, 6*, pp. 21-28, 1981.

Frugé, E., and C. Adams, Chronic Illness and Family Systems, *Teaching More Than Medicine: Psychosocial Considerations in Pediatric Oncology*, J. Van Eys, D. R. Copeland, and E. R. Davidson (eds.), The University of Texas, M. D. Anderson Cancer Center, Houston, 1992.

McGrath, P. J., J. Dunn-Geier, S. J. Cunningham et al, Psychological Guidelines for Helping Children Cope with Chronic Benign Intractable Pain, *Clinical Journal of Pain, 1*, pp. 229-233, 1986.

VOLUME 2–PART B

Helping Dying Children and Adolescents

CHAPTER 10

Palliative Care for Children Dying of Cancer: Psychosocial Issues

Michael M. Stevens

INTRODUCTION

This chapter describes issues encountered during management of children dying of cancer. Guidelines are provided to assist caregivers with the psychosocial management of such children and their families.

The initial treatment goals for a child with cancer are almost always curative in intent. Considerable advances in surgery, radiotherapy, and particularly chemotherapy have occurred over the last forty years. The advent of multi-institutional randomized trials of therapy for pediatric cancer in the United States, the United Kingdom, and elsewhere has led to encouraging improvements in the cure rate for many types of childhood cancer. Overall, approximately 70 percent of today's young patients with malignant disease will be cured. The remainder will ultimately die of their disease and need palliative care.

At diagnosis, the child should be referred to a pediatric institution offering skilled multimodal cancer therapy. Occasionally, children may be very ill at the time of diagnosis and almost immediately may enter the terminal phase. However, for most children the emphasis of initial therapy will be strongly directed toward cure.

When a child develops cancer, there are various phases in the illness. The first begins at diagnosis and extends through treatment. This phase ends either with completion of therapy and follow-up of the presumably cured survivor, or with the passage through one or more relapses. If relapse occurs, therapy may be intensified with cure still the goal. If the disease progresses despite further therapy, a decision will become necessary to cease curative treatment and alter the emphasis of therapy to palliation. The family then experiences a passage into palliative care which extends on to the child's death and beyond.

FOUNDATIONS FOR EFFECTIVE PALLIATIVE CARE IN EARLIER MANAGEMENT

Each family will have distinct patterns of communication, behavior, roles, rules, and expectations. The experiences that each family encounters and the challenges generated also vary considerably.

The family's successful transition to palliative care is strongly affected by its experiences earlier in the child's management. Attention to earlier aspects of the family's management does much to help the family cope with the child's palliative care and death. The quality of the family's experience in the earliest phase of the child's illness, during the first few weeks after diagnosis, is particularly important in determining later adjustment to palliative care, should that become necessary.

Communicating with the Child's Parents at Diagnosis

Communication with parents of children with cancer is challenging because of the anxiety and stress that they experience. Successful communication at diagnosis strongly influences the family's attitude and coping throughout treatment and beyond [1].

In interviews with twenty families of children who died of leukemia, many parents described the events at diagnosis as the hardest they had to bear throughout the course of their child's illness. All families expressed appreciation of the frankness and honesty of initial discussions with the treatment team, and eight specifically identified them as one of the major sources of help [2].

Disagreements and misunderstandings due to poor communication between children with leukemia, their parents, and physicians may lead to unusual or maladaptive coping by parents or families [3].

If information, friendly encouragement, practical support, and hope have been made freely available by the treatment team from the time of diagnosis, parents will be more likely to cope successfully with later crises or palliative care. Parents feel most secure when one senior medical member of the caregiving team assumes responsibility for their child's treatment and for communication with the family.

Pointers to Good Communication

- Ensure that both parents are present for the initial consultation. This recognizes the importance of both parents and makes it less likely that one partner will misinterpret information.
- Interview parents in a quiet, comfortable room, with everyone seated.
- During important discussions, allow the parents to include a close friend or relative, who may recall information that parents forget.
- Have another member of the caregiving team, e.g., the nurse, present to help identify areas for discussion.
- Give parents a clear description of their child's illness; identify the illness as cancer; use plain English.
- Emphasize that the parents did not cause the disease and could not have prevented it; that the disease is not hereditary (if that is so); that the diagnosis has been made without undue delay; and that effective therapy is available that has cured other children.
- Provide enough time so that parents can ask questions and not feel rushed. Encourage them to write down any points of concern as they occur for discussion at the next consultation. Seek feedback about what parents have understood from each consultation.
- On receiving the diagnosis, parents always assume that their child is going to die, and soon. Aim to readjust their expectations to a hopeful level, in keeping with the child's actual outlook.
- A written summary or tape-recording of the discussion may be helpful.
- With parental approval, involve the child in some of the early discussions to lessen his or her anxiety.
- Parents will be shocked initially and even disbelieving, then angry, guilty and depressed. This limits their ability to absorb and retain information. Repeat information patiently over several consultations. In the beginning, do not provide detailed technical information that the family may misunderstand or forget.
- At an early stage, spend time with the patient's siblings and grandparents and liaise with the child's school to help allay anxiety and reduce family members' stress.
- Have the family meet a child with a similar diagnosis who has done well.

Longer Term Pointers

As the child's therapy progresses and the parents meet more caregivers and other families who corroborate what the family has been told, parents develop trust in the treatment team and willingly cooperate.

- Be easy to contact by parents.
- A patient-held medical record [4] provides the family with readily accessible information about their child's progress.
- Regular seminars, support meetings, and newsletters for parents of surviving and deceased patients improve parents' knowledge and help them feel supported.
- Have parents attending the treatment center elect a liaison committee to assist in optimal patient management. The liaison committee is a group of elected members of the parent body who act as conductors of information between the oncology staff and the patients' families. This is achieved through a quarterly magazine, an annual parent seminar day, casual wine and cheese nights in different parts of the city, and meetings with the oncology staff during which the committee can act as parent advocates.
- Always allow parents hope, no matter how poor the outlook. Support the family in their current hope and help them maintain a realistic focus on what their child can still do.

Who are the Families at Risk?

Families will be encountered that experience significant difficulties, for one reason or another, during their child's illness. For example, families at risk include those already coping with physically or intellectually handicapped children, single-parent families, families where parents are separating at the time of the child's diagnosis, and families struggling because of financial difficulties, unemployment, or cultural or language difficulties.

Such families require extra help at diagnosis and during therapy to lessen the likelihood of additional crises, other than those unavoidably linked to their child's diagnosis and treatment. If excessive criticism of health professionals has already been encountered earlier in the child's management this indicates poor adjustment and the need for additional support. The family that places unreasonable demands on the treatment team needs to be recognized, since compliance with all the family's requests may lead to conflict later. Some early agreement about level of service should be tactfully negotiated with such families in order to avoid problems.

THE TRANSITION TO PALLIATIVE CARE

The recognition that a child's leukemia or cancer is entering a terminal phase after one or more unsuccessfully treated relapses heralds the onset of renewed stress for all concerned. Prior to this, the child will have been receiving chemotherapy and supportive treatment in a planned and methodical attempt at cure. During this time the child's cancer will have been under control and the child will have been reasonably or completely well. The family's shock, grief, and depression present at the time of diagnosis will have eased, although anxiety about the implications of relapse is constantly present in both parents and patients, even in those very long-term survivors already declared cured. Relapse and the eventual advent of palliative care plunges the family into renewed crisis.

All the reactions present at the original diagnosis resurface with heightened intensity, now overshadowed by the loss of hope implicit in relapse. The parents experience feelings of hopelessness and helplessness, coupled with grief, fear, depression, anger, and denial. Parents who constantly dread relapse and terminal care may express some sentiments of relief that the worst has occurred at last.

There is no easy way to convey bad news. All aids to communication employed at diagnosis and discussed previously become more important now. Matters are made even more difficult when the family involved has been referred during remission by another treatment team, for example, following a family's move from overseas or another state. Such families will not have built up the trust in the new treatment team that can only develop effectively at diagnosis.

The pediatrician in charge of the child's cancer therapy should accept the responsibility for these painful discussions. One must be honest, frank, gentle, and sympathetic. This requires a certain degree of empathy and therefore, pain for the caregiving team.

Options for Continuing Management

There are several paths that may be followed for the child who is fatally ill at diagnosis or who has failed curative therapy and is entering a terminal phase [5].

One option is to give no medical or nursing treatment at all, other than to enhance the physical, personal, and social comfort of the dying child. Comfort measures, such as a manageable diet, pain control, and prevention or treatment of skin breakdown, are the only form of medical or nursing care provided. This plan may be difficult for the caregiving team to accept because it implies that the caregivers, as well as their treatments, have failed. Unfortunately in some instances, the transition to appropriate palliative care may be very delayed, or not occur at all, because of a treatment team's bias to persist with aggressive therapy well past the point where such therapy is appropriate for the child in question.

A second plan is for palliative care which places the highest priority on the control of pain in its broadest sense. Certain medications, chemotherapy protocols, irradiation, and even surgery may eventually result in a higher quality of remaining life for the child, even though extension of life is not the goal of palliative care. The treatment team must consider carefully the enhanced quality of life following such palliative procedures when measured against their inherent discomfort. Recovery time must not consume long periods of the child's remaining life.

The third and most controversial plan is to administer investigational treatments which offer only a slight chance of cure and very frequently cause a significant increase in the pain and morbidity suffered by the child. This option is the only one that offers any chance at all of cure.

Keeping the Child's Best Interests Foremost

In explaining the implications of the terminal nature of the child's illness, the pediatrician already will have made a judgement that further therapy directed against the underlying cancer is not appropriate. This places a responsibility on the doctor to be fully informed of all recent advances in treatment, particularly those involving investigational agents or techniques of unproven activity against the disease involved. A decision by the child's pediatrician to change to palliative care should only be taken after full discussion of possible treatment options with the other team members. Occasional conflict will arise within the team over whether to proceed with investigational therapy or change to palliative care. While the need for trials of investigational therapy is not disputed, foremost consideration must be given to the anticipated benefits and disadvantages of the proposed therapy for the particular child. The need for a sensible advocate for the child within the treatment team is vital.

Surprisingly, most families make the transition from curative to palliative therapy smoothly and effectively, even though it is an extremely demanding time for them. The time taken in earlier phases of a child's management to establish a trusting relationship between the child and family and the staff will be invaluable in helping them through this crisis. The caregiving team can help the family make this transition more successfully by providing the necessary information and support to assist in the family's decisions. Most families are able to retain sufficient equilibrium to deal with the situation effectively. Information is most commonly relayed from the treatment team to the parents, who then convey it to the other members of the family. Maintenance of confidentiality at this stage is even more important than at diagnosis in order to allow the family to retain some control over how widely information is disseminated.

Working Through the Transition

Parents need a careful and sympathetic explanation of the situation, including available options for further therapy, so that they can participate in the decisions being made. It is necessary that parents, and ultimately the patient and family, adjust to a shift in emphasis from cure to relief of symptoms. In acknowledging that the underlying disease will not be successfully eradicated, the goal of further treatment becomes that of ensuring optimal comfort and quality for each remaining day of the child's life.

The parents must be reassured that treatment failure is not their fault, as there will be considerable guilt about previous minor and insignificant non-compliance with medication schedules. An estimate of how long the child is expected to live will be sought and should be provided. This may be only a matter of days when there is rapidly progressing infection or metabolic disturbance, or several months in a well child with a slowly growing tumor. A summary of the plan for the child's management during the terminal phase should be presented to the family and subsequently discussed with them by members of the treatment team, all of whom play a role in the child's palliative care. Such a plan requires personal knowledge of the individual child.

It is best to inform the parents first and give them time to adjust to the new situation before consulting directly with the child. The patient's siblings, grandparents, other relatives, and friends are also involved in the crisis. A brother or sister of the patient, who has acted as a donor for a bone marrow transplant, will face special difficulties, as will single parents and families hampered by cultural or language barriers. Allowance must be made for a wide range of reactions from families of different cultural backgrounds. Such reactions should not be allowed to prejudice the caregiving team's treatment of the child.

Refusal to Accept the Transition

Occasionally, a family will refuse to accept the transition to pallia-tive care. Such families will continue to insist that "everything possible be done" and may seek alternative sources of therapy which may be of unproven benefit or even potentially harmful. The best approach is to continue discussing the issues objectively and patiently, emphasizing what is best for the child. Parents in such families may need to confront and acknowledge fears and other negative emotions relating to the potential loss of their child that may have been denied at diagnosis or in earlier phases of treatment.

HOME CARE VERSUS HOSPITAL CARE: MAKING THE DECISION

As the child's palliative care commences, liaison must occur both within the treatment team and between it and the available support in the community. All members of the treatment team should be informed of the child's continuing condition and the plans for palliative care. Community resources must be mobilized to ensure that much of the child's care can be based at home. This is particularly important for families in isolated areas, where considerable distances exist between the family's home and local caregiving agencies and the palliative treatment team's hospital. As the program of care commences, the parents will require further education about the ill child, particularly in practical matters such as maintenance of central lines and the nursing and biomedical equipment used in symptom control.

As the emphasis of treatment shifts from cure to palliation and making the best of what time remains, care of the child at home becomes a priority for the family. Returning a terminally ill child to the home keeps all family members together, allows everyone to share in the child's care, and provides mutual support. The home care program needs to be flexible to meet the needs of individual families. Parents will need reassurance to help them cope with the fears of having their child at home. Careful preparation and planning as well as securing lines of communication usually help allay these fears. The parents and older brothers and sisters will become primary caregivers in the home and will need much support and encouragement from the treat-ment team.

The Value of Respite Care

With the change in emphasis from complex therapy to supportive care, the family physician may become more closely involved in management and provide much of the emotional support needed. Where possible, regular home visits by members of the treatment team (e.g., the community nurse consultant, the social worker, and the child's oncologist) will help to ensure that care is optimal. Regular telephone contact to discuss day-to-day difficulties also assists the parents in coping. Even with the best planning, care of the child at home may become too difficult because of parental exhaustion, stress, or development of symptoms requiring hospital admission (e.g., bleeding or refractory seizures). The child may express a desire to return to the security of the hospital and the closer support of the medical team. Under these circumstances, a return to the treatment team's in-patient facility for respite care is preferable. A few days may be all that is required to allow the parents to rest. Longer periods of respite may be necessary according to the wishes of the child and family.

From a family's perspective, it is not easy to care for a terminally ill child. The strain and loneliness can be great. The advent of free-standing children's hospices, initially in the United Kingdom and more recently in Canada and Australia, provide a welcome alternative to hospitals for respite care for children and their families. A home-like atmosphere can be maintained more successfully in a hospice than in a hospital, while the burden of responsibility for the child's care can be temporarily transferred to hospice staff.

Benefits and Disadvantages of Home Care

Care in the home offers the family the advantage of being together in a secure, familiar, and comfortable environment. There is less disruption to family life. Nursing the child at home is perceived by parents as a positive experience. Siblings can participate in the child's care and their needs can be met more easily. The child's food preferences can be catered to more readily. There is greater privacy and freedom from the hospital environment which holds unpleasant associations for the child. There is ready access to parents, brothers and sisters, friends, possessions, and pets. Visitation by family and friends can be more flexible as well as regulated by parents depending on their child's condition. The parents will feel more in control since all the family can participate in the child's care. More time can be spent with the child. By witnessing the child's gradual deterioration they may be able to face the approaching death more realistically. Family members are more likely to be present at the time of death and to grieve afterwards in an unhurried manner.

From the parents' perspective, the commonest difficulties of home care are: watching the child's physical decline, coping with nights, handling fears of what will happen at the time of death, dealing with medical complications such as haemorrhage and seizures, and coping with domestic difficulties, including care of siblings.

Care in the hospital offers a greater degree of security for management of potentially frightening complications such as hemorrhage or seizures. However, the hospital may not be able to provide the same degree of privacy and informality that is available in the home.

A recent study of families attending the Women and Children's Hospital in Adelaide, South Australia, found that nearly half of a group of children with cancer were using one or more alternative therapies. Less than half of the parents of children who were using alternative therapies had informed their children's doctors that the children were receiving them [6].

Providers of alternate therapy, at the family's request, may be actually involved in the child's management. Their influence on the family may be substantially greater after the child's care is transferred from hospital to home. Sadly, this may not always be in the child's best interests. One of the author's patients was dying at home from an illness which had started twelve months ago. A person who had been providing dietary and other therapy for the child and family for some time became more controlling of the family's routines and the child's diet after home care began. The child's bed was aligned to the earth's magnetic field. All who visited the home were required to wear cotton rather than nylon underwear. Visitors were also instructed to discharge any accumulated static electricity prior to entering the home by stamping their feet in the garden beds. Three days before he died, the boy lamented to his nurse that he was not permitted to eat his favorite breakfast cereal, a well-known brand of chocolate-coated puffed rice, because it infringed his "diet." Fortunately, the nurse reported this to the hospital-based treatment team, and for the short time remaining, the boy was given free access to his favorite cereal.

Evaluation of Hospital-based Care

An inquiry into the management of dying children and their families was recently conducted by the patient care review committee of a large Australian pediatric teaching hospital [7]. Parents whose children had died in hospital and clinical staff were able to offer the committee many valuable and practical suggestions. These included the following:

- provision of better facilities including quiet rooms for communication, private grieving, rest, reflection and privacy,

- provision of more sensitive arrangements for body viewing and transport to the mortuary,
- provision of a more sensitive approach to requests for autopsy and assistance with funeral arrangements,
- provision of a more accessible chapel,
- relocation of telephones to ensure privacy,
- provision of better accommodation facilities for parents, better facilities for brothers and sisters, hot food available out of working hours, improved car parking,
- provision of facilities appropriate to adolescent patients,
- provision of better in-service education for staff, and information for families,
- development of stronger links with palliative and hospice care teams, general practitioners, and community nurses.

Evaluation of Home-based Care

Those working in pediatric palliative care commonly advocate the advantages of home care over hospital care for dying children. However, to date, there is little published information about how parents themselves actually perceive the care and support that they receive in this situation. A recent Australian study provides information obtained from parents whose children died after receiving care at home [8]. Recommendations for improved care of such children based on the parents' suggestions are as follows:

- Families need to be able to opt for home-based, hospital-based, or hospice-based care for their child and receive adequate professional support to validate their choice. If circumstances change, the family needs to be able to change freely from one option to another. An integrated, coordinated program of palliative care is required that offers these options.
- Professional support needs to be available on a twenty-four hours a day, seven days a week basis, so that medical and nursing needs of children receiving palliative care at home can be met at all times.
- Parents providing care at home need to receive sufficient information about drug treatment and about what to expect. Adequate opportunities for communication with, and feed-back from, parents must be provided prospectively during home visits by members of the caregiving team.

- Parents often benefit from speaking to another parent who has had a similar experience. Opportunities for such contact should be offered.

- Parents require assistance with routine home duties to enable them to spend more time with their dying child. A coordinated volunteer service will fulfil this requirement.

- Relief for parents at night is required to ensure adequate sleep. The presence of a non-professional volunteer may suffice, but in some cases professional nursing skills will be required. Relief for parents by provision of respite care in hospital or hospice should also be available.

- Readmission to hospital, when necessary, should be expedited. Parents, if they desire, should be permitted to remain the primary caregivers while their child is in hospital.

- Local doctors and community nurses assisting families may need additional information about aspects of symptom control or nursing that are essential for successful management. This information can be provided via a case conference for all involved, by written instructions, and by ongoing contact between caregivers.

In the author's view, the current advocacy for home-based care is strong, particularly in North America. However, professional caregivers should remember that hospital-based care for a particular child and family may be a better option. Making a recommendation for hospital-based care does not necessarily indicate a lack of awareness of the potential advantages of home-based care. Unless the treatment team can be confident beforehand that services and staffing to support the child and family are sufficient to ensure adequate home-based care, it is inappropriate for that family to be entered into a home-based program of care when, for that case, hospital-based care would be better.

THE SICK CHILD'S PERCEPTION OF DEATH

Children suffering from a life-threatening illness acquire a concept of death in very different circumstances to children who are well. A review of the chapters in Volume 1 of this series, which focus on how a concept of death develops in well children, may be helpful before considering how terminally ill children come to think and feel about death.

Although the survival rates for a variety of chronic illnesses have dramatically improved over the last thirty years, many children still do not survive. Thus knowledge about their concepts of death is still pertinent. Anxiety about death is an issue for all chronically ill children, particularly those with leukemia or other malignancies whether or not they eventually survive. Most significantly, children who are dying will have acquired awareness and concepts far advanced of what one might assume from their age.

Prior to 1970, most caregivers believed that unless a child was over ten years of age, he or she was incapable of understanding death and therefore, did not experience anxiety about death. It was felt that children did not need information about their disease and that they would be incapable of coping with the distress and anxiety of knowing they were dying. A closed protective approach was advocated [9-12].

Key Studies Establishing the Sick Child's Awareness of Death

In the late 1960s and early 1970s, pioneering work by Vernick and Karon [13, 14], Waechter [15], and Bluebond-Langner [16] prompted a complete revision of this perspective. In 1971, the views of those advocating a closed protective approach were challenged bluntly for the first time by the late Eugenia Waechter, who reported on sixty-four children between the ages of six and ten that were divided into four groups of equal size: those with a fatal disorder, children with a chronic non-fatal disease, those with a brief illness, and well elementary school children who were not in hospital. A General Anxiety Scale for children, measuring concerns in many areas of living, was administered to each child. A set of eight pictures was also shown individually to each child and stories were requested in order to elicit fantasy expression of the child's concern regarding present and future body integrity and functioning.

Parents of children in the first three groups were interviewed to assess how the quality and quantity of their children's concerns about death were influenced by any previous experience with death, the religious devoutness within the family, the quality of maternal warmth toward them, and the opportunities they had had to discuss their concerns or the nature of their illness with their parents, professional personnel, or other meaningful adults.

Although only two of the sixteen fatally-ill children had been told their prognoses, the generalized anxiety was extremely high in all sixteen cases; almost double that of the two comparison groups of children in hospital, and three times that of healthy children. The children threatened with death discussed loneliness, separation, and death much more frequently in their fantasy stories. Waechter's most striking finding was the dichotomy between the children's degree of awareness of their prognosis, as inferred from their imaginative stories, and the parents' beliefs about their child's awareness. Only two of the sixteen fatally-ill children had discussed their concerns about death with their parents, yet 63 percent of stories told by these children related to death. The children often gave the characters in the stories their own diagnoses and symptoms; they frequently depicted death in their drawings and occasionally they would express awareness of their prognoses to persons outside their immediate families. Waechter concluded that denial and protectiveness by adults may not be entirely effective in preventing these children from experiencing anxiety or in keeping their diagnosis and probable prognosis from them. She recommended that the child's questions and concerns be dealt with in a way that did not further alienate and isolate the child from parents and other meaningful adults.

In the early 1970s, Myra Bluebond-Langner, an anthropologist, confirmed and extended Waechter's research by conducting long-term and detailed observations of leukemic children, their parents, and the various health professionals caring for them in the hematology/oncology clinic and ward of an American hospital. Her observations and conclusions, published in 1978 [16], have been pivotal, together with those of Waechter, in changing the establishment's views on how to work most effectively with dying children.

Although parents and staff provided little or no information to the children about any aspect of the illness in the hope of lessening their anxiety, it was found that over time such children acquired information about their disease in stages, and that particular experiences (diagnosis, remission, first relapse, later relapses, learning of the death of an ill peer) were critical to passage through these stages. As the children passed through these stages, their self-concept altered progressively from "I was previously well but am now seriously ill" to "I am always ill and will get better," and lastly to "I am dying." The children's personal experiences were a much more significant determinant than age or intellectual ability in determining concepts of their sickness. Thus, a three or four-year-old child might know more about their prognosis than a very intelligent nine-year-old.

An evaluation of anxiety and withdrawal in children, aged between six and ten years who were terminally ill with leukemia, was conducted in 1974. It found that these children appeared to be aware of the seriousness of their illness (even though they might yet not be capable of talking about this awareness in adult terms); expressed more anxiety than controls; and, of greater concern, perceived a growing psychological distance from those around them [17, 18].

A contemporary study of concepts of death, illness, and isolation in twenty-one children with leukemia, aged between four and nine years, was conducted in the United Kingdom [19]. Some of the perceptions of these sick children, about themselves in hospital, were worrisome. The children's feelings of being alone, even with ample company, suggested deprivation of another sort. There was a large variation in the concept of death between individual children, especially in those under eight years of age.

The implications of these revised views of sick children's awareness of death are discussed later in this chapter.

The Terminally Ill Child at School

Children with cancer, as a result of their illness, will have acquired concepts and experiences of pain, loss, and grief which will have changed them and distinguish them from their peers. Children who receive treatment for cancer encounter a loss of self-esteem. Their unusual situation requires them to deal with new and significant issues, occasionally with some anxiety, so that they may have less attention and energy for the day-to-day matters of school. They will be less assertive. They will be more reluctant than their healthy peers to attempt new concepts in which failure is possible because of the risk of losing more self-esteem through failure. Schooling for these children should always start out from areas and levels of competence in which they feel absolutely comfortable [20].

Children who are terminally ill from cancer may be continuing with further treatment, and in many cases will remain well enough to attend school for many months. Even though they may be in an advanced stage of their disease, it is very important for children's self-esteem and sense of mastery over a deteriorating situation to continue to attend school when they wish to, if only for a few hours a day.

An explanation to the class about the child's illness will have been given by a member of the treatment team earlier in the course of the illness, usually soon after diagnosis. At the outset, classmates are most frequently concerned about whether or not they can catch the disease from the patient.

In the event of the child becoming terminally ill, the child's teacher will have to confront and deal with the impending death of the child and the resulting effects on the classmates, other teachers, and students at the school. Under these circumstances, it is wise to have made some preparation beforehand. Discussion at a staff meeting might take place involving other teachers and the principal to examine their attitudes to death and dying. This would enable staff to formulate an appropriate plan which the teacher could then implement with the class. The teacher should also confer with the child's parents, who need to be involved in these plans.

The child's treatment team, particularly the hospital school teacher, will liaise with the school and the child's school teachers to maximize the child's educational opportunities. Terminally ill children may wish to be included and need to be treated as normally as possible. A bean chair or similar comfortable support in the corner of the classroom close to the focus of interest may provide many hours of satisfaction to such children, even though they may not be able to participate actively in all lessons.

Deterioration is usually gradual and death is not expected to occur suddenly or unexpectedly, for example, during class. If the terminally ill student deteriorated rapidly or unexpectedly collapsed, there still would be sufficient time to take the child home or to the hospital with the parents and family.

Saying Goodbye: How Does the Child Prepare for His or Her Death?

Children who are terminally ill will commonly take steps to put their affairs in order. During her preparation for a mismatched bone marrow transplant, one of the author's patients completed tapestries bearing personal notes of thanks for the author and another doctor. These were presented after her death by her parents, who reported that she had discussed her funeral with her friends, requesting that her two closest girl friends sing a favored hymn.

Another patient, a teenage boy dying of progressive non-Hodgkin's lymphoma, summoned each of the ward staff to his room to say goodbye. Later, with many of his friends present, he bequeathed one of his possessions to each of them, including his most cherished possession, a CB radio.

Another patient, aged thirteen, with relapsed acute myeloid leukemia, underwent mismatched bone marrow transplantation during second remission, with her mother as the donor. She died five weeks after the transplant. Her mother reported that during the last few months, her daughter spoke more about the possibility of death and of the need to plan for the disposal of her material possessions. After her relapse, she frequently spoke of not wanting to die, mainly confiding her thoughts to her mother. She attended three healing masses and was noted to have fewer periods of depression afterwards. Her mother reported her child's great self-control as she planned for the possibility of not surviving the transplant. She requested that the family have a holiday together before the transplant. She asked if she owned her bedroom furniture and her piano, and about her right to make a will. Those attending her funeral were to wear bright colors. The service was to be held in her school chapel and the madrigal group, of which she was a member, was to sing a favorite hymn. She chose a white coffin, selected the clothing for her burial ("not a nightie, under any circumstances"), and asked that a family photograph, a bible, and her rosary beads be placed in her coffin. She purchased a remembrance gift for her parents and wrote them a personal letter. She recorded herself playing a special piece of music on the piano. She asked her parents not to remain sad, to be kind and loving to each other, and always to stay together. These examples show that dying children may respond in a manner well beyond their years.

Terminally ill children often know when they are about to die and may even share this information with their parents. One of the author's patients, a nine-year-old boy, died suddenly shortly after the abrupt onset of severe interstitial pneumonitis, eight months after bone marrow transplantation. His family owned one of a number of shops clustered in a marina and their son was well known to the other tenants. After their son had died, the parents learned that he had spent time chatting with each and every tenant in the marina, on the day before his death. Another of the author's patients, a five-year-old boy with terminal acute lymphoblastic leukemia, died at home. On the night that he died, he came into his parents' bedroom. He explained that he didn't quite know what to say to them and instead, sang a familiar children's song, "I can sing a rainbow."

GUIDELINES FOR WORKING WITH THE DYING CHILD, PARENTS, AND SIBLINGS

Guidelines for Working with the Dying Child

Seriously ill and dying children are much more aware of their illness and prognosis than it is comfortable to acknowledge. They know a great deal more about their situation than might otherwise be thought. Attempts to conceal the situation from them have proven to be ineffective and damaging. Dying children invariably know the true situation from their past experiences in the treatment unit. Their own bodies provide strong additional clues that death may be imminent. They are known to harbour anxiety about their situation and are helped by the provision of age-appropriate information. Equipped with this knowledge, the caregiver certainly can be more attentive to the child's verbal and non-verbal communications and seek, where possible, to lessen the child's anxiety.

Dying children have the same emotional needs as all children regardless of their health. In addition, they have needs which result from their reactions to illness and hospital admissions, as well as those arising from their concept of death.

It is essential to involve the child in at least some of the discussions about further management. With the consent of the parents one should consult directly with children over five or six years of age at this important phase of their management. A tactful but honest explanation as to why specific therapy is being discontinued should be given and ample opportunity for discussion of the implications provided. Children older than six or seven are often very matter-of-fact in their approach to their own situation.

The child's perception and understanding of death will be influenced by chronological age, developmental level, individual personality, past experiences with death and loss, and the family's religious beliefs. It may be difficult for young children to express their fears. In particular, they fear separation from their parents and loved ones and sense and respond strongly to the level of anxiety surrounding them. They have a continuing need for reassurance and security. Expressive play with art or music will assist them in working through their concerns. Children who do not wish to discuss painful matters and seemingly put on a brave front may, in fact, be seeking to protect their parents from further emotional turmoil for which they may feel responsible.

Helping Seriously Ill Children Communicate their Feelings

The following guidelines, provided by Adams-Greenly [21] can be used to help seriously ill children communicate their inner experiences related to their illness:

- Before proceeding with communication, ascertain the child's own perception of the situation, taking into account his or her developmental level and experience.
- Understand the child's symbolic language. Children often experience emotions without being able to put them into concepts or words. Young children can use symbolic language to communicate their worries.
- Clarify reality and dispel fantasy. Children often have difficulty distinguishing between reality and fantasy and between actions

and thoughts. A common fantasy of sick children is that of being responsible for the illness. Thus, admission to the hospital and medical procedures are interpreted as punishment.

- Encourage the expression of feelings. When children are allowed to express their anger, sadness, and anxiety they are able to examine these feelings, place them in perspective, and gain control over them.
- Promote self-esteem through mastery. The self-esteem of the child with cancer is threatened by pain, frustration, deprivation, changes in body image, and the possibility of death. As a result, his or her school attendance and peer relationships may both suffer. School is the ideal setting in which to encourage the child to communicate about his or her illness in a way that will promote self-esteem through mastery.
- When approaching the child with cancer, make no assumptions about what the situation will entail. Be open to what each encounter can teach. Do not underestimate the child's ability to master life's challenges creatively and with humor and dignity.

If a child asks "Am I going to die?", the wisest and best response is to be honest and confirm that such is the case. How one replies and the words one uses will vary greatly because the details of each child's situation and management, and the relationship with the caregiver asked the question, make every case unique. The important thing is to be honest, confirm that the answer to the question is "yes," and stay with the child to deal with whatever specific concerns he or she may mention next.

Remember that a child who asks this difficult question has already picked the person to ask and is merely seeking confirmation that it is safe to discuss the issue with this person. Failure to be honest deprives the child of a valuable opportunity for communication. Like adults, children are concerned that they will be comfortable, safe, and not alone. Before one answers the question, it could be helpful to try and ascertain the specific issues that are concerning the child [22]. Some approaches used as initial responses to direct questions about dying include: "What makes you ask me that right now?" "Are you feeling worse?" "That's a very hard question. You and I know that you're very sick right now. Are you unsure about how things will turn out?" "It sounds like you might be very worried," or "You know that your tumor has come back." Once the conversation is started, careful listening can ascertain the young person's concerns. The important thing is not to be evasive and to answer questions honestly.

The Role of Expressive Therapies

Art therapy and music therapy are forms of expressive therapy that can be used for effective communication by the child. Both can also be used as effective measures of the child's psychological adaptation. Children are natural artists and can express themselves with few inhibitions. The child's art may communicate what words cannot. While the therapist needs to understand the images produced by children, interpretations of the children's work are most reliable when provided by the children themselves. Music therapy is also effective in uncovering and working through fears and anxieties related to death and mourning. It offers the opportunity for creative acts. Music therapy may energize or relax, promote thought or distract, and provide an opportunity for expression. A variety of music therapy techniques, including song-writing and selection, lyric substitution, improvisation, and guided imagery, can all be used to encourage the child to release his or her fears through a creative act.

For the infant too young to have a concept of death, one should aim to provide maximum physical relief and comfort. The child two to seven years of age will fear the separation from parents and other loved ones that death entails. Such separations should be minimized during palliative care. The child aged between seven and twelve years will fear abandonment, destruction, and body mutilation. One should be open and honest and provide truthful explanations of symptoms and their management. Access to peers should be maintained and the child's sense of control over his or her deteriorating body should be fostered.

The dying adolescent represents the greatest challenge to the caregiver [23]. It is necessary to reinforce the adolescent's self-esteem and body image, and allow adequate opportunity for ventilation of anger. The adolescent needs privacy and his or her sense of independence should be preserved as much as possible. Access to peers should be maintained and contact with mutual support groups may be helpful.

Some members of the treatment team may feel less equipped to work directly with the dying child. Such members can direct their skills to working with the child's parents, helping them to cope more effectively with the situation. If one is uncomfortable working directly with the child, another caregiver that the child trusts should be involved. Honesty and compassion somehow must be combined to alleviate the child's anxiety and preserve hope.

Guidelines for Working with the Parents

Sources of distress that parents face include the following:

The Parental Role

Parents must face not only their child's imminent death but also the perceived loss of part of themselves. They must cope with the feeling of having failed as a parent. Feelings of loss of self-esteem are common.

The Unnaturalness of a Child Predeceasing a Parent

There may be strong feelings of guilt associated with surviving when the one who is perceived as being "more worthy of life" is dying prematurely.

Societal Reactions to a Child's Death

The approaching death of a child is unnatural and threatening to parents of other children. Fearing the loss of their own child, they withdraw thus leaving the parents with little of the social support that may be helpful in coping with the stresses of palliative care.

Loss of Support of the Spouse/Partner

The threat of impending death strikes both parents simultaneously. Each is preoccupied with his or her own grief and is unavailable to support the other. Each becomes vulnerable to feelings of anger or blame displaced by the other. One partner may misinterpret the other's withdrawal and depression as rejection.

Parenting of Healthy Children

The parents are obliged to continue in the very role that they are attempting to grieve for and relinquish. Healthy children serve as a painful reminder of the dying child. Feelings of hostility may be displaced on to these children, leading to deepening guilt.

Identifying the issues above and discussing them will help parents focus on, and talk about, their feelings and deal more effectively with the difficulties that are confronting them.

The employment of one or both parents may be put at risk during the child's final stage of illness. Simple liaison with the employer by the treatment team may be all that is required for the parents to obtain compassionate leave. The family may experience significant financial difficulties at this time because of loss of work and the increasing demands of the child's care. The assistance of supportive agencies and funds can often be obtained for the family to help make ends meet and have important bills paid on time. Practical difficulties arising from managing other children and the household may be significant.

Grandparents or other members of the extended family may be available and willing to assist parents with the care of the other children and management of the household during this time. Also, volunteers from supporting agencies may be available to assist with the day-to-day tasks of routine home care.

The family will need adequate breaks from the stresses of caring for their dying child. Parents exhausted by care at home may benefit from the child receiving periods of respite care in a children's hospice or hospital. The family may simply "need permission" to take a break.

Occasionally, significant behavioral disturbances will occur in families attempting to deal with the stresses and threats of a terminal illness. The caregiving team must be alert to early signs of decompensation and intervene as required.

The Child's Impending Death– Planning for the Funeral

Some time should be spent with the parents gently discussing the practical implications of the child's impending death. Family members will feel a need to make their final farewells to the child and should be encouraged to do so in whatever way each feels is appropriate. The child's condition usually deteriorates gradually and the parents are often considerably reassured to know that the death, when it occurs, will almost always be peaceful and free from fear and distress for the child. At this time, the child will become more withdrawn and detached from those providing care. The family may need reassurance that this detachment is a normal part of the distancing and separation that occurs in the dying process.

As the child's death draws near, the question of an autopsy should also be raised. There is considerable fear of, and misconception about, autopsies and parents usually welcome information that will assist them in making a decision. Further, if there are significant and unanswered questions about the child's illness, an autopsy may provide information that will be of assistance to parents during their bereavement. If an autopsy is planned after a death managed at home, provision must be made for removal of the child's body from home to hospital.

Parents should also be encouraged to give some thought to the child's funeral. They will be required to decide whether the child's body is to be buried or cremated and will need to be in touch with a funeral director who will make the necessary arrangements. Although seemingly difficult subjects to broach with the family, a small amount of planning in advance will later be regarded as valuable by the parents.

After death, the parents may benefit from a quiet time with the child's body. Hasty attempts to have the body removed by well-meaning, but uninformed, relatives are not to be encouraged. Brothers and sisters should be asked if they wish to see the child's body and allowed to do so. Family members who are excluded are deprived of the opportunity of "saying goodbye" and may harbour distressing fantasies of how the deceased looked after death. Such issues may lead to considerable additional emotional disturbance during the period of bereavement. In effect, it is necessary to relearn practices which were considered perfectly familiar and desirable in earlier generations.

Guidelines for Working with the Siblings

A useful study has documented the following reactions seen in brothers and sisters of pediatric cancer patients [24]:

- Siblings may have their own private version of the causation of their brother or sister's illness.
- There may be misconceptions about the nature of the illness because of the lack of a visible focus of disease (e.g., in leukemia as compared with an amputation).
- There may be misconceptions about the hospital clinic and the treatment program.
- There may be fear of developing the same illness.
- There may be guilt and shame related to relief for not developing the illness, ambivalent feelings about their sick brother or sister (envy or resentment over the family's preoccupation with the patient), and shame over the ill child's disfigurement which marks the family as different.
- There may be compromised academic and social functioning because of preoccupation with the stress of illness.

These emotions may lead siblings to exhibit irritability, social withdrawal, academic under-achievement, enuresis, and acting-out behavior.

Well children who act as donors for their brother or sister's bone marrow transplant feel a responsibility for the outcome of the procedure. At the outset they are required to undergo a bone marrow harvest, a painful procedure which is not primarily in the donor's interest. If complications such as graft-versus-host disease arise and particularly if the transplant fails, the surviving donor will feel guilty for playing a seemingly easily identified role in the patient's death, especially if the death is due to severe graft-versus-host disease. Such children require additional counseling and support to reverse and preferably prevent such misapprehensions.

Recommendations for Parents and Caregivers

Suggestions which may help parents to assist siblings of the ill child include [25]:

- Treat children equally by taking into account each child's special needs,
- During hospital stays with the ill child, keep in contact with the siblings,
- Spend time alone with each sibling, even if it is very limited,
- Permit siblings to continue with their lives as normally as possible.

Specific recommendations for caregivers in counseling the sick child's siblings during the phases of palliative care include:

- Give children a clear and unambiguous concept of their brother or sister's illness and its cause.
- Encourage siblings to dispense with any erroneous concepts of the cause of the illness.
- Allow siblings to visit the clinic, meet staff caring for the ill child, and witness the treatment program.
- Assign helpful tasks to siblings during home care.
- Whenever possible, reassure siblings that they will not develop the same illness.
- Provide siblings with appropriate opportunities to ventilate their feelings of resentment toward their parents and/or ill brother or sister.
- Liaise with staff at the siblings' schools.
- Provide an opportunity for siblings to "say goodbye" as their brother or sister's death approaches.
- Allow siblings to attend the funeral along with the rest of the family if they choose to do so. Children should not be forced to attend such events. They need the freedom to participate to the degree that they feel comfortable.

Support groups or discussion groups for siblings of children with cancer offer another source of support for working through difficult conflicts.

Many of the emotional reactions of the family of the terminally ill child are manifestations of anticipatory grief. It is well documented that the grieving process may commence prior to the child's death. Anticipatory grief is characterised by depression, a heightened concern for the ill child, rehearsal of the death, and attempts to adjust to the consequences of the death.

Parent support groups which have been of value in earlier phases of the child's illness may assume special importance during the child's palliative care. Other parents who have experienced the loss of a child may provide compassionate understanding and support which can help parents deal with the approaching death of their own child. These groups may also provide practical assistance with cooking, house-keeping, shopping, child-minding, running errands, and other similar day-to-day tasks that would otherwise tax the ill child's family.

How Cultural Differences Influence the Palliative Care of Children

Little research is yet available on how cultural differences influence the palliative care of children and on how a child's concept of death is affected by the family's culture and environment. However, there is a recurrent theme in the death literature that the way in which parents and others discuss death within the family will have a significant effect on the child's developing concept.

Virtually all the literature encourages openness, honesty, and opportunities for the child to talk about death. Some predictions that could be tested by research can be attempted based on knowledge already available about how various cultures handle serious illness, dying, death, and mourning. For instance, the Buddhist regards illness and death as a natural part of life whereas the Australian Aboriginal regards death as punishment, or the result of evil magic. It is likely that the Buddhist child would have a different concept of death to the Aboriginal child and would be less afraid of it, accepting it more as a part of life. Some cultures, for example, the Lebanese culture, are rich in mourning rituals but have a closed attitude to discussion of death. It is not yet known how Lebanese children, who attend a relative's funeral or who are seriously ill themselves, deal with the sudden massive displays of emotion that they witness, without the benefit of discussion or explanation from other members of their family.

In any culturally diverse country, customs and expectations sur-rounding the events of serious illness, dying, death, and mourning will vary. Members of a given culture will often maintain religious beliefs which differ from those of the host country's predominant culture. Usually, there will be a strong overlap between religious and cul-tural practices, often with no distinction between the two made by the members themselves. Traditional practices within the culture will have been modified by the effects of mixing with other cultures, by the laws or practices of the host country's culture, and by the requirements of modern society. Staff should ask the family in question about their particular beliefs and needs. Cultural requirements tend to be altered or relaxed by families in the case of an ill or deceased child in comparison with an adult.

IMPLICATIONS FOR CAREGIVERS

It is important to preserve hope at all stages of the illness, including the terminal phase. To take away all hope will destroy a child's ability to live on from day to day and will foster feelings of hopelessness and helplessness. No matter how grim the situation, one should always strive to deal with issues in a positive manner. The focus of hope changes over time, for example from hope for cure to hope for a longer remission than last time, to hope that the child can be cared for at home, to hope that the child will die without pain. It is necessary to acknowledge the gradual accumulation of losses and the change in the focus of hope. The family should be supported in their current hope and helped to maintain a realistic focus on what the child can still do [26].

Those providing care to dying children and their families face the prospect of repeated losses associated with the deaths of many of their patients. Caregivers must recognize their own limitations and avail themselves of appropriate support within their treatment team or institution. A well-balanced and effective level of care can only be maintained on an extended basis by provision of adequate and regular periods of leave and by fulfilling interests outside the work-place.

It is often asked how one can work in such an emotionally charged field. The response (as those who work in this field will confirm) is that one enjoys the work and considers working with children and their families rewarding, fascinating, frequently unpredictable, never boring, and always a privilege.

A mother addressing a recent information day for oncology parents, organized by parents and staff from the author's department, spoke of the difficulties faced by families on treatment and the need to preserve hope. "My youngest son Thomas was ten and a half months old when he was diagnosed with a liver tumor," she said. "We were initially told that it might not be operable and if it was that he might not survive the operation. Well, he did and we did our time in Camperdown. He's now a wonderful, beautiful, gorgeous, healthy almost six-year-old. Now I look back on those days with very mixed emotions. But I have very, very fond memories of the encouragement and support that was given to us by so many people, and especially the marvellous oncology staff who showed so much empathy and gave us what I think was the most important gift of all, and that was hope—even in those very early days, when I thought there was none."

She continued, "I have two very lasting memories that I keep with me all the time from our early traumatic days. I'll address these to the people whose children are currently on treatment, because I'm sure you'll identify with them. They are comments that my other children made at the time. One day they came into hospital to visit us and we'd been there for a very long stay and they looked particularly sad and perplexed and they said, 'You know, we think our baby Thomas has forgotten how to smile.' And my second little boy, who was just four at the time, told his grandfather, 'My mummy has a pain in her heart.' "

She said, "I read a really nice quote recently by John Steinbeck which said: 'There are those of us who live in rooms of experience that no one else can enter.' I'm sure all of us here have felt that at some stage, although we all share a common bond. Sadly, there's nothing we can do to alleviate the pain in your heart. But if there's any way, any way at all, that we can lighten your load, please let us know" [27].

Just as this mother and other parents like her offer emotional support to parents facing similar difficulties, so too must we as professional caregivers be just as willing to stand by these children and families in their need, not only to open the doors into their rooms of experience but also to step across the threshold.

ACKNOWLEDGMENTS

I thank Margaret Burgess and Rhondda Rytmeister for their helpful comments and all staff of the Oncology Unit for the care they provide to our patients and their families.

REFERENCES

1. M. Stevens, Improving Communication with Parents of Children with Cancer, *The Medical Journal of Australia, 160*, p. 325, 1994.
2. C. M. Binger, A. R. Ablin, R. C. Feuerstein, et al., Childhood Leukemia: Emotional Impact on Patient and Family, *New England Journal of Medicine, 280*, pp. 414-418, 1969.
3. R. K. Mulhern, J. J. Crisco, and B. M. Camitta, Patterns of Communication among Pediatric Patients with Leukemia, Parents and Physicians: Prognostic Disagreements and Misunderstandings, *Journal of Pediatrics, 99*, pp. 480-483, 1981.

4. M. Stevens, "Shuttle Sheet": A Patient-held Medical Record for Pediatric Oncology Families, *Medical and Pediatric Oncology, 200*, pp. 330-335, 1992.
5. C. C. Synder, Nursing Care of the Child with Cancer, in *Oncology Nursing*, C. C. Snyder (ed.), Little, Brown, Boston, pp. 247-297, 1986.
6. M. G. Sawyer, A. F. Gannoni, I. R. Toogood, et al., The Use of Alternative Therapies by Children with Cancer, *The Medical Journal of Australia, 160*, pp. 320-322, 1994.
7. M. A. Ashby, R. J. Kosky, H. T. Laver, et al., An Enquiry into Death and Dying at The Adelaide Children's Hospital: A Useful Model? *The Medical Journal of Australia, 154*, pp. 165-170, 1991.
8. J. J. Collins, M. M. Stevens, and P. Cousens, *Home Care for the Dying Child: the Parent's Perception*, submitted to Australian Family Physician, 1995.
9. A. G. Knudson and J. M. Natterson, Participation of Parents in the Hospital Care of their Fatally Ill Children, *Pediatrics, 26*, pp. 482-490, 1960.
10. J. R. Morrissey, Death Anxiety in Children with a Fatal Illness, in *Crisis Intervention*, Family Service Association of America, New York, pp. 324-338, 1965.
11. J. M. Natterson and A. G. Knudson, Observations Concerning Fear of Death in Fatally Ill Children and their Mothers, *Psychosomatic Medicine, 22*, pp. 456-465, 1960.
12. J. B. Richmond and H. A. Waisman, Psychologic Aspects of Management of Children with Malignant Diseases, *American Journal of Diseases in Childhood, 89*, pp. 42-47, 1955.
13. J. Vernick and M. Karon, Who's Afraid of Death on a Leukemia Ward? *American Journal of Diseases of Children, 109*, pp. 393-397, 1965.
14. J. Vernick and M. Karon, An Approach to the Emotional Support of Fatally Ill Children, *Clinical Pediatrics, 7*, pp. 274-280, 1968.
15. E. H. Waechter, Children's Awareness of Fatal Illness, *American Journal of Nursing, 71*, pp. 1168-1172, 1971.
16. M. Bluebond-Langner, *The Private Worlds of Dying Children*, Princeton University Press, Princeton, New Jersey, 1978.
17. J. J. Spinetta, D. Rigler, and M. Karon, Personal Space as a Measure of a Dying Child's Sense of Isolation, *Journal of Consulting and Clinical Psychology, 42*, pp. 751-756, 1974.
18. J. J. Spinetta, D. Rigler, and M. Karon, Anxiety in the Dying Child, *Pediatrics, 52*, pp. 841-845, 1973.
19. C. Clunies-Ross and R. Lansdown, Concepts of Death, Illness and Isolation found in Children with Leukaemia, *Child: Care, Health and Development, 14*, pp. 373-386, 1988.
20. M. Stevens, Cancer in Childhood, in *Physical Disability: A New Reference for Schools*, Special Education Directorate, NSW Dept of School Education, 1995, in press.

21. M. Adams-Greenly, Helping Children Communicate about Serious Illness and Death, *Journal of Psychosocial Oncology, 2*, pp. 61-72, 1984.
22. G. V. Foley and E. H. Whittam, Care of the Child Dying of Cancer: Part I, *CA-A Cancer Journal For Clinicians, 40*, pp. 327-354, 1990.
23. M. M. Stevens and J. C. Dunsmore, Adolescents who are Living with Life-Threatening Illness, in *Helping Adolescents Cope with Death and Bereavement*, C. A. Corr and D. E. Balk (eds.), Springer Publishing Company, New York, in press, 1995.
24. B. M. Sourkes, Siblings of the Pediatric Cancer Patient, in *Psychological Aspects of Childhood Cancer*, J. Kellerman (ed.), Springfield, Illinois, pp. 47-69, 1980.
25. B. Davies and I. M. Martinson, Care of the Family: Special Emphasis on Siblings During and After the Death of a Child, in *Pediatric Hospice Care: What Helps*, B. B. Martin (ed.), Children's Hospital of Los Angeles, Los Angeles, California, pp. 189-190, 1989.
26. E. M. B. Davies, Personal communication, February 1991.
27. Proceedings 1994 RAHC Oncology Unit Parent Information Day, reproduced with permission.

CHAPTER 11

The Impact of the Hospital System on Dying Children and Their Families

Mark L. Greenberg

INTRODUCTION

In recent years, a substantial shift has occurred in the prevailing view of the appropriateness of the hospital as the context for the process of a child dying. This paradigm shift has seen the emergence of a strong commitment to the principle that home is the right place for a child to die. There can be no question that, for a substantial majority of children and their families, home is the right place for this terminal transition phase to occur. But there can also be no doubt that for a considerable minority of patients, home is not the right place. This minority of children and their families include single-parent families, immigrant families with little community support, families dealing with other contemporaneous crises, (either health related or socially based), and children and families with cultural or personal reasons.

For these families, the hospital must play its traditional role—the role defined for it in medieval times as the place of respite for the weary, the wounded, the injured, and the dying. It is particularly important in our society, driven as it is by peer pressure, that families for whom the hospital is the right place for a child to die do not feel that opting for a hospital-based death process constitutes failure, inadequacy, or abdication of duty. If they are forced to feel this way, the surviving family members will bear the burden of an ill-founded judgmental view imposed upon them by society for the remainder of their lives. The death of their child will become a double tragedy— the absence of the child and the presence of guilt and shame. That combination is a potent predictor of poor long-term adaptation after the death.

The corollary of the foregoing is that the hospital must be geared to cope with this subset of children and families who opt for terminal care in the institutional setting. In fiscally constrained times, this is a progressively harder task to undertake. However, a hospital that has as its mission, tertiary, quaternary, and even secondary care, must include in its strategic planning consideration of the requirements for the provision of optimal palliative care. Just as these institutions strive for state-of-the-art curative therapy for those children who will live, they must also strive to provide state-of-the-art palliative care to those children who will not. Thus, it behooves health care professionals to consider, in some depth, the physical, familial, sociological, and demographic issues that will bear upon the provision of optimal palliative care in an institutional setting.

In so doing, it is important to retain the perspective that, just as palliative care is a dynamic and changing process along the continuum of the child's life, the context in which dying occurs may need to change over time. Dying does not occur in any given instant—it is a process and components of it may occur in different contexts. Continuity in this process is critical. For families who have received their care with curative intent in a particular institutional setting the link to that institution often remains of key importance in the palliative phase. The interaction between home and hospital must be maintained, even if the dying process is happening at home. There must always be the option of moving from the home to the hospital, either for respite or when particular physical or circumstantial issues make home management untenable. There must be the facility to move from the hospital to home when circumstances change, tilting the preferences in favor of home-based dying. In other words, a decision to traverse the dying process in either the hospital or the home context is not irrevocable and options must be retained to reverse that decision. In this context, the use of an agency and individual capable of linking home with hospital is a critically important component. The "Interlink"[1] nurse concept champions the idea that an individual versed in and connected with the hospital, but based in the community, enables the expertise of the hospital to be transported into the home and enables the status in the home to be conveyed to the hospital in a very direct and expert fashion. This two-way communication by a doubly-based individual promotes and

[1] Interlink Community Cancer Nurses, 620 University Ave., Suite 701, Toronto, Canada M5G 2C1.

encourages continuity and familiarity, and is a concept well worth the fiscal expenditure it demands.

In planning for hospital-based terminal care, it must be understood by administrators and hospital financial officers that terminal care is not a cost-effective process. Terminal care is a slow, labor, resource, and care-intensive phenomenon. Children and their families may spend long periods of time in the hospital and will require specialized care that includes particular attention to their physical and emotional needs as well as their need for privacy and dignity. The price of these requirements is not small, but this function of the final succor of the dying child is a commitment as ancient and sacrosanct as the founding principles of hospital care.

THE BACKGROUND AGAINST WHICH THE HOSPITAL TERMINAL CARE AND THE HEALTH CARE SYSTEM IMPACTS ON DYING CHILDREN AND THEIR FAMILIES

The fundamental task of a child is growth which encompasses cognitive, emotional, physical, and spiritual development. The growth of a child mirrors and catalyzes the growth of the family. Parents experience the expansion of their identities as individuals, the dynamic of family interaction grows and burgeons, and the family experiences the joy and the challenge of change, expansion, and redefinition.

Times of growth demand adaptation and change, and times of adaptation and change are times of relative instability. These are times when intimacy between parents and within families is of key importance. These are also times of vulnerability. When a life-threatening illness and progression to death are superimposed on a changing, growing system, the participants in the system are particularly vulnerable to catastrophic effects.

In the life cycle of events, there are developmental phases that permit more or less adequate coping with equilibrium shattering events. For this reason, dealing with the death of parents or the processes of illness fit more comfortably in the more mature phase of individual and family life cycles and fit poorly with the stage of the life cycle that most families of dying children are in. Consequently, these families face special demands and special risks.

The family confronting terminal care for their child has transited a process of cure-oriented health care delivery and, thus, are not naive when they enter the terminal phase of coping with their child's illness. They bring with them the experience of living with their child's illness, surviving in the health care system, and being caregivers. In addition, they have the knowledge, support and expertise of those in their extended circle who have shared their experience. There is no question that what they have encountered influences the reactions and competencies of both parents and child and must be considered in planning by health care providers.

DEFINITION OF THE OBJECTIVES AND OPTIMAL OUTCOMES OF THE DYING PROCESS

Just as clear-cut goals, objectives, and cost-benefit analyses are deployed in making curative and therapeutic decisions, goals and objectives for the care of a dying child and the family must be formulated. In attempting to decide whether a child with a limb tumor should have an amputation, a rotation-plasty, or a joint fusion, the treatment team considers the type of tumor, the child's nature, his or her hopes and aspirations, and the context in which the child lives. The objectives are to decide which procedure best meets the needs of a particular child. Similarly, objectives for optimal outcomes for the following three distinct categories of participants involved in the care of the dying must be defined.

The Child

The objective of caring for the dying child must be to provide the child with maximum quality of life for as long as possible, followed by maximum quality of death. This implies pain-free, discomfort-free living, and a pain-free, discomfort-free, emotionally calm death in a loving, supportive context.

The Parents

For parents, the death of a child constitutes inversion of the natural order, violation of the rules of the world, and death of hope as they customarily define it. Parents invest dreams of their past and hopes for their future in their children. The death of their child may constitute the death of hope for the future. The objective for parents must be to permit them to transcend the death, to retain self-esteem and self-value, and to be supported in a way that will permit the re-definition of hope and the future.

The Caregivers

The objectives for the caregivers must be to ensure that, at the end of the process, they believe that they have delivered their professional expertise in the most effective manner possible, that their professional functioning was a success, and that, despite the sadness of the death, both they and the parents are satisfied with their professional participation.

THE PARTICIPANTS AND THE CONTEXT

Overview

All phases in the evolution of an illness are transitions. These may include transitions from health to illness, illness to recovery, recovery to relapse, relapse to palliation, and palliation to death. This last transition is influenced by the nature of the prior transitions, by the participants in the prior transitions, and by the experience gained in and from these transitions. At the epicenter of the whole process is their child and his or her characteristics. The parents form a protective umbrella over the child. This umbrella is heavily influenced by the nature of the relationship between the parents, by whether or not this is a single-parent family, and by the strengths and weaknesses of parents, individually and conjointly. The parents are molded, influenced, and impacted upon by the cultural, sociological, and ethnic characteristics that have defined them all of their lives; these now take on particular significance. Cultural and ethnic determinants tend to be maximally evident around critical life cycle events—tribal and religious practices find their maximum expression at times of birth, puberty, marriage, and death.

Similarly, the extended family and social circle of the family exerts significant influence, both directly on the child and upon the parent couple, thereby affecting the characteristics of parenting. Caregivers also impact both directly and indirectly on the child via influences and interactions with the parents. All of this complex interaction occurs within a prevailing institutional milieu under circumstances of impending hospital death. This institutional milieu exerts a critical influence upon all participants, a fact easily apparent when it is recognized that each institution creates an individual and very particular, although often not well defined, culture. An attempt to graphically represent the circumstances and their influences can be found in Figure 1.

Equally important to the circumstances is the nature of the dying process. This, in turn, is influenced by the nature of the disease process. Disease-specific variables exert significant influence on the attitude of parents, children, and the family unit toward death, and on the preparedness for handling death. Parents confronting an illness

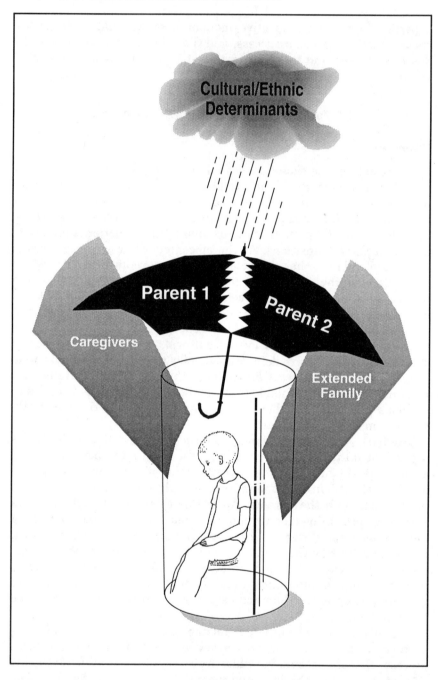

Figure 1. Relationship between human and social influences on the ill child.

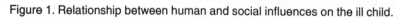

with a sudden onset and catastrophic course, such as a motor vehicle accident, have a very different approach to parents who have experienced a long, drawn-out illness with a series of transitions. Parents whose children have had illnesses that have steadily eroded their quality of life have different attitudes to those whose children may have had chronic disease, but with good quality of life maintained throughout. Thus, the quality of the dying is influenced by the quality of the living and the nature and pattern of the disease variables. Examples of such disease variables are depicted graphically in Figure 2.

The Child

To provide truly focused care for the dying child in hospital, there must be an understanding of some of the determinants of the child's experience. Critical to this is the caveat that the child's experience must be understood from the child's perspective. Although the analysis of the child's needs and experience must be through the objective eye of the professional, the perceptions must be through the eyes of the child.

The standard image of the dying child is one of a sad, miserable, crying child in pain and distress. Those who work with dying children know that they are as variable in their dying as they are in their living. This variability resides, in part, in the individual characteristics of the child and, in part, in the level of developmental maturation of the individual child. It is fundamentally important to focus on the characteristics of the individual child rather than assigning characteristics to the category "the dying child."

This phenomenon is well illustrated by the story of two children of identical age, dying of neuroblastoma within months of each other. Both had widely metastatic neuroblastoma. Until two hours before her death, Tiffany, who had amongst other sites a metastasis to the eye orbit that had produced severe proptosis, was playing on her mother's lap, smiling and responding amiably to social contact. By contrast, Monica, who was as far as could be ascertained pain-free, lay passively in her very anxious mother's lap, curled into the fetal position for six days prior to her silent, sad death. Simone, a paraplegic paralyzed and dying due to a metastatic osteogenic sarcoma, responded until the day of her death to questions about how she was feeling by replying, "Much better today, thank you." Laurie, also dying of a metastatic bone tumor, became progressively withdrawn, panicked, and spent several horrendous days fighting her impending death, until she required sedation to cope with what was coming. Given these variations, it is not possible to prescribe a particular way of handling the child, other than

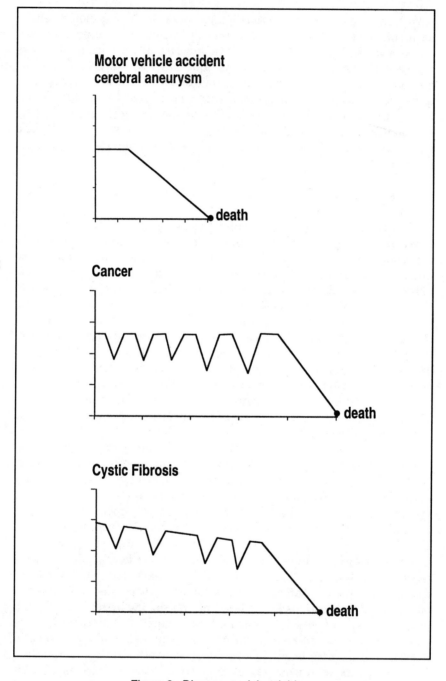

Figure 2. Disease model variables.

to recommend responding to each particular child's characteristics and behaviors.

As they approach the end of their lives, dying children retain the same normal, basic needs as well children. They also have specialized needs and sometimes these predominate, making it easy to lose sight of the very important role that "normal" needs play in a child's happiness. A child needs laughter and play in the face of death as much as during normal life. Their absence implies disruption of normality and familiarity. Comfort and equanimity for the child are wrapped up with familiarity; and quality of life and quality of death are both negatively influenced by the loss of familiarity. Along similar lines, the need to comfort a child with respect to routine everyday discomforts is often lost in the overwhelming context of comforting the child in the face of impending death. The small day-to-day needs of a child must continue to occupy the same level of importance as they do in normal living.

One of the roles that parents and adults fulfill in the life of a child is to impose order upon his or her life in a world that is sometimes chaotic. This takes place by virtue of the setting of guidelines and the imposing of discipline. In this fashion, security is imparted to the child by the knowledge that someone has control over the way the world works and will guide the child through new and challenging experiences. At a time when the world is turning upside down, it is particularly important that a child does not feel abandoned and that parents continue in the normal parental role as guide and protector. This may be especially difficult in the context of the hospital, as institutions have their own rules. A balance must be struck between institutional rules and parental and familial rules.

Particularly challenging for parents is the need of many children to express sadness and anger and to engage in confrontational behavior. In attempts to comfort children, there is often a tendency to neutralize the expression of extremes of emotion and to equate equanimity with peace. Comforting and calming must be practiced, but the expression of sadness and anger may be a necessary component of behavioral development, as well as a component of coping and adaptation.

The age of the dying child exerts significant influence on the evolution of care patterns. Age determines cognitive differences that relate not only to children's perceptions of death, but to their capacity to process information and articulate their needs and demands. Caregivers must be alert to conceptual and cognitive peculiarities of individual children and of particular age groups of children and determine how these influence their ability to communicate their needs. Particularly difficult in this context is the discord between children's physical maturity and their cognitive level and their cognitive level and their level of emotional maturity. Thus, physically bigger and more mature children are often assumed to have equivalently advanced cognitive development. Similarly, children who are bright and intellectually advanced are assumed to have levels of emotional maturity concordant with their cognate capacities. In point of fact, there is often significant discrepancy between levels of physical, cognitive, and emotional maturation. Predicating interventions and explanations on levels of physical and cognitive development will often lead to an overestimate of children's emotional capacity to deal with information. A patient of the author's, a tall eleven-year-old girl with early sexual maturation, was considerably less socially and cognitively mature than suggested by her physical appearance. She was handled by the staff in accordance with her physical appearance rather than her emotional and cognitive level. At one point, she confided that she wished she would not be treated like a big girl, since she did not understand what was being said to her most of the time. Such mis-assessment of developmental level can only lead to a child's feeling isolated and lonely.

Particular challenges are afforded by adolescents who are dying. Even dying adolescents continue to feel the need to individuate and establish independence. At the same time, however, they are confronted with a need for dependency and a powerful desire to revert to an earlier time in which comfort came more easily. Adolescents are often in conflict with parents and express their rebellion through anger and confrontational behavior. This may be focused on the parents, but also may be focused on caregivers. Adolescents have a great need to be able to make decisions and parents may have particular difficulty allowing their adolescent to make decisions during this difficult time. Denise, a sixteen-year-old dying of non-lymphoblastic leukemia, was fiercely independent and wished to stay involved in her regular activities away from the control of her parents. She required platelets to prevent bleeding, but was determined that she would define when she needed platelets and when she did not. Often, she would deliberately delay coming to the hospital to receive them until long after she should have, in order to demonstrate to her parents that she was in charge. Jordan, a fifteen-year-old with osteogenic sarcoma on continuous infusion of morphine, would turn off his infusion pump and tolerate increased pain in order to ensure that he was in control, and that the staff understood that he was in control.

Other difficulties that adolescents pose are related to the closeness in age between the older adolescent and the young caregiver. The caregiver often feels a particular identity with the older adolescent and identifies in a very personal way with the mortality and personal dissolution that the adolescent mirrors for him or her.

In the context of a hospital environment that has clear-cut rules and dictates, adolescents must be permitted to participate in decision-making and indeed, to have ultimate authority in a proportion of the decisions. This group in particular requires caregivers to appreciate the dilemma that there is no right and wrong in the process of dying. The challenge is to provide maximum comfort for adolescent patients as much of the time as is possible.

The Parents

Oriented as they are toward growth, expansion, and hope for the future, parents confronted with a dying child face an overwhelming task in transiting the crisis of the child's death. The child's death will irrevocably impact on the parents' lives, and the nature of the experience of the death process may dramatically increase the negative impact of the actual death. If the negative impact is compounded by a difficult experience, the perceived meaning of the life of the parents will be severely compromised and the memory of the child, instead of becoming hallowed, will become hollowed. Thus, there is a particular responsibility to optimize what is intrinsically a negative experience. Consequently, insight into some dimensions of the parental experience is important.

Despite the common myth that all children are equal and occupy equivalent places in the family hierarchy, the reality is that each child has a particular significance to each parent. Any given child has a specific impact on any given parent, determined in part by the developmental stage of the parent, the age of the parent, and the need that the child fulfills for that parent. For example, one of the author's patients was the product of the first and only pregnancy of a thirty-eight-year-old single mother and clearly carried the hopes of the mother for her old age and immortality on his shoulders. His death signified a life of absolute loneliness for her. A sixteen-year-old son of two elderly Portuguese immigrants provided the only linguistic and cultural channel into an alien society for his parents. His death consigned them to an isolated life on the fringe of society.

Significant influence on family dynamics is exerted by the time the family has become accustomed to the child. A child who has been terminally ill, virtually from birth, has not had the opportunity for protracted periods of healthful, joyous growth, whilst the child who has been sick for many years may have the experience of good times which are obscured by protracted, difficult times. Parents, who have endured the illness or death of another child, bring into relationships with the current child, a substantially different set of experiences than a family dealing with the issues for the first time. It is imperative that care-giving staff familiarize themselves with the circumstances that surround each individual family constellation and the impacts those experiences might bring to bear on the handling of the family.

Under normal circumstances, parents practice their parenting in the context of the privacy of their own home. They establish patterns by evaluating which forms and modes of discipline work and which do not, by exploring patterns and methods of child rearing, and by retaining that which works and rejecting that which does not. For such a process to occur, privacy and intimacy are critical. In the context of handling a dying child in an institutional setting, parental behaviors and patterns are, or are perceived to be, under continuous scrutiny by external agents. Adults who normally live independent, self-sufficient lives perceive themselves to be under evaluation and, indeed, they often are. Physicians, nurses, social workers, and other professionals constantly evaluate the efficacy of the parenting role and may even make suggestions as to how to better execute it. There is a very real sense of being graded as a parent as one grades a school child. This is demeaning and awkward.

Outside the institutional setting, parents are responsible for the routine care of their children. Such processes as feeding, bathing, and changing diapers are part of the normal, daily routine that establishes and perpetuates a parent-child relationship. In the institutional context, professional staff have a great tendency to assume these minor tasks and functions, since that fits well with hospital routine. It is of utmost importance that this displacement of normal parental function be avoided, since the assumption of normal parental duties by professional staff renders parents impotent and removes from them one of the few remaining anchors of normality.

In parallel with the loss of normal parenting functions, parents in an institutional context suffer the loss of normal coupling functions. It is particularly difficult to maintain intimacy in a context of constant public exposure. The mutual support and succor that results from regular, intimate interaction of a couple can be severely compromised. Not only can the role of parent be subsumed in the hospital context, but the role of spouse, with its attendant implications of mutuality, re-invigoration and sexuality, is compromised.

One of the hallmarks of growth and maturation of parents as individuals, and as a couple, is the assumption of control over one's life. Thus, through the stages of development of a couple, assumption of control over the couple's affairs is succeeded by assumption of control over the family's affairs. One of the defining characteristics of successful parenthood is being in control of the circumstances that surround a child's life. The process of a child dying wrests control completely from parents and forces them into the mode of coping with what is happening to them, rather than setting their direction for life. They are, in a very real sense, dependent on external influence for the well-being of their child and family. There is an enforced development of dependence on a health care system and on caregivers within that system. Much of the dependence is voluntary and reflects the need of parents to receive guidance and assistance from individuals with particular areas of expertise. However, much of the dependence is involuntary and may engender hostility toward the system in general and toward caregivers in particular. Thus, parents confront a conflict between their need to depend and their hostility toward the system upon which they must depend. One family cared for by the author, whose child had a protracted and difficult death from medulloblastoma with progressive neurologic deterioration, was very appreciative of the care and support given by hospital staff when their child became paraplegic. They openly expressed their belief that they could not have coped if the child had not been surrounded by competent, caring professionals. However, as the illness dragged on, considerable anger at the dependency of both child and family upon the caregivers began to emerge. By the time of the child's death, hostility toward the system that had trapped them had overwhelmed their gratitude. Their experience of care and compassion became one of charity and dependence.

Both hostility and dependence may be affected by caregivers through the attitudes and skills they bring to the family. Caregivers who require absolute control over the behavior of parents induce undue dependency, while those who are inconsistent and poorly responsive to the needs of parents and children may induce hostility. Caregivers, as a group, must examine regularly whether they are inducing undue dependence and whether they can modulate their behavior to minimize both dependence and hostility.

Hospitals are systems and systems are designed for the general rather than the specific case. Hospitals are bureaucracies with rules of governance, frameworks, policies, and procedures; they thrive on conformity and congruity. Families of dying children do poorly when confronted with hospital expectations of conformity and congruity. A *rapprochement* must be found whereby only those rules that must apply are enforced and others are waived. Co-existence should be negotiated and it is the obligation of the institution and the caregivers to adapt their institutional norms to the needs of parents wherever possible.

Parents are generally viewed as a dyad and parental wishes, desires, and needs are viewed as unitary. In point of fact, each parent may perceive him/herself as the ultimate protector of the child. The parent feels the need to act with absolute integrity in what he or she perceives to be in the child's best interests. Not infrequently, differing perceptions of the child's best interests result in conflict that is difficult to resolve. As a result, hospital staff may be drawn in. For instance, when Lindsay, a child dying of a brain tumor, experienced considerable distress from an attempt by the physiotherapist to help her regain mobility of her paralyzed arm, her father believed that this was a futile exercise. He demanded that the physiotherapy be stopped, while her mother, with equal conviction, demanded that it continue, since discontinuing it would be tantamount to abandoning hope, which she was not yet ready to do. Several members of the ward staff involuntarily became involved in this conflict. What began as differing views of the child's best interests escalated to an acrimonious clash between each parent and their supporting staff. Such conflicts are extraordinarily difficult to resolve, since each parent believes, with absolute conviction, that his or her view reflects the child's best interests.

The Impact of Parental Behavior on the Dying Child

Operating as an interdependent system, parents and child impact substantially on each other's behaviors during this difficult time. The parental influence on a child's coping capacity is substantial and the impact of individual behaviors is profound. It is, nonetheless, very difficult for parents to alter their behaviors as they have not had the opportunity to practice them prior to the real event.

Some parents are unable to deal honestly with their children, most often out of a mistaken belief that protecting them from the truth and reality will avoid undue distress. There are no rules as to how bluntly or directly children should be told that they are dying—the most consistent and compassionate pattern to follow is to listen attentively to the child's questions and answer them honestly. There is no place for forcing unwanted information upon children, but equally, no value in withholding information they wish to hear. Most often, parents who choose not to deal honestly and openly with their child's expressed desire for information are reflecting their own inability to confront the impending death for fear of breaking down emotionally and not demonstrating "bravery." This is a potentially destructive behavior, since the child needs permission to break down, if that is what is necessary. A child who does not benefit from open communication ends up isolated and unable to share his or her central fears. John, who was dying of a lymphoma, was the only son of an elderly couple. His parents absolutely insisted that at no point was he to be told that he was dying. Five minutes prior to his death, he called his physician over and whispered, "Don't tell them I'm dying, Doc, they'll be too upset." Joanne was a child with acute lymphoblastic leukemia whose parents refused to share the initial diagnosis with her. She spent two weeks curled up in bed in the fetal position. The child in the room next door to her had died the day Joanne was admitted to hospital. Joanne subsequently went on to die herself, and her parents still had neither shared the diagnosis nor her imminent death. Joanne was silent and withdrawn throughout, and the picture of these three human beings sharing a primal event, each in complete solitude, was convincing evidence that honesty is imperative.

Parental attitudes based on culture or tradition may transmit a very clear message to children that may not be appropriate and may seriously impact on their ability to deal with their situation. In many Mediterranean contexts, impending death is handled by the drawing of curtains and the donning of mourning weeds, long before the event has occurred. A child confronted by a darkened room and family members wearing mourning weeds must perceive impending doom, sometimes when there is still room for life.

Parental attitudes to pain may also impact on the child's comfort level. Most often, parents are rational and empathic with regard to their child's pain. Occasionally, however, a parent will perceive that "giving into pain" is hastening death and therefore, will attempt to withhold adequate pain control. Most often, this represents an attempt to exert control over a process that they cannot control. Periodically, such withholding of pain control is based on religious beliefs. Whatever the reason, parental attitudes toward pain control find their expression in the level of pain that their child must tolerate.

Religious belief systems impact significantly in other ways on the experience of the dying process. Occasionally, devout practitioners of orthodox belief systems will take the position that only a higher being can determine when active treatment should be withheld. Their view is that God provided the opportunities for active intervention and therefore, active intervention is divinely ordained and must be carried out. In this view, discretion of either parent or physician is not an option and aggressive treatment must carry on to the end. Genevieve, who was dying of Burkitt's lymphoma, was the daughter of a devoutly pious lay Catholic. She had proved resistant to all therapy, had severe complications of treatment, and had experienced severe, uncontrollable pain, which had just come under control. Her father insisted that further chemotherapy be attempted, since God alone would determine whether or not the chemotherapy would work. Genevieve's pain and suffering increased as a result of this attitude.

The Caregivers–The Impact of Personal and Professional Characteristics on the Process

In obvious contradistinction to death at home, families experiencing death in an institutional context are very directly impacted by the caregivers, their personal characteristics, and their collective attitudes. These characteristics and attitudes may either enable the practice of compassionate care or exert potentially negative, often covert, influences on care. There is great value in labeling and identifying some of these issues to permit understanding and pre-emptive response.

Perhaps more than in any other practice domain, the borders between the professional and the care recipient blur in the context of care of the dying child. There can be nothing but compassion, condolence, and empathy for those in the process of being bereaved. There is virtually no practicing professional who has not been touched at a personal level by bereavement. Separation of empathy at the personal and professional level is difficult to achieve. This may be particularly true for younger members of the caregiving team, particularly medical students, and newly graduated physicians, nurses, and social workers. There is a fundamental difference between professional advice and care and the compassion of a friend or relative—and that difference must be recognized and maintained. The risk of loss of objectivity by the caregiver may lead to crossing of boundaries that may render the caregiver professionally ineffective. Compassion must be retained at all times, but compassion is only one part of the professional function.

As professionals, a variety of experiences and contexts define our personal approach to professional function. In the context of caring for the dying child, the following are relevant.

Medical Disease Variables, Caregiver
Personality Variables and Their Interaction

The characteristics of care required for different categories of medical illness vary. Children being cared for in an intensive care unit require short-term, high-intensity interventions. The caregiver contact in this kind of illness is circumscribed and time-limited. By contrast, children with chronic illnesses or acute-on-chronic illnesses require longitudinal care, with a baseline, low-intensity level of care punctuated by periods requiring short, intense care. The caregivers working in this context have a more longitudinal exposure to families.

Individuals with different personality characteristics are drawn into specific disciplines within medicine, in part, because of the fit between their personality and the type of care required in the discipline they select. Thus, there are differences in personality types between those who become operating room nurses and those who become nurse coordinators in cystic fibrosis, hemophilia, or oncology clinics. The fit between personality type and the type of caregiving required determines, to a certain extent, the effectiveness with which health care professionals function in the context in which they have chosen to work. It is particularly relevant in the context of caring for dying children that the health care professionals identify their own capabilities in respect to their satisfaction with providing comfort and symptom control, rather than providing active intervention. They must also accept that peaceful death is the end point of their professional ministrations rather than a failure. Discord between personality type and illness characteristics leads to ineffective care.

Personal Experience

All caregivers bring into the caregiving context their own stressors and decompressors. The personal circumstances of the caregivers engaged in the care of dying children is particularly important. Family circumstances, the existence of a support structure outside of the institution, the ability to disconnect from families and children, the ability to separate personal experiences of death and chronic illness, and the ability to circumscribe personal, religious and cultural belief systems from impacting on children and families, are all factors that bear upon the ability of caregivers to effectively care for vulnerable families experiencing a primal event.

Stage of Professional Development

Negotiating the intricacies of caring for dying children and their families is a challenge at any stage of professional development. It may be particularly challenging to young and relatively inexperienced caregivers, as the scope of demand and the intensity of the experience requires a significant degree of maturity. The balance between maturity and enthusiasm may be transparent to families and impact significantly on how families perceive and receive caregivers. Familiarity with the processes involved in providing care to dying children and their families has obvious advantages, but it is very important that each family perceive itself as unique and not part of a stereotyped pattern. The more junior members of the team may be perceived as young and inexperienced or as enthusiastic and resourceful, while the more mature members of the team may be seen to be seasoned and experienced or burned out and empty. Maintaining a positive view of what each stage of career development offers is important for both members of the caregiving team and its leaders.

Particular Circumstances

When there has been a run of deaths on the ward, the capacity of the caregivers to deal with yet another impending death may be impaired. It is important, under such circumstances, to recognize the need to increase support for the staff.

Families with long histories of confrontational behavior with caregiving staff do not change when they enter the terminal care phase. This poses particular challenges because the expectation that a relationship that has been confrontational and combative will change to one that is gentle and supportive is unrealistic. Melanie's parents had long-standing marital difficulties. Her father had a history of alcoholism and confrontational and combative behavior long before she became ill. During the course of her illness, he antagonized the nursing staff, physicians, and hospital administration. When Melanie was admitted for terminal care, the prevailing attitude on the ward was one of wariness, protectiveness, and hostility from both Melanie's father and the ward staff. It was not possible to resolve the hostility, and as a result Melanie's death was handled with great distress by the staff.

Occasionally, complex familial circumstances surrounding dying children pose unmanageable problems for staff and compromise effective care. Christopher was dying of Burkitt's lymphoma, complicated by an interstitial pneumonia. He had been placed on a ventilator. When his two-month old sibling developed meningitis and had a cardiorespiratory arrest, he was admitted to the bed next to Christopher. When Christopher's ventilation was discontinued, the nursing staff found themselves overwhelmed by the two siblings dying at the same time. They were ineffective in meeting parental needs or providing effective professional support.

The Need to Shift Gears from Curative to Palliative Intent

Palliative care in the context of an acute care hospital requires formal consideration of the need to shift gears and adjust the mind sets of caregivers. Most caregivers are committed to the concept of cure and see, as their mission, the achievement of cure at almost any cost. Thus, the orientation is toward aggressive intervention. In some contexts, the problem of switching from curative to palliative intent is so vast as to preclude effective palliative care by the same treatment team that has been operating with curative intent. However, there are significant advantages to involvement by members of the same team, providing sufficient resources and skills are added to meet the necessary standards required for palliative care. Continuity of care is a fundamental desire of many families. When the family must face the hardest times, the value of the trust and understanding that has been built up over the months or years of active treatment should not be lightly dismissed. The process of active treatment generates a relationship that is both intimate and contractual, and provides families with the security of knowing that the treatment team has the child's best interests at heart. It may be inappropriate for care to be transferred at such a critical time in the evolution of the illness.

Children too, often express the need for familiarity and are reassured by their continued relationship with the health care team that they have come to trust over the course of their illness. Under some circumstances, however, it must be recognized that a shifting of the mind-set from curative to palliative intent may not be achievable and, under those circumstances, transfer of responsibility of care to a palliative-oriented group may be necessary.

The shift to a palliative mind-set has some very specific implications for the medical care and interventions, including the need to discontinue:

• Routine monitoring of physical signs
• Routine blood work
• All oral medications except those that are essential or necessary for the child's comfort.

Comfort, not routine, should dictate care at this point.

CAREGIVERS, PARENTS AND CHILDREN– THE INTERFACE

The nature of the relationship between the child, the parents, and the external participants can be conceptualized graphically as three concentric spheres (Figure 3). The child is in the center sphere occupying the central role. The child is surrounded on all sides by the sphere provided by the parents and, in a sense, is cocooned by the parental sphere. That cocooning is the normal function that parents fulfill for their children—protecting them from the outside world. This function has many attributes and many advantages for both the child and the parental dyad, but makes enormous demands on the parental dyad.

Outside the concentric parental circle lies the circle of the caregivers, the extended family, the community, and the institution. All access to the child in the inner circle is via the parental circle. Thus, each parent must function as an individual, dealing with individual crises, and as part of a dyad dealing with spousal crises. Each must serve as a gatekeeper at the interface, controlling and modulating access to the child and soliciting and promoting positive influences. The interface is broad and multifaceted and parents and caregivers must interact over a wide range of issues. The wider the range, the greater the potential for discord and conflict.

As the age of the child in the central sphere increases, the integrity of the parental concentric sphere is penetrated more and more by the outside world. The natural evolution of the child into adolescence requires loosening of the concentric sphere and thus access to the dying child is more direct for caregivers and other external influences. This imposes upon the caregivers a greater responsibility to ensure that any direct interaction that they may have with the child is in the child's best interests.

As noted previously, there is a difference between professional advice and competence, and the compassion of a friend. In order to function effectively, professionals must have an organizational

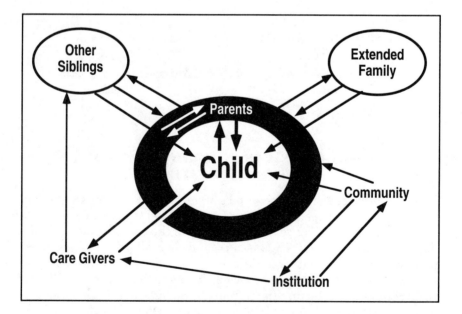

Figure 3. Interaction of participants.

framework within which to work. These organizational frameworks are developed by empiric observation and reformulated into patterns of behavior and routines. Patterns define the general case, not the specific, and carry the great danger of force-fitting the particular to the generic. Professionals are most often used to devising plans, implementing actions, and taking control. The framework within which they work must be constantly examined to ensure that it is adaptable, adaptive, and serves the function for which it is designed. Such routines as ward rounds, medical student teaching at the bedside, and nursing schedules may have to be re-examined in the light of differing functions required in ministering to the dying child as opposed to providing active treatment.

Points of Conflict

In an intense relationship in which there is constant contact between the caregivers and the family, some particular issues that may provide flash points of conflict are identifiable.

Cultural Characteristics

Cultural influences shape attitudes of both providers and parents. Where those cultural backgrounds are widely discrepant, conflict is more likely. Cultural characteristics impose traditional behaviors and social norms on their adherents that are instinctively practiced, but differ widely. For example, Caribbean parents frequently are very directive and often quite physical in their disciplinary behavior with respect to their children. This conflicts sharply with North American views of what is appropriate disciplinary behavior and what constitutes child abuse. In the context of the dying child, this cultural divide is accentuated. Similarly, the cultural mourning practice of loud wails and ululations that is practiced by the Romany and by some Mediterranean groups is very disturbing to caregivers who are used to an Anglo-Saxon practice of grief, especially prior to the child's actual death. As alluded to above, the practice of some cultural groups to perform mourning rituals prior to a child's death when staff is still trying to bring enjoyment into the remaining survival time is capable of generating significant conflict.

Religious Influences

Religious influences differ from cultural influences because they have a belief system attached to them as opposed to a tradition. Belief systems have important intrinsic values in sustaining both caregivers and parents in the difficult task of dealing with the dying. They have the potential, however, to create conflict when individuals attempt, consciously or unconsciously, to impose their religious beliefs upon others. Religious beliefs that bestow serenity and comfort upon one individual may stir anger and distress in another. It is very important that participants in this process not proffer their own religious beliefs as the solution to coping with the process of a child dying, lest it be perceived as an intrusion into a private domain.

Personal Agendas

As discussed earlier, children may fulfill different purposes in parents' lives. For this reason, some parents may manifest behaviors different from the norm and behave differently than caregivers expect. This may cause surprise, consternation, and distress. However, caregivers must accommodate to these behaviors, provided that they do not threaten the well-being of the child. Michael was a five-year-old dying with non-lymphoblastic leukemia. His mother was a forty-one-year-old naturalist who had never weaned him, and at age five, Michael was still suckling. This caused anger and disgust in some of the younger nursing staff. They attempted to change this behavior in the last days of Michael's life. Their efforts were not successful and his mother became extremely distressed.

Decision-making

Decision-making by parents for dying children may involve two potential areas of conflict. One occurs when parents must vest responsibility for the care of their child in caregivers with a resulting loss of the power to make decisions. Frequently, the routines of both the caregivers and the institution preclude routine decision-making by parents about matters that may be viewed as minor, but important. For example, these may include decisions about when to feed their child, and whether or not their child should bathe. The removal of the capacity to make such decisions generates great frustration and particular attention must be paid by caregivers to allow parents to participate in decision-making opportunities whenever possible.

By the opposite token, a culture that has evolved more latterly suggests all points of action are points of decision and parents are viewed as having to make decisions every time there are choices. Parents are often ill-equipped to make complex choices with regard to medical investigations and treatment, especially when the impact of those interventions may be irrevocable. Parents often require clarification as to when they have true choice, and when there are no choices, since the consequence of making a choice is living with the result. Parents who believe that their child suffered unnecessarily due to an incorrect decision they made, will live out their lives with the unnecessary burden of guilt and responsibility.

Ultimately, there needs to be a balance between the needs of children and the needs of the systems that surround them. These include the health care institution, the caregivers, and the familial system. Children have no choice but to be part of the systems that surround them. The obligation of the participants is to ensure that the needs of children are met and not forgotten or submerged in the needs of the systems.

STRATEGIES AND APPROACHES TO MAXIMIZE EFFECTIVE COMPASSIONATE PROVISION OF CARE TO THE DYING CHILD AND FAMILY IN THE HOSPITAL ENVIRONMENT

Fundamental to all strategies and approaches to the care of dying children is the need for caregivers to recognize the pain of parents, the needs of the child to enjoy life to the greatest extent possible in the time remaining, and the necessity to reduce suffering to the absolute minimum. Dying can rarely be an entirely comfortable process, but for a vast majority of children and their families it can be made peaceful and dignified. Parents may need to be advised that some physical characteristics that they perceive to be associated with pain, in fact are not—such knowledge often helps to alleviate subsequent agonizing over their child's final moments. Phenomena such as inspiratory rattling and Cheyne-Stokes breathing ought to be anticipated and explained before they are encountered by the parents.

Strategies and Approaches

1. The early definition of a clear and understandable outline of roles and responsibilities is invaluable. In a sense, this constitutes a contract between caregivers and parents and helps to define the expectations of both sides and what the hierarchy of responsibility will be. While there must be room for extemporaneous development of plans and strategies, parents find it very helpful to have the person in charge identified as the one who should be asked about who will provide which components of information and care. Early in the process it is also helpful to identify limits as to what is or is not possible because defining limits becomes progressively more difficult as death approaches.

Also, it must be understood that rules may change over time. There should be a clear-cut line of responsibility with definition of the most responsible physician and nursing personnel. But it must be understood that as needs change, team members may assume different responsibilities.

Parents must feel comfortable defining their expectations, their needs, and the needs of their child, and the approaches that are acceptable to them. However, they will not be able to define all of these before they have experienced them. The communication must be open enough to permit identification of limits in both directions at any time during the process.

2. There must be respect for difference, and acceptance of divergence by both parents and staff. Quite often, the expectation by the institutional staff is for the child and parents to conform to preconceptions of appropriate behaviors and expectations. There must be room for divergence, both between parents and between caregivers and parents. Quite often in the process of terminal illness, parents begin to diverge from one another. If this is highlighted or emphasized, the possibility exists that the divergence will continue after the child's death and produce separation in a family that might not have otherwise separated.

Divergence between caregivers and parents on the basis of cultural, ethnic, religious, or traditional beliefs must be labeled, identified, and dealt with. It is unreasonable to expect parents to accommodate their traditions and beliefs to the institution's requirements at a time of crisis, unless those beliefs impact destructively on other patients or lie beyond the limits of tolerability that society imposes. One of the most frequent causes of conflict between caregivers and parents is the traditional role of male dominance in many socio-cultural groups. Caregivers experience difficulty when fathers, who have had limited involvement in the care of the child, enter the picture in the dying phase and dictate approaches to care. It must be understood by the caregivers that long after they have been involved with the family, socio-cultural norms may dictate continuation of such behavior and any attempt to modulate it in a time of crisis may render the crisis less tolerable.

3. Areas of potential conflict should be identified early and preemptive action taken to avoid such conflict. Multidisciplinary team discussion involving all levels of medical, nursing, and behavioral professions will most often identify the bulk of potential conflict points and permit strategizing to prevent or temper them.

4. A mechanism for screening and monitoring staff for subsequent burnout and situational stress must be in place. Not all professional

staff can handle ongoing exposure to the dying child and the family with equanimity. Like visiting the sick, handling the dying effectively is comprised partly of learned skills and knowledge and partly of intuitive characteristics. It must be accepted that not all individuals have this intuitive skill and those who do not, should not be compelled to enter into this situation. Even for those who have the skills, situational stress may supervene and after repeated situational stress, burnout may occur. Supervising staff must be watchful for this and receptive to parental feedback. At the same time, it must be appreciated that the needs of parents and dying children are often a bottomless pit that cannot be filled, no matter how many resources and how much skill is utilized. Inability to fill this pit is not necessarily a professional failure, but may be an occupational hazard. Parents, too, have an obligation in this context—to accept what is offered for what it is, appreciate it, and ensure that whatever is positive is allowed to soothe and comfort, and that which is not positive is allowed to slide off without causing undue irritation. Obviously, it is not possible to achieve this ideal at all times, or even at most times. Nonetheless, it is the ideal to strive for.

5. Staff must be helped to tolerate a parent's anger, especially when they believe that it is unjustifiably directed against them. Ongoing assistance in understanding and redirecting anger is of great value, and can facilitate longer tolerance of a difficult, emotional situation. However, it is also acceptable for staff to define their limits and not tolerate aggressive, vituperative, or personally-directed, angry behavior.

6. Staff must not be permitted to introduce personal, religious, or philosophical beliefs into a context of vulnerability. Staff should understand that they are at liberty to use whatever belief systems they wish to maintain their own equanimity, but should not proffer or impose those belief systems on vulnerable parents and family members. Great and continuing resentment can ensue from this.

7. Ongoing decompression opportunities must be provided for staff. They must be encouraged to identify when they are reaching their limits of tolerance and should know that such identification will lead to a change in assignment. The involvement of a behavioral professional to deal with the fears, hopes, and personal difficulties that this kind of intense care raises for staff on a continuing basis, is invaluable.

8. There is great value in identifying for parents the areas and decisions in which choices are possible and those in which there are none. It is a myth of our times that there is always choice and that parents who are provided with adequate information can automatically make a rational and ordered decision. In some contexts, it is preferable

to provide information with a clear recommendation of what is the best course of action. Thus, parents are allowed the option of disagreeing, but are not forced into making a choice or believing that they have made a choice, the consequences of which may be far-reaching and impact on their subsequent adaptation for a long time.

9. The services provided must be multidisciplinary, drawing on the expertise and spheres of knowledge of different disciplines. Perhaps as important as multidisciplinarity is interdisciplinarity—the skill whereby the expertise of one discipline is melded into the expertise of others. Thus children and their families do not suffer as a result of overlapping and repetitive interventions and services. Dying children and their families are vulnerable to the best intentions of many different disciplines who proffer help—it is the responsibility of those disciplines to ensure that their help is complimentary and neither competitive nor overlapping.

The overall goal of the care of the dying child and his or her family is to obtain a balance whereby the comfort and peace of the child is preserved until the moment of death, the hope and self-esteem of the parents is preserved and enhanced, and the potential exists for the testament to the child to become a source of growth and development of the family. From the ashes of the tragedy of a death of a child must come some warmth and substance that will positively influence the lives of the survivors. Optimally, the efficacy and compassion with which terminal care is provided will positively influence the process of healing and growth.

CHAPTER 12

Lessons on Living from Dying Adolescents

Joan M. Auden

While writing this chapter, I found myself immobilized at times by the flood of memories of the many vibrant young people that I have come to know through my work as a pediatric oncology social worker. At first, I reasoned that my immobility was solely the result of grief associated with the loss of those who died. I soon realized that grief was only a partial answer. In fact, I was still absorbing and assimilating the intense life experiences that I have shared with these young people and their families. The lessons are on-going; the learning is continuous and poignant. The meaning of life is gradually unfolding before me. I feel honored.

The provision of psychosocial support for dying adolescents requires an understanding of the complexity of the dependence/independence continuum from birth through adulthood. As well, we must understand and accept the concept of death as the end point of the developmental process, common to us all. If we have not come to terms with our own mortality, we will be limited in what we have to offer.

I have found a number of guidelines helpful over the years in assisting me to remain focused on my role as a consultant and provider of support to young people as they face their illnesses and deal with their limited futures. These guidelines are the outcome of observations from a continuously evolving practice as well as from professional discussions, clinical readings, and conversations with patients. They reflect my approach to social work and provide me with a framework for my participation in the psychosocial care of dying adolescents.

ADOLESCENTS, EVEN WHEN ILL, CONTINUE TO TACKLE MOST OF THE TASKS ATTRIBUTED TO NORMAL ADOLESCENT DEVELOPMENT

The road to independence is a pathway that begins at birth and ends with the attainment of a self-sufficient adulthood. At the culmination of this continuum, the mature adult is able to function with self-reliance in emotional, intellectual, physical, and spiritual spheres. As parents, our role is to prepare our offspring to live independently. In adolescence, parents and other trusted adults become consultants and role models—even when teenagers think and act in direct opposition to the adults in their lives. When an adolescent is dying, the striving for independence does not stop, only the process is altered. While physical dependence is increased, movement toward intellectual, emotional, and spiritual independence continues with the added urgency of the need to complete developmental work in the limited time available.

Intellectual Growth

Intellectual growth is described by Erikson as the "conquest of thought" [1, p. 85]. The young adolescent is capable of using mental operations that are characterized by logical thought, such as formulating hypotheses and constructing strategies, that are not directly derived from personal experience. Yet, adolescence also provides a period in which thoughts, beliefs, and perceptions are tested in the world around them. Adolescents believe that they can attain perfection and that all can be cured. Their own mortality is a distant and even unlikely event. Those who are dying are faced with a premature reality of the world's imperfection. They and their peers are confused by the contrast between their reasoning and previous experience and the present lack of control over the direction of their lives.

Emotional Maturity

Common to all adolescents is the emotional maturity associated with the acquisition of a conscience and moral values. Emotionally mature adolescents have moved away from the self-centered focus of childhood and are now able to consider the feelings and viewpoints of others. For dying adolescents, it is important to recognize that emotional independence may be achieved apart from increasing physical dependence. Acknowledging and fostering emotional independence assists the dying adolescent in achieving emotional maturity, a major milestone of life. In the case examples that follow, Alex and Andrea demonstrate two different perspectives of emotional maturity.

Although, at times, Alex had pushed his parents away in order to fight his health battles himself, he called them to his bedside less than an hour before he died. He asked his mother to lie beside him and to rub his back, just as she had done so many times when he was a child in order to help him go to sleep. He told his father that he could not "do it alone" and asked to be held. In a short time, with his arms around his father's neck and his mother rubbing his back, he relaxed and died. His final step seemed like a very dependent process, but by permitting his parents to participate in this last intimate time with him, Alex demonstrated a reflection of his understanding of their need for this final memory of him—an indication of his emotional maturity. He included their needs with his own in his final step toward ultimate independence.

Andrea was twelve years old when she died. Independence and self-reliance were valued in her family and from early childhood she had insisted on doing everything for herself. She had not slept well for several days prior to her death. At two o'clock in the morning, she sang a funny song that amused her mother, father, and the hospital staff. She then told her parents that she would be fine and asked them to go home for a good night's sleep. Both parents felt uncomfortable with her request but respected her wishes. Ten minutes after they complied, Andrea died. Her chosen method of leaving was one that Andrea had decided would be the most loving and considerate for her family. She knew that this approach was the best one for her parents. Andrea also knew that they would remember her with admiration for her independence of spirit.

Andrea's independence and Alex's dependence both reflected emotional maturity, although they chose opposite ways to portray it.

Spiritual Maturity

Spiritual maturity is perhaps the most difficult aspect of adolescent development to define. The dying adolescent seems to quickly reach conclusions at an intellectual and emotional level about questions relating to death. They gain their understanding of death through normal developmental growth as well as through direct and indirect personal experiences. Direct experiences of death relate to the death of someone they have known, or their own observations of a dead pet or animal. Indirect experiences have been gained through the influence of books, television, movies, newspaper reports, overheard conversations, religious teachings, and parental attitudes. Consequently, all adolescents entering their own dying process, have a unique concept of death. For this reason, even for adolescents who have had strict religious teaching, the concept of death is complex. It behooves us as caregivers to understand and accept this complexity. By the time children have reached their teen years, they understand intellectually that death is irreversible, universal, and inevitable. Yet vestiges of thought processes attributed to children three through eleven years of age, are retained within the spiritual context. These may include such concepts as reversibility associated with the belief in an afterlife, magical thinking (hope for a miracle), and fears associated with the dark, sleep, mutilation, and suffocation. When the complexity of coping patterns are added to beliefs and experiences, it is no wonder that the spiritual domain is so often avoided. In my experience, few adolescents wish to discuss death directly, but when others close to them die, they may need to talk about their thoughts and feelings with someone they trust. Trina was no exception.

> Trina was a young teenager who had difficulty discussing any aspects of her impending death, but was able to discuss the deaths of other patients. For example, Trina cried intensely when Luke died. Both had been diagnosed about the same time and had been hospitalized frequently for extended periods. They had become close friends who could share their thoughts and feelings. When I perched on the end of Trina's bed to talk with her about Luke's death, she threw her arms around my neck and sobbed, "I didn't think Luke would die—now I know I can die too." I asked her to tell me what she thought Luke was going through before he died—what he was thinking and experiencing. I assumed she would be speaking her own thoughts but nevertheless I was surprised by the clarity of her quick response. "I thought Luke was like me—he could handle pain and suffering—and so he would live."

She was voicing her new realization that coping with the disease heroically did not necessarily result in physical survival. She had not been prepared to address this possibility before Luke's death. We were then able to discuss Trina's strong religious beliefs, and her own "knowledge" that Luke was in heaven. During our discussion, I introduced the topic of Luke's spirit living on in us through our memories of him. Trina wrote about Luke in her diary that night. In the morning she told me that there were three memories she had about Luke that were the "essence" of his spirit—he did not take medication without a fuss, he did not want his friends from outside the hospital to see him sick, and he did not complain about pain. I told Trina that if I was to describe her spirit, I would say that "you do take all medicine without a fuss, you put on the cheeriest, happiest smile for your multitude of school friends, and even when you're very ill you keep going." Trina thought a moment, smiled broadly and added, "Yes, and I'm musical, artistic, funny, sweet, good—oh yes, include modest with that too."

ADOLESCENTS RESPOND MOST FAVORABLY TO PEERS, FAMILY MEMBERS, CAREGIVERS, AND OTHERS WHO THEY PERCEIVE TO BE COMPETENT AND HONEST

The most important aspect of psychosocial intervention is the nature of the relationship between dying adolescents and ourselves. As caregivers, we usually meet these young people and their families at the time of diagnosis. We further our relationship during subsequent clinic visits and admissions, thus providing opportunities to understand the interaction patterns of families, to ascertain the ways in which they deal with crises and stress, and to determine the level of maturity of each family member.

When adolescents die, they often make adults, particularly young adults, think about how and when they may die themselves. As caregivers, we are no exception, and when adolescents die, our awareness is heightened. Each death of an adolescent patient becomes unique, special, and emotionally taxing for us as well for the family. When adolescents are dying, I have learned that I must be generous with my time for them and their families. These young people and their families benefit when they are offered options to consider but not decisions, so that they can handle the experience in their own way. Based on knowledge about the disease process, what has transpired during treatment, and what may lie ahead, a helpful approach focuses on anticipating and eliciting questions, helping them to examine problems, and assisting them in selecting the most appropriate ways to alleviate or resolve difficulties. At all times, the domains of parents and adolescents must be respected. Caregivers need to maintain a professional manner and remain honest with young people and their families by admitting mistakes, misunderstandings, or gaps in knowledge.

> Mac was a teen who was newly diagnosed with Hodgkin's disease. I had been in attendance when Mac and his mother were informed of the diagnosis and treatment protocol. Within hours of this news, I went to visit Mac in his room. As I opened the door he asked, "Am I going to die?" "Of course not," was my quick reply.
>
> I immediately realized my error but decided to take some time to work out how to change my answer while still maintaining the high degree of hope associated with this disease. The next morning, I again visited Mac. The following conversation occurred. I asked, "Remember when you asked me yesterday if you are going to die?"

Mac nodded. "Well I answered very badly—can we go back to that statement and let me answer it better?" Again, Mac nodded. "Well, you have a disease call Hodgkin's disease—it is a kind of cancer and you would die if you didn't have treatment. There are now good treatments and very few people die from Hodgkin's disease. At this point it looks as though your chances of living are excellent." "I know," he said, "I had an uncle who died when he was a teenager from Hodgkin's disease because there was not good treatment then." That conversation was eight years ago. Mac is still alive and well. He has since told me that my first answer caused distrust. When I went back, he knew I had been caught off guard and was merely "human." The correction of my error was the beginning of a close relationship between Mac and myself. My honesty also had the effect of teaching others (in this case, other staff members and Mac's parents) a useful and successful method of resolving conflicts associated with misunderstandings or misinterpretations.

Adolescents spend more time in contact with their friends, in person or by telephone, than with adults. Peers are important sounding boards for dying adolescents and so the observations and comments of peers have important implications for the handling of issues such as body image including factors such as hair loss and variations in weight. Peers also can be perceived as competent and honest. As an example, let me tell you about Marcie.

Marcie had a strong group of friends at school. They spent leisure time together in sports activities and "hanging out." She had participated in conversations about hair, weight, clothes, and physical difficulties. Marcie knew very well what her friends did not like or would laugh at. She knew what not to be if she was to be accepted by her friends. What she did not know was how to be accepted upon her return to school. She had changed so much. Now she walked with a limp, had one arm in a sling, and her face drooped on one side. She had also gained weight and lost all her hair.

Marcie was afraid of the rejection by her peers. Only one former friend continued to visit during her hospitalization, furthering Marcie's impression that she was now unacceptable to her former group of friends. I asked Marcie to consider the possibility that it was their own discomfort with what to say and do in the alien environment of the hospital, rather than a rejection of her personally, that had kept them away. With this insight Marcie developed her own plan to help her friends feel more comfortable with her. First, Marcie called her closest friends and asked them to visit her at home so that they could help her return to school. Only one did not comply. The others arrived as a close-knit group of four. Immediately Marcie told them, "Even though I look different on the outside, I'm the same inside." She then asked her friends to help her figure out the best way to protect herself from being made fun of by others. She listened while her friends tossed ideas around.

One suggested that Marcie go to school with them as a group and visit with each of her teachers so they would be comfortable with the changes they observed. She would then return the next day with her friends to begin classes. Another pointed out that their classmates needed education about cancer so that they would not be afraid of "catching it" or fearful of Marcie suddenly dying in class. A third posed the idea that Marcie and her friends could counter any hurtful remarks with comments that would educate their fellow students. All of her friends thought that taking advantage of the school re-entry program[1] to educate teachers and students would be an excellent approach. They joked comfortably about a few wilder suggestions.

Marcie felt supported in choosing the options she wanted. Integrating all of the suggestions worked well at school and increased communication between Marcie and her friends. This communication continued through relapse and Marcie's eventual death. This group of peers, together with Marcie's parents and some hospital staff, became her trusted and competent confidantes. Marcie was able to discuss her own funeral, her fears, and her losses, and she left a legacy of understanding with her friends. By sharing her growing maturity with her peers, Marcie enabled them to understand their own fears and mortality. At the same time, they enriched their own lives by using their talents and empathy to help her. Marcie moved rapidly through her own developmental stages, and brought her friends with her on the journey. None of them will ever forget her.

SEXUALITY REMAINS AN IMPORTANT ASPECT IN THE LIVES OF DYING ADOLESCENTS

One of the important tasks of adolescence is to attain sexual maturity, not just physically but also socially as part of their desire to form a meaningful relationship. Both the illness and therapy impact on adolescents' perceptions of themselves as sexually attractive beings. However, as we have observed in previous stories, the person

---

[1] See Bibliography for information regarding school re-entry programs.

on the inside remains the same. Adolescents retain the same hopes, dreams, and aspirations as other teens, modified by the limited time available to achieve them. Often a social worker who is comfortable in discussing sexuality with these young people will obtain a positive response from adolescents who cannot share these dreams with anyone else.

> Sophia was approaching her fifteenth birthday when she was told that the treatment was no longer effective and the cancer had metastasized to her lungs. One of her first remarks to her mother, after leaving the clinic that day, was one of despair concerning the reality of the limits on her future. She told her mother, "This means I'll never have kids—I always wanted to have kids." By the end of the week she had decided that there were other, more immediate experiences that also seemed to be beyond her realization. Her wish list included three items: tickets for a particular rock concert complete with arrangements for a private meeting with the lead singer; driving a car—not on an empty parking lot but on the street with other drivers; and to date an eighteen year-old neighbor who had, "turned me on from a distance for at least three years." Although she really wanted to make love with him, Sophia did not verbalize this wish but stated instead that she would be satisfied with a date.
>
> By this time Sophia was pale, thin, and bald. She felt very unattractive and believed that she needed a broker to make her wishes come true. Sophia's mother approached the young man and found the attraction had been mutual but he had been too shy to ask Sophia out. A date was arranged. Sophia and her admirer had dinner, went to the concert and met the lead singer. Three days later, the police and motor license bureau collaborated with Young Drivers of Canada to enable Sophia to drive on the street and proudly say, "I'm a good driver."

Just prior to Sophia's death six weeks later, she confided that she had done everything in life that was important to her. She said she had only missed out on having children and a career. Sophia minimized these issues in her own mind by explaining that chemotherapy had probably sterilized her and that she had not even considered a career direction since her diagnosis.

A REVIEW OF LIFE IS IMPORTANT IN THE DYING PROCESS

The word "palliative" refers to the provision of as much comfort as possible during the dying phase of life. I have found that dying adolescents who share stories of their lives through discussion, photo albums, artistic expression, and other media are comforted by the experience and feel more comfortable with themselves. Families who share in the experience may also find meaning in their son's or daughter's life that is heightened by a permanent record, symbol, or collection of special memories.

> When I explained to John that two of his friends had called me because they were afraid they would say or do something that would hurt him, he echoed Marcie's words to her friends. "There are a few things I don't think about any more and there are a few things I don't care about. I don't think about what I'll be when I grow up and I don't care what people wear or look like. But I still have my memories of the good times that I had with my friends."
>
> I relayed the message to John's friends that he would appreciate a visit and that pictures or memories of what they had done together would be the best going away gift they could give him. After a ninety minute visit, John lay back on his pillows exhausted from laughter and reminiscing. He told and retold their stories and smiled until he died three weeks later.

I recognize that it was John who taught me about the importance of reviewing life as part of the dying process.

> A year later, Melissa, aged thirteen, was only days from death. Since she was very agitated, I suggested to her parents that it might be helpful if they told her stories of her childhood. They did, and her agitation subsided. The reviewing of these memories was beneficial to her parents also as it helped them to recognize that they had done the best they could for Melissa, and to understand that her impending death was not their fault. Over the next few days, Melissa talked during every waking moment. At times, she came out of a semi-comatose state to make such statements as, "When I went skiing with Uncle Harold, he put a harness around my waist so I wouldn't go too fast" and "You know Mom, I hated carrots but you were right to make me eat them."

Melissa had made it clear to me that she did not want to discuss "you-know-what." I respected that the topic of her death was not open for discussion, it was the life she had lived that was important. By reviewing her life experiences she was able to help her family accept how valuable her life had been.

SHARING STORIES AND/OR HISTORIES IS AN INTENSE AND EFFECTIVE WAY TO JOIN WITH ADOLESCENTS IN THEIR CURRENT EXPERIENCE, AND TO GAIN MUTUAL TRUST AND RAPPORT

In my work setting, I am fortunate to have the opportunity to follow patients from diagnosis through death and the family's bereavement. This perspective provides the opportunity to develop rapport over an extended period by discussing interests and sharing personal stories.

I am not suggesting that social workers should get into conversations about their personal lives or problems, but a few personal, casual, comments may be helpful. For instance, to the sibling of a dying ten-year-old, I mentioned that my own brother had died when he was ten. To a thirteen-year-old boy, I said, "You must be in grade eight? My son is twelve and he is in grade seven." To another young patient whose mother had died, I commented about my own mother having lost her mother at the same age and how fortunate I was to have had parents living until I became an adult. Through these comments, I join with them in their experiences as a person who has some understanding of their present situation.

During my involvement, I also make use of experiences from the lives of other patients and families. I have learned that their experiences may be especially useful to those who have reached the point where no further treatment will be helpful, as demonstrated in my work with Allison.

> Allison asked me what she could do now that her disease was resistant to every available treatment. Her question reflected both despair and a recognition that she needed coping strategies different from those used throughout her childhood. In reply, I recounted the stories of several young people who has previously faced this trauma. As I explained to Allison, Peter had decided that he wanted no more chemotherapy so that he could feel well during his few remaining weeks. He wanted to paint in water colors. A family friend who taught painting gave him private lessons. Although he was only twelve years of age, Peter displayed mature talent. He had always liked to draw, and his decision to fulfill this dream before he died enabled him to express his hidden creativity.
>
> I also described another situation where Marianne had decided that she was not going to die crying—she had already cried enough. She consulted with a friend who was a movie lover and she watched funny movies for the next few weeks. Without chemotherapy and with lots of laughter, her energy increased enough to enable her to participate more in family activities. Another patient, Susan, used

visualization techniques to imagine herself as a healthy person. She went back to school and became very engrossed in her studies. A return to the magical thinking of childhood helped her to create the life she wanted for herself, however brief.

For Allison, the stories I shared helped her to make her own decisions about what she wanted to do with her remaining time. Adolescents who are facing the failure of treatment continue to use patterns of coping with loss which are the result of their earlier experiences. The caregiver who has become a trusted friend can assist these maturing adolescents to reassess their behavior and seek alternatives when previous approaches are no longer helpful.

CAREGIVERS CANNOT SUCCEED BY IMPOSING PERSONAL VALUES OR EXPECTATIONS ON ADOLESCENTS

Adolescents, who are fully informed of the progress of the disease from diagnosis to palliative care, feel most empowered and are able to attain the greatest level of independence. However, it is important to recognize that adolescents, who have become helpless and frustrated due to the stress of their illness, cannot always be reached, despite the efforts of skilled and supportive staff.

> Moira was a seventeen-year-old adolescent who gave up once she learned her diagnosis. Although she had walked into hospital two days earlier with symptoms that did not appear to be immediately life-threatening, she turned her head to the wall and responded with anger to questions or attempts by staff to care for her. Within three weeks, after refusing treatment, she died of an infection.

Many of the caregivers felt upset by what they judged to be Moira's refusal to even try to fight off her disease. Others expressed despair that she was not communicating in the same manner as adolescents with whom they had worked. Their own expectations resulted in personal feelings of rejection and criticism of Moira rather than an acceptance of her reaction to her own frustration and helplessness.

THE QUESTION BEING ASKED MAY NOT BE THE QUESTION BEING ASKED

The expectation that questions seldom reflect what adolescents and their families want to know is a tenet upon which caregivers should base most of their interactions with them.

For Paula, the question "Am I going to die?" represented a search for a competent and truthful caregiver. When Paula suddenly asked me this question on the second visit, I was tempted to reply, "Of course not." Instead, I told Paula that she did have a life-threatening disease but that she was not ill enough to die at that time.

Three years later, upon relapse, Paula confided in me that she was really asking me if I was honest. Fortunately, I passed the test.

Andrew, on the other hand, asked the same question when he was very sick. For Andrew the question "Am I going to die?" meant "How sick am I?" When I rephrased the question as "Are you asking me how sick you are?", room was left for hope. By reframing, an answer was given that satisfied Andrew's need for hope without deviating from the need to provide him with an honest answer.

WE CAN BE HONEST AND STILL OFFER HOPE THROUGH OUR RESPONSES. WE MUST RESPECT DYING ADOLESCENTS' CHOICES

How can we offer hope when an adolescent is actually dying? Glib answers like "Everyone is going to die" or "I could get hit by a truck any day" are not helpful and underestimate the capacity of most young people to deal realistically with their remaining time.

Mark's leukemia relapsed after he had already battled a second cancer, a brain tumor. This time, remission could not be reached without great difficulty. Consequently, a bone marrow transplant donor had been found. Mark was given his options by his parents. These included: to receive intensive chemotherapy, probably accompanied by long hospitalizations in order to achieve remission for up to a year; to have a bone marrow transplant from an unrelated donor which offered a poor survival rate; or to go home with no further treatment. Mark's parents told him they would support his decision.

Mark chose the third option believing that none of the options would give him long-term survival. He had decided that he wished to enjoy himself. Throughout the last three months, he made comments such as "If I am still here . . ." and "I want you to have your Christmas present now in case I am not here at Christmas." He was well aware that he was dying, but for each day that he lived, he still had hope. Mark had worked with ceramics and pottery, and made gifts for his mother, father, siblings, and extended family. He also wrote a will, filled with thoughtful gestures, that brought tears to the eyes of many. He shrugged off their tears with, "I know you love me and will miss me but I want you to wait until I am gone before you cry."

Each day, Mark set the pace of hope and challenged his family and friends to respond to his wishes. He rewarded them by savoring each day as it came and looking no further than one day into the future. Mark's response was very different from Patrick's.

> Patrick was angry. At sixteen, he was told that his cancer had spread to his lungs. His family's way of dealing with the news was to assure him that he would be going to a better life. They totally refused to discuss the reality of his impending death. Cut off from any control over his life or opportunity to share his feelings, Patrick spent the next six months in angry protest. His only outlet was the writing of stories that were full of the anger and resentment which he was not otherwise permitted to express or to resolve through taking charge of his life.

CONCLUSION

The guidelines described in this chapter are just that—guidelines. They reflect the need to respond to the individual qualities of each dying adolescent. The stories in this chapter give credence to my observation that adolescents are developmentally capable of using their intellectual, emotional, and spiritual maturity to face their own death. These stories also demonstrate the ability of dying adolescents to form relationships that provide support for them throughout the dying process. At the same time, they reflect how difficult it is for adolescents to speak directly about how they think and feel concerning what is happening to them and about their deaths.

I am often asked how I can bear to work amidst so much suffering, grief, and loss. I see my role as empowering dying adolescents to complete their developmental tasks in the brief time available to them. I never cease to marvel at the strength, courage, and maturity that is demonstrated by so many.

I believe that the lessons I have learned from the adolescents who have died are lessons in living. I thank each adolescent I have known for contributing so much to my life.

REFERENCE

1. D. Elkind, Egocentrism in Adolescence, in *Adolescents: Readings in Behavior and Development*, E. D. Evans (ed.), Dryden Press, Inc., Hinsdale, Illinios, 1970.

BIBLIOGRAPHY

Candlelighters Childhood Cancer Foundation Canada, *Candlelighters School Re-Entry Resource Manual*, Toronto, Canada, 1993.

Chambers, A., A. Klinck, and D. Rynard, *Helping Schools Cope with Childhood Cancer: Current Facts and Creative Solutions*, Children's Hospital of Western Ontario, London, Canada, 1992.

CHAPTER 13

Imagery for Children in Pain: Experiencing Threat to Life and the Approach of Death

Leora Kuttner and Cynthia A. Stutzer

As life draws to an end, therapeutic imagery is a gentle, non-intrusive, child-centered, and energy conserving option for children and adolescents in pain and distress. It is said that a picture is worth a thousand words. So too, an image, for those with few words, can convey a great deal when energy is diminished and time is precious. Imagery also offers a meaningful alternate experience when the present reality is fraught with pain, anxiety, fear, and tension. Absorption in an imagery experience can sustain inner strength and self-esteem, and lessen pain, anxiety and terror. It can help a child manage an intolerable situation, and aid in the process of letting go—even in the face of death. Hyde and Watson write:

> Imagery has a power and a gentleness that are consistent with the psyche's best ability to heal itself. Used effectively, imagery is not merely a technique or tool, but indeed is a part of the fabric of psychotherapy, because it is an aspect of the self that (each person) brings to the work, as much as are her words, her feelings and her thoughts. And she learns over time to feel empowered by and even take delight in the creative and healing use of her own images [1, p. 165].

When used for pain control, imagery works synergistically with analgesics to reduce pain and discomfort [2]. As the child's attention and absorption in the imagery increases, the capacity to increase comfort, disassociate from the pain, reduce anxiety, or alter the pain sensations and perceptions becomes greater [3-4]. Olness, an eminent pediatrician and researcher writes:

> Unlike the average adult, the young child may be consciously aware that he can confront, challenge and dispel images of fear through play. In controlled studies our research has documented the abilities of children to control voluntarily certain physiological processes previously believed to be autonomic (such as transcutaneous oxygen, peripheral temperature, and brainstem auditory evoked potential) [5, p. 173].

She continues:

> As children succeed in accomplishing the desired control, they often describe spontaneous images which they used to effect the changes. Images vary from child to child; they are unique and unexpected. We are convinced that understanding the source and nature of the images that trigger the neuro-humoral cascade is more important than the machines to which the children are connected.

As yet, we do not know how imagery effects changes in pain and other physiological factors, but our clinical experience indicates that it is a highly effective way of providing therapy for children and adolescents in distress. In this chapter, through case examples, we will provide general guidelines to describe different ways of using imagery with children who are facing life-threatening illness, are in pain, or are dying.

GENERAL GUIDELINES

Relationships

It is best not to bring in a new health professional during terminal care, but to maintain contact with the people with whom the child is not confortable. An established relationship built on deep understanding and respect, will provide the foundation to choose images that best fit the child's current needs. Be guided by your personal knowledge and previous experience with each child. Allow the methods and styles to vary with developmental age, taking into account cultural and ethnic factors. It is important that flexibility and sensitivity to the child's desire, style, and energy level be maintained throughout the encounter. Non-intrusive support frees the child to enter the experience more fully, without explanation or interpretation.

With continuing illness and fatigue dying children tend to draw into themselves. As they draw inward, reliance on parents often becomes stronger. The working relationship can then shift so that the clinician facilitates the parent-child relationship. For parents who do not know what to say or do when their child is in pain or dying, imagery can provide a framework within which they can communicate, decrease their feelings of helplessness, and create memories to treasure after their child's death. It is a playful, intimate, and life-affirming way of relating to a child when his/her energy is low and when he/she finds it difficult to muster any strength for interactional play. At these times, guided or interactional imagery can be highly nurturing.

We have guided parents in doing imagery, very simply and directly, with their sick child, as illustrated in the following example:

> Tammy was an eight-year-old girl dying of Duchennes Muscular Dystrophy. She was at home throughout the terminal phase of her illness. Several days before her death, Tammy was cranky and restless. Her mother thought she was in pain but did not know how to make Tammy more comfortable and at peace. Over the phone, she was directed to increase the sustained release morphine. Also, Tammy's mother was carefully instructed on how to use deep breathing and images of their previous family camping trips to direct Tammy's attention to a happier time, away from her constant pain. Gradually, Tammy's anxiety began to lessen. Her mother felt relieved that she was still able to help her daughter. The imagery provided a bridge for the mother to then say what she had longed to say to her daughter: "We will always remember you . . . We will always love you . . . You will always be a part of our family."

Assessment

It is important to conduct an ongoing and thorough assessment of the child's clinical condition, including altered levels of consciousness and receptivity. Although imagery can be used even when consciousness is clouded, remaining responsive to these differing states is important because they are diagnostically relevant. This includes paying close attention to the child's facial expressions and body movements throughout the imagery experience.

An assessment should also include particular image experiences that the child prefers, dislikes, and wishes to avoid. For example, if the child is afraid of the water, movement imagery such as "swimming with the fishes" would be counter-productive. Information from the parents or other family members can help the clinician gain a better understanding of the images that will enhance meaning and provide therapeutic impact.

Starting Out

Imagery is a natural process for all of us, but particularly for children aged three to seven whose cognitive boundaries between fantasy and reality remain quite fluid. These children move easily into, "Let's imagine . . ." or "Let's draw a picture . . . ," as easily as they move into playing, "Let's pretend . . ." These familiar and comfortable introductions make it easy to engage this age group in imagery.

Older children may need a little more formal introduction or invitation, such as, "Let's go into your imagination . . . ," or "Let's use your imagination to . . . ," or "Do you want to try to use your imagination to change what is happening . . ."

It is advisable to choose a quiet place and ensure that there will be no interruptions during the session. There are three ways in which imagery can be initiated:

1. Imagery can be spontaneous—generated freely by the child, or by asking:
   "What would you be doing now if you were at home?"
   "I'd be playing baseball."
   "You can play baseball right now in your mind . . . close your eyes . . . that's it . . . tell me what's happening?"
   "I'm taking my time up at bat . . ."
2. Imagery can be controlled by taking the spontaneous image and using it in a more controlled way to free or release the child. (Refer to page 259 for the example of the boy who could not talk.)
3. Finally, the clinician can suggest a specific image or scene in a guided format. Children can choose to go along to experience, discover, and develop a clearer relationship with their inner world. As an example:

   > In her final hours of life, Tracy, a seven-year-old girl, was in a light coma. Although her pain appeared to be well managed, Tracy's facial expression indicated pain and anxiety—her brow was wrinkled and her mouth was open and turned down. Knowing that "taking her to the beach" was an image that had, in the past, evoked a strong relaxation response and reduced her anxiety and pain, Tracy was invited to "come to the beach and feel the easing warm sun . . ." As the familiar image unfolded, Tracy's facial expression relaxed. Her brow smoothed out, her mouth closed, and her lips turned up. She retained that peaceful expression until her death, five hours later.

The Therapist's Position

In working therapeutically with children, the image and analogy that Kay Thompson [6] proposes offers us a helpful image to hold on to. She suggests that therapists think of themselves as automobile mechanics and their patients as "cars brought in for repair." This image enables the therapist to work with what the patient brings. The task is to promote and enable smoother and better performance. She elaborates:

> Mechanics listen to the car and then fine-tune it, not taking anything away but working with and modifying what is there—perhaps using different lubricants for different speeds, reducing discords, or removing the grating of metal on metal . . . We can teach the owner how to remove rust and put in softer upholstery . . . But, as the image implies, after all the skilled service is completed, "it is still the client who ultimately will drive the car and determine the desired destination" [6, p. 249].

The confidence to drive will come from guidance, frequent practice, feedback, and adjustment to increase the level of competency. The more competent the patient feels in driving her own car, the more responsibility she will take, and the greater the therapeutic benefit.

When imagery is developed during earlier admissions to hospital, it becomes a source of competency and strength for the child facing life-threatening illness, and can become an extra therapeutic aid during more difficult times:

> Mary was diagnosed at thirteen years of age with acute myelogenous leukemia. In the beginning, she experienced severe side-effects from chemotherapy, including extreme nausea and abdominal pain. She loved Pachelbel's Canon, which she associated with her mother who had died two years previously. As the music played, Mary was invited to settle in her bed, close her eyes, breathe deeply to release any tension, and then leave the hospital "to go to the sea, where the rhythms of the waves, like her breath, allowed the pain in her tummy to settle like the sand at the bottom of the ocean." She softly said that she was feeling closer to her mother. Mary's anxiety and nausea subsided quite rapidly, despite the fact that, to her distress, she had envisioned herself on the beach with no swimsuit on! In subsequent encounters, through further chemotherapy and a bone marrow transplant, her music and sand and sea imagery continued to calm and comfort Mary and fuel her confidence.

This imagery provided Mary with a framework for coping with future painful and distressing experiences. When a septic infection sent her to the intensive care unit, she stated, boldly and openly, that she had a vision of heaven complete with white light and angels. It was clear to us that this image brought her great strength as she faced her bone marrow transplant. Her music along with her imagery of sea and heaven became an established part of how she managed her day, even when she was sent to the intensive care unit for the final time.

Getting the Most out of the Experience

If skillfully and sensitively handled, imagery is rarely, if ever, frightening or disturbing. The child's experiences can be surprising, helpful, illuminating, and informative. For the dying child, in particular, the discoveries can be transformative and powerful in shedding the apprehensions that are common to families and children who are profoundly ill.

In our clinical experience, the child who is dying appears to be particularly receptive and responsive to imagery. In order to draw the most out of the imagery experience the following four factors are important.

1. Draw on All the Senses

For example:

visual — "I wonder what you can see when you turn the corner?"

auditory — "Notice what sounds there are here" or "Now listen to what this person is going to say to you."

olfactory — "There is a strong familiar smell, a smell you know so well, what is it?"

gustatory — "There may be a taste there too, what does it remind you of?"

touch — "How does it feel?" or "What is going on in your body right now?"

2. Guide the Image

Gathering the child's experience can be left to the end of the session for "debriefing." Alternately, it may be helpful to the process to invite the child to describe what is happening as inner events unfold. This allows a gentle, slow-paced dialogue to be woven into the imagery experience, and can be encouraged through questions such as, "And what is happening now?" If further elaboration of the event is needed, you can ask, "What do you hear, see, smell, or taste now?"

If the child, for one reason or another, prefers not to talk, this must be respected. Flexibility and sensitivity are essential in providing support to the child.

3. Monitor the Impact of the Imagery Intervention

The child's desire, interest, style, and energy level must be maintained throughout the encounter. It is advisable to pay close attention, since both the child's nonverbal and verbal behaviors are equally important. Behaviors include facial expressions, position, and movements of the child's body throughout the experience. From the previous example, Tracy provided only nonverbal clues to her inner experience. Monitoring her physical changes indicated her increasing involvement in the imagery and the relief that it provided. If there is the sense that something is amiss, check with the child: "Is this okay with you?" or "Is this how you imagined it to be?" The supportive interaction provided by the clinician frees the child to enter the imagery experience more fully and obtain relief.

4. Use Dreams

Days, weeks, or even months before their death, children who are dying often have vivid dreams. Sometimes these dreams are images of heaven, God, or angels. Descriptions of near death experiences by children corroborate our experiences [7]. These dream images can be used in a controlled way to lead the child to greater peace as death approaches. Sometimes children experience frightening and dark images. By accepting these and working with them the child's fears are expressed and he/she becomes more open to possible resolution.

> David was thirteen years old and dying of a bone tumor. Though he had not talked much about his impending death, he started having dreams one month before he died. He dreamed of heaven, "all white, even the trees . . . even a white hot tub!" He revealed this image only to his mother who related it to the staff. David was also troubled by darker dreams, "something bad happens to my family—I don't know what." When the clinician broached these dreams with him, he firmly stated, "I don't want to go back into that dream!," and refused to talk. It was suggested to his mother that, on those nights when he had difficulty sleeping, she gently ask him about the heaven images so that he knew they were acceptable. Although David never talked about the darker dreams again, he seemed to derive some comfort from his mother's invitation, and experienced no further disturbing dreams. At a later time, the

clinician drew on these darker, scary images to explore David's fears of dying (see page 260).

How to Prepare Yourself

Working with dying children can be immensely rewarding, but it can take an emotional toll. The challenge rests in balancing your therapeutic responsiveness to the needs of the child with the personal grief that this experience evokes. During this process track the reactions of the child and family—as well as your own. Choose an appropriate time and situation in which to express and explore the impact of your experience and emotions with your colleagues. Carrying an emotional burden can hamper your therapeutic effectiveness—work to keep a balance.

We have noted that there are particular times when the dying child is more open to confiding in a trusted professional as he/she grapples with life-death concerns. These "windows" are not predictable; they may be fleeting and infrequent. Since they may be your only opportunity to respond to and address such profound issues, it is important to gently meet the challenge, even if you may not feel "ready."

Because hospitals tend to be noisy and filled with many distractions, it is important to establish a place and set aside time that are free of distractions and interruptions in order to do the imagery work. We have found that it is best if one does not feel too harried or distracted by other matters. The ability to concentrate on the child and the unfolding experience, as well as to center oneself in that process, is paramount in creating full therapeutic benefit for the child.

Imagery within a Busy Hospital

A hospital can be a very non-restful place for children and adolescents and can interfere with their ability to cope. In the following example, imagery became the route to creating a restful environment for one adolescent in pain by providing her with a meaningful focus and a way of actively participating in resolving what was happening.

Fifteen-year-old Jamie was having a difficult time sleeping in the hospital though she was on appropriate intravenous analgesics. The bone pain from her Ewings sarcoma, intravenous pumps with alarms, bright lights, interruptions at night, and her own active mind, all contributed to her insomnia. She was apprehensive about imagery, but agreed to discuss its possibilities. After exploring several options with her, Jamie agreed to listen to relaxing music to help calm and focus her mind and to see what images came to her. She saw her hip as a throbbing red fire-ball, hot and burning, emitting spurts of fire down her leg and across her pelvis (this is nerve pain). Together we chose this imagery: We imagined making snow balls and throwing them on the fire . . . one after the other. The quenching of the pain began slowly. Her growing comfort was enhanced by the clinician massaging her feet so that she could focus on the pleasant non-painful sensations in her body. After approximately ten minutes the combination of pain-relieving methods began to work for Jamie. The session was audiotaped for her with the music she had chosen playing in the background. Jamie used the tape throughout her hospitalization and at home. She told us that it took her away from the hospital, its noises, and her "achiness." After many weeks it worked so well that she often fell asleep before she was aware of any images.

Imagery in Difficult Situations

There are occasions when clinicians must make assumptions about a child's experience, because the child is unwilling or unable to communicate. In these situations, foreknowledge of the child and his/her behavior is imperative in order to use imagery as a means of connecting and helping the child transform his/her distress.

David, the thirteen-year-old who was dying of a bone tumor, had battled cancer for eight years: first, a rhabdomyosarcoma in the right maxillary sinus, and subsequently, an osteosarcoma in the radiotherapy field. He had always been a quiet boy, picking and choosing his confidants, but never revealing too much of his innermost thoughts and feelings. Over the course of eight months, David's tumor remained localized but expanded over his face, pushing his right eye outward, and growing down through the hard, and later soft, palate. Toward the end of his life it was virtually impossible to understand him when he talked. Until the day before he died, David chose not to discuss any aspect of his impending death. It took these eight months to build a trusting relationship with David, answering the few questions he posed, giving information when necessary, and supporting him as his symptoms, especially pain, worsened. As his last hours approached, David's fear and anxiety overcame his natural reserve. In an emotional display of tears, David requested to see the clinician. Realizing that the more conventional way of allowing the child to express fears, anxieties and, later, therapeutic images would not work with him, the clinician drew on her knowledge of the needs of dying children, her experience and, most importantly, her relationship with David:

CS: I heard you wanted to see me.
D: (nod; closes eyes)
CS: You look tired, David.

D: (nod)

CS: But it seems like there is something else going on. Is there?

D: (nod; tears fall from his one eye)

CS: Do you want to talk to me about it?

D: (nod; says something that the clinician cannot understand)

CS: Are you afraid, David?

D: (nod)

CS: Are you afraid of dying?

D: (nod)

CS: Do you want to try some things to help you relax; to help make the fear go away?

D: (nod)

CS: I know you have some music that you have been listening to. Shall we put that on?

D: (nod; clinician plays David's soft music)

CS: David, I want you to close your eyes and listen to the music.

D: (Closes his eye. Facial expressions are difficult to read since the tumor has invaded most of his face. His brow is furrowed, one side of his mouth is turned down, his eye is closed. He is lying on his side, knees and arms drawn up.)

CS: Are you feeling the fear now, David?

D: (nod)

CS: Sometimes when we feel fear, our bodies feel it too. Sometimes our stomach feels like it is in a knot. Does yours?

D: (nod)

CS: Sometimes our muscles get tight, so tight they almost ache.

D: (nod)

CS: . . . and our head hurts. Are you experiencing these things David?

D: (nod)

CS: Picture your fear as a big ball in the pit of your stomach, a black one.

D: (frowns)

CS: Is that how you imagine your fear to be?

D: (Shakes his head)

CS: Tell me how the fear looks to you, David.

D: Like a cloud, a dark storm cloud.

CS: So, the fear is like a dark storm cloud. Does it fill up your body?

D: (nod)

CS: And, does it make all the muscles tense and does it put knots in your stomach?

D: (nod)

CS: Well, David, you know that clouds have no substance; they're not solid at all. They are just wisps of air, really! You are stronger than those wisps, David. And wisps can't hurt you. I want you to close your eyes and picture dark, ugly storm clouds in the sky. Picture a bright blue sky, with the storm clouds coming closer. You know there are two ways to get rid of storm clouds. One way is for the wind to blow them away—one wisp at a time. You can break up those storm clouds, David. Let the music be carried on the wind. Let it enter your body and carry those wisps away. Let the music surround your body, and lift it up, and carry your body. Can you feel it enter your body?

D: (nod)

CS: David, let it enter all the places where the fear is and allow the music to blow the fear clouds away. (Pause for almost a minute). Can you feel the music enter your body and surround your body?

D: (nod)

CS: Are some of the fear clouds gone?

D: (nod)

CS: You know there is another way that clouds in the sky disappear. When the sun shines on them, they evaporate. Picture in your mind a soft, bright white light entering your body and evaporating the fear clouds. The light shines on you and in you. It feels warm, and soft, and good. And wisp by wisp, it evaporates the fear clouds while the music blows some more wisps away. Can you feel that?

D: (nod)

CS: You are stronger than the wisps of clouds, David, and you are stronger than the fear. Fear and clouds cannot run your life. You are stronger than they are. David, what has happened to the fear now?

D: Gone.

CS: David, you are stronger than the fear. Listen to the music for a while and let it carry you . . . relax into the music and the light.

The Diagnostic Value of Imagery

Over time, children who have used and relied on imagery to ease their discomfort often develop a strong "inner sense" and great sensitivity to their body signals. They use imagery as an internal scanner, building up greater self-reliance in coping with their failing bodies. This is certainly not for every child or adolescent, however, for those who need greater self-control, this method will foster that goal. For example:

Diagnosed three years ago with Ewings Sarcoma, fifteen-year-old Judy had a difficult course of medical treatment, including surgery to remove a cancerous rib, chemotherapy, and a recent bone marrow transplant that she found to be a harrowing experience.

Through these years, particularly while in isolation during the transplantation, she developed her ability to relax and use sensory-based imagery. She would lie down, focus on her breath, and study it with all of her attention as it moved in, circled around her body, and then moved out. She did this until she was able to allow the pain in her body to become more distant from her mind. At that point, she would begin to go from the top of her head, down her scalp, and systematically through her body, focusing on each part that needed easing and release from the pain. She had practised and perfected this simple technique which she called "my scanner." Judy would insist on a quiet room, no interruptions, and the freedom to do it by herself. She loved the feeling of independence during this process and how it calmed her. One of the benefits of this self-regulatory technique was that she became very aware of how each part of her body felt, the typical body sensations, and what they meant. This enabled her to speak, with greater authority, to the staff. On one occasion, she came into the clinic and said that she had back pain:

LK: What kind of pain?

J: It feels like a deep aching kind of pain.

LK: Have you ever felt it before?

J: I've felt this kind of pain before, but not in this part of my back and it's . . . scary.

LK: Why does it feel scary, Judy?

J: Because it feels different.

LK: Let's check it out using your scanner.

J: (laid down on the bed, closed her eyes, and exhaled)

LK: Judy, take your time and ease into that familiar comfort zone that you know so well. Let me know when you are ready to use your scanner.

J: (after a few minutes, nods her head)

LK: Take your scanner through your body, checking and easing, and let me know when you get to the troubling part in your back. Tell me what you sense and see.

J: It's different, sort of dense . . . I don't know . . . hotter and swollen . . I don't like it.

For Judy this discovery was very frightening. Her oncologist saw her and immediately ordered a bone scan. To the surprise and dismay of the whole team, metastasis to her lumbar spine, well below the original surgery site was found. Judy continued to use her relaxation and imagery in a quiet and personal way throughout the remaining eighteen months of her life. Her technique had become fully integrated into her way of coping, calming her, and helping her maintain self-control.

Imagery work will be effective only if the therapist is able to stay out of the child's way. In the words of Naida Hyde:

> The therapist who needs to understand, control, lead, direct and make sense out of everything presented by the client will soon shut down the process, being left with a rebellious client, an overly compliant client, or no client at all. The therapist must have a deep and sustaining belief in the client's right to her own self-discovery—and must practice this belief! [1, p. 171].

In particular, this respect is called upon when a child or adolescent is struggling with his/her impending death.

Expect the Unexpected

When using imagery with children, it is helpful to remain open for surprises. Sometimes the images may inform you of something other than what the child has been saying, and in those instances, can lead to a greater understanding of the real story.

> Angela, a bright twelve-year-old, had cystic fibrosis. On opioids for a high level of pain, and in distress, Angela spoke of all she had to live for and how much she believed that she could fight this disease and live. She wanted to use imagery to help her mobilize, keep active, and as well as possible. I invited her to close her eyes and make herself comfortable — to take three cleansing breaths and let the breath go through her body.

> LK: Let's go to a comfortable place, a place where you can let go, and be comfortable, and at ease. Nod your head to let me know when you are there.
>
> A: (nod)
>
> LK: Good. Notice clearly where you are, what is around you, what sounds you hear, and what smells there may be. Let that become clearer and stronger for you in this, your comfort place. Take your time and let it become clearer to you. When that happens, nod your head.
>
> A: (nod; her respiration becomes slightly deeper and more regular)
>
> LK: Now, it will be very easy for you to let me know where you are in this place, your comfort place. Where are you, Angela?
>
> A: I'm sitting on the pavement.
>
> LK: You're here on the pavement and what is nearby or around you?
>
> A: There are some big high gates . . . right here . . . I'm sitting here next to them.

> LK: What is the color of the gates?
> A: They're white.
> LK: How is it for you here?
> A: Okay . . . I'm just waiting.
> LK: Waiting for . . . ?
> A: The gates to open . . .

An image is worth a thousand words. The image of Angela's body sitting on the pavement in front of the big white gates said much more about the truth of her inner experience than any discussion about how she was facing death. It also revealed more than Angela was consciously aware of at that point in time. Her imagery wiped away all her words of protest about fighting her disease and wanting to live. Her waiting posture said that she was expecting to die quite soon and that she was psychologically, spiritually, and physically ready to make that transition. Her imagery clarified that her earlier statement, "I want to fight," may have been what she thought she had to do, or what was expected by the hospital staff and her family—but not truly what she felt able or willing to do.

Her imagery was implicitly religious in that it represented the popular Christian image of Heaven's pearly white gates, and conveyed that her religion was giving her comfort now. "It was okay," she added. She expected that soon "the gates would open" and she would be allowed in. Death was not scary for her, it was a natural transition into heaven.

IN CONCLUSION

Imagery is a gentle, yet powerful way of joining with a child or adolescent in the process of managing a life-threatening illness or helping the child approach death. It is not as intrusive as direct, continual questions or discussion with a child who is tired, yet wanting some contact with others who are close. If used frequently, it becomes a special kind of contact between the clinician and the child. It can also be a source of play, and provide comfort and nurturance at a time when activities are restricted and the child's energy is diminished.

Imagery is more than pictures in one's mind. It can be elaborated and enhanced by the senses of smell, touch, hearing, and taste and lead to journeys of discovery and delight. Imagery can make the losses, such as the need to use a wheelchair, or the transitions, such as hospitalization, easier to handle for children who are gravely ill. As a link with the child's inner process, imagery can release the kind of energy that lifts the spirit even as death awaits.

REFERENCES

1. N. D. Hyde and C. Watson, Voices from the Silence: Use of Imagery with Incest Survivors, in *Healing Voices: Feminist Approaches to Therapy with Women*, T. Laidlaw and C. Malmo (eds.), Jossey-Bass, San Francisco, California, 1990.
2. P. A. McGrath, *Pain in Children: Nature, Assessment, and Treatment*, Guilford Press, New York, 1990.
3. L. Kuttner, Favourite Stories: A Hypnotic Pain-Reduction Technique for Children in Acute Pain, *American Journal of Clinical Hypnosis 30*:4, pp. 289-295, 1988.
4. L. Kuttner, Management of Young Children's Acute Pain and Anxiety during Invasive Medical Procedures, *Pediatrician, 16*, pp. 39-44, 1989.
5. K. N. Olness, Little People, Images and Child Health, *American Journal of Clinical Hypnosis, 27*,3, pp. 169-174, 1985.
6. K. Thompson, Metaphor: A Myth with a Method, in *Brief Therapy: Myth Methods and Metaphors*, J. K. Zeig and S. G. Gilligan (eds.), Brunner-Mazel, New York, 1990.
7. M. Morse and P. Perry, *Closer to the Light: Learning from Near Death Experiences of Children*, Villard Books, New York, 1990.

BIBLIOGRAPHY

Dienstfrey, H., *Where the Mind Meets the Body*, Harper-Collins, New York, 1991.
Epstein, G., *Healing Visualizations: Creating Health through Imagery*, Bantam Books, New York, 1989.
Gersten, D. J. (ed.), *Atlantis*, The Imagery Newsletter, 4016 Third Ave., San Diego, California, 92103, 1988 to present.
Leick, N. and M. Davidsen-Nielsen, *Healing Pain, Attachment, Loss and Grief Therapy*, Tavistock/Routledge, London and New York, 1991.
Murdock, M., *Spinning Inward*, Shambhala Publications Inc., Boston, Massachusetts, 1987.

CHAPTER 14

When Truth Hurts . . .

John T. Maher and Eleanor G. Pask

> Tell all the Truth but tell it slant—
> Success in Circuit lies
> Too bright for our infirm Delight
> The Truth's superb surprise
> As Lightning to the Children eased
> With explanation kind
> The Truth must dazzle gradually
> Or every man be blind—
> —Emily Dickinson, *Poems*

A BRIEF HISTORY OF TRUTHTELLING

Long before, and certainly during the period of so-called "modern medicine," lying was a common and well-accepted practice by those who exercised the healing arts. In the western world, kings, generals, and clergy dominated a populace in which superstition and ignorance bowed to the directives of alchemists, barbers, shamans, and herbalists. It was well understood by these medical forefathers that words could wound as surely as any blade, and that belief in proferred cures was often the key to efficacy. In short, what was said mattered as much as what was done.

The assumed importance of withholding terrible news from a patient is well illustrated by the fact that "Died of Fright" persisted as a common medical diagnosis through to the nineteenth century [1]. There was no doubt among physicians that information should be withheld if harmful consequences could be anticipated. Ignorance, it was believed, sustained patient hope. Limits on disclosure also meant that the physicians could preserve their own personal comfort and avoid the unpleasantries and added professional demands that attended honest revelation.

As we moved into the twentieth century new pathophysiological discoveries altered the view of medicine. For example, the emergent "germ theory" led to a narrowing of medicine's focus; disease models evolved which regarded illness as being causally independent of emotions and feelings. This was, in effect, a movement away from the seemingly naive "holistic" perspective that had guided medicine for centuries. As a consequence, some concerns related to the dangers of truthtelling were pushed aside [1].

The conceptual separation between mind and body did not significantly alter day-to-day communication patterns; physicians still treated patients with due appreciation of the likelihood that state of mind somehow affected disease outcome in more than insignificant ways. They continued to lie but their justifications were now slightly different. It was claimed that patients could not understand the new and sophisticated information, and that doctors still knew best how to protect them from unnecessary worry; benevolent paternalism perdured.

The 1950s appear to have been the decade when some physicians began to challenge what was euphemistically known as "therapeutic privilege." Generally, the patient's desire to know and the physician's decision to inform were thought to be contingent upon the nature of the patient-physician relationship, the patient's mental or physical state, the physician's personal "style," and the presence of problems within the family.

By the 1960s, truthtelling, though still not widely practiced, was viewed as a more acceptable option for many physicians [2]. Western society (especially in North America) has since witnessed a sustained evolution in truthtelling philosophy and practices in the adult domain; lying to patients is now more the exception than the rule.

The more contemporary policy of honesty within medical culture represents a complex shift that is inextricably linked to broader social and scientific values. In part, it relates to the emergence of a consumeristic and humanistic ethos that challenges paternalism with claims of patient rights and autonomy, both being rooted in a respect for each patient's intelligence. The new policy also relates to the growing interest in, and demands of, medical ethics [3].

Improved technologies, better understanding of disease processes, and most significantly, new treatment options forced this issue even further: patients must be informed in order to make decisions along the illness trajectory.

We now have some relatively sophisticated sociological and psychological tools that have been used to garner information concerning patients' desires for truthful information, and their preferred patterns of disclosure. These same tools have been used to determine whether truthtelling is psychologically harmful; it almost never is.

Despite the fact that we are now better able to offer answers to the questions concerning psychological harm, some questions related to physical harm are re-emerging with a new vigor. Adult patients generally want and cope well with the truth, but does what others say determine whether, or how fast, they heal? Our knowledge of placebo effects, our growing understanding of the biology and biochemistry of mental states, and the work of newer subspecialty disciplines such as psycho-neuro-immunology, will continue to influence how health professionals communicate with their patients.

The social backdrop to all of this physiological and clinical research is the resurgence of holistic medicine and its attendant philosophy that forcefully reminds us of the dangers of a false dichotomy between mind and body.

THE FOCUS OF THIS CHAPTER

Do we tell the truth to dying children? In the remainder of this chapter the reader will find some relevant theoretical considerations, and arguments and evidence in support of truthtelling. You will not find a detailed formal ethical analysis of truthtelling; such theoretical work has been better done elsewhere. However, there is some discussion of four useful ethical principles, more by way of illustration than as part of a sustained philosophical argument. The chapter also contains a review of some pragmatic concerns and concludes with advice on how to tell the truth.

This chapter does not deal directly with any of these issues: child competence, pediatric medical decision-making, informed consent (or assent), or conflict between the wishes of caregivers and children. Indirectly, however, it addresses all of these matters insofar as they are rooted in common issues of communication and information flow.

Also excluded is any formal discussion of family system dynamics in relation to truthtelling. This important piece of a comprehensive exploration of the topic merits its own thorough treatment in a separate chapter.

For someone who is new to the issue of truthtelling it is hoped that there will be some food for thought. For others who have already struggled with this matter and adopted a position, it is hoped that you will be supported or challenged.

A WORD OF CAUTION

This chapter frequently uses the terms "lie" and "liar." It is important to note that the colloquial use of these terms carries an inescapably negative connotation that the academic use may not. It must be made clear that an objective description of an act of lying tells you nothing about whether the act itself is good or bad. What is needed to determine the morality of the act is an ethical analysis of intent, context, and outcome. For example, a person who lied to would-be murderers about the whereabouts of their intended innocent victim may have performed a morally good act. The question here is whether parents who lie to their children may, in a similar manner, be performing a truly virtuous act.

In seeking to tackle this difficult question head on, there is a risk of alienating some readers. There is a natural hesitancy to label a loving or good act as a lie; yet there are no other terms available that accurately identify the acts that need to be analysed. Therefore, in this debate, caution, and a clear understanding of the moral neutrality of the terms are required in order to avoid the danger of prejudiced labelling of parents.

ABOUT INFORMATION

Truthtelling is contingent on the flow of information, and we all know that information can be used to do harm or good; its use is a therapeutic option [4]. We offer clinical information to reduce uncertainty (and its attendant anxiety), to provide a basis for action by the patient/parents, and to improve the therapeutic relationship between the health professional and patient/parents [3]. As Cassell suggests:

> Information has many facets—it has an amount, it can be spare or full. It has a kind—technical information, information about the future, information about medication. There is a degree of detail—how specific, how minute the detail to be provided. There is timing—when is information provided? It could be given at a time when a patient is unable to hear it because of his sickness or for other reasons, or it could be provided at a time too late to allow the patient to act. It has truth content—but truth content is only one aspect [3, p. 126].

WHAT DOES IT MEAN TO LIE?

If the information you offer someone does not have truth content, then either you are mistaken, or you are lying. Classically, lying means having a particular thought or belief in one's mind and uttering another with the intention to deceive. However, it is a moral act that can take many forms and these should be recognized by health professionals. Some forms of lying are:

- withholding information that the patient has a right to hear or wants to hear (lie of omission),
- delaying the provision of information knowing that such a delay may affect the outcome of the decision,
- giving true information in such a way that you know it will be misunderstood by the listener (i.e., jargon, euphemisms),
- giving incomplete information (i.e., evasiveness, lack of adequate detail, not educating the patient to the necessary level),
- offering probable information as certain fact (or vice versa),
- providing information at a time when you have reason to suspect the patient may be mentally or emotionally impaired,
- presenting all the relevant information accurately, realizing or suspecting that the listener has not understood, and then doing nothing to further clarify the situation,
- using tone or authority to inaccurately characterize information (e.g., presenting subjective value judgements as though they were objective medical judgements),
- providing a hopeful statistical prognosis to the exclusion of a dire personal prognosis [5].

It is also important to note that the distinction between truth-telling and being truthful is the difference between content and intent. For example, a person can tell the truth with the intention of accomplishing some broader deception; this is frequently referred to as manipulation.

Ethicists distinguish between lying (i.e., saying something false) and intentional deception (i.e., withholding information) [6]. Some maintain that doctors should not lie but may knowingly deceive in other ways. However, if the intended outcome is the same, then these might be viewed as morally equivalent acts that merely have been expressed in different ways [7]. From a consequentialist perspective, the most significant difference between the two is that lying, if discovered, will likely undermine trust more than withholding information, and accordingly, is more dangerous from a relationship maintenance viewpoint.

A DIFFERENT CONCEPTUAL SLANT
ON TRUTHTELLING

What follows may be obvious to health professionals immersed in their practices. Regardless, it needs to be stated that the academic literature heretofore has argued the ethical question from a perspective that was too narrow.

The traditional view of an act of truthtelling is the delivery of a discrete packet of information using words as the primary medium (i.e., statements). We believe or pretend that it is a framed event, isolated in time, and independent of all but immediate context. But the real world should not be approached in this manner. The moral target in clinical settings is never just a single endpoint. Rather, it is a series of interim points that are on a broad and contextually modifiable pathway.

One lie makes you a liar, but one truth does not make you a truthteller. Truthtelling is a continual flow or process whose expression takes on many forms: words, touch, body language, and absence. Truthtelling is not "all or none" but rather "some and some more."

Understanding and adaptation occur over time, and within and through a complex network of relationships [8]. Most significantly, truth is, in part, a self-supplanting subjective construct born out of, and into, a unique personal history [4]. That is to say, we each make and re-make our own truths.

SHOULD CHILDREN BE TREATED
DIFFERENTLY?

Children are not just "small adults." They should be treated differently because they have distinct moral status by virtue of their different intelligence levels, maturity, and functional competence.

In everyday life, children are excused or protected from adult pressures or concerns. Why would we look at medical information and therapeutic decisions differently? Adults may have an obligation to know the truth, but do children, especially when they are not allowed to make their own medical decisions, even if they are informed?

As a society we systematically and selectively support certain benevolent lies to our children (e.g., Santa Claus and the Tooth Fairy). Does this mean that we may lie to children generally? Clearly not, but as adults we give ourselves permission to lie to young children when they cannot understand complex information or when the lie produces an obvious benefit. Younger children seem more appropriate and easier targets of deception because of their limited competence. As they mature, a parent's duty is to inculcate values of honesty that they must endorse by word and example. Yet, even if we agree that we should tell the truth to older children, the question that still remains is whether we might lie with impunity, particularly to sick or dying children.

The inherent vulnerability of sick children seems to count as justification for withholding information, or even lying to them for their protection. The three common reasons offered for lying to children are: 1) they will be harmed by the truth; 2) they are unable to understand the information; and 3) they do not want to hear the truth.

If lying is acceptable then presumably the most successful approach should be used. This might entail health professionals lying to parents in order to eliminate the possibility of inconsistent parental behaviors or to prevent unwanted revelations to the child. But why does no one seriously argue in favor of lying to parents? Some theorists and practitioners of family medicine have argued that the whole family is the unit of care, and that therapeutic goals are best achieved through consistency and intervention with entire family systems rather than just selected individuals.

Sometimes death is seen as changing the rules of the game; what was unacceptable before may be acceptable now. Why should this be? This seems counter-intuitive to our healthy state belief that the imminence of death should make us cut through the social facades and deal more honestly with one another because time is short.

Traditionally in pediatric health care, the physician decided what was in the best interests of the child and family, and very little was questioned. Over the past two decades this paternalistic approach has been replaced by one that encourages active participation by the family in decision-making concerning the child's medical care. Enhanced parent participation has been paralleled by increased participation by the child. It is now generally recognized that parents and professionals have a duty to share the responsibility for involving the child in treatment planning.

THE RIGHT OF CHILDREN TO KNOW THE TRUTH

Children have rights. Among these are the right to protection, education, housing, and health care. Parents have an obligation to respect and maintain these rights. Do dying children have a right to know the truth? Do parents have a reciprocal obligation to inform them?

It would be far too simplistic to say unequivocally that children have the right to know they are dying. Compassion, understanding of children's concepts of death, religious beliefs, cultural values, hope, and trust in parents and professionals all contribute to, and shape the need for, and perception of, truth.

At the very least, when long-term survival is no longer possible children have, if not a right, a strong ethical claim on being informed that they will not be alone, their pain and discomfort will be controlled, and their families will be present.

Some individuals maintain that children have the right not to know they are dying. Presumably, this desire for restraint in others can only be expressed through some highly unusual advanced directives exercise, or by children who actually decline offers of information. Either instance presupposes that the decision to tell has already been made.

WHY WE SHOULD TRY TO
TELL THE TRUTH

Telling the truth is one of the first moral practices for which we received repeated and direct guidance as children. It is a practice that has been entrenched through social convention and each of us has a clear idea or strong intuition about what it means to tell the truth. In daily life we repeatedly act on this understanding as we determine how much information is necessary to constitute "the truth." The limits were established, in part, because we saw that the bald, hard truth could do great harm [3]. Total honesty with friends, family, or colleagues would produce unpleasant personal and social consequences. Usually we try to select those pieces of information which we deem necessary at a particular moment, but which do not undermine trust.

We value the truth until we are confronted with telling someone, especially a child, that he or she is dying. Then the truth becomes much more difficult to impart. Western culture hides death from children, and in fact, many parents have grown up with little or no direct experience with death. Buckman has said that "we live in a society in which dying is not part of the business of living" [9, p. 3]. This makes the task more difficult.

In situations where a child is terminally ill, or has experienced a protracted illness in which death is the likely outcome, professionals and parents usually have talked together about the likelihood of death at an early stage in the illness. From the time of diagnosis, the typical well-founded response to the child's question about death is that "some children with the same disease do, in fact, die, **but** (and this is a big 'but' in the minds of those addressing the child), the doctors and nurses are using the best treatments and research to help you get better." At some stage in the child's illness this response will no longer represent the truth. When further treatment does not result in a cure, the

decision must be made about what the child needs to know and understand in order to enhance his quality of life and begin any preparations
for death.

The most difficult pieces of information to pass on to a dying child
are found in the following six core items:

"Your diagnosis is . . ."
". . . can be (is) a fatal disease."
"I don't know the answer to your question."
"The treatments are not helping you to live longer or better."
"You will probably die soon."
"Nothing more can be done to control your symptoms."

With respect to the last item, the importance of good palliative
care cannot be over-emphasized. It must be noted that some of the
worst news of the past (i.e., the prospect of intractable pain) need no
longer be conveyed. Realistic options for therapeutic intervention can
sustain hope, and when acted upon, provide great physical and emotional comfort. Yet, a terrible and difficult psychological shift still
remains for parents as they move from the goal of cure to one of
symptom control [10].

Parents and caregivers who concur about the truth, how to talk with
the child, and how to support the child once that truth has been given,
can set the stage for a shared and more emotionally balanced dying
process. In such instances, some tension tends to dissipate and a
greater sense of calmness pervades. This mutual sharing among
parents, caregivers, and children enhances the quality of the time
remaining.

The imminence of death need not destroy hope, nor should truthtelling. Hope cannot be sustained adequately by being evasive or lying.
Rather, such strategies increase the stress of uncertainty and powerlessness [3]. It is not what you do not know that hurts you, but rather
the wallowing in suspicion that takes its toll [7]. Some children never
learn the actual truth and some of these children die under the added
weight of an unnecessary burden.

In a deceptive situation, children's fears may be exacerbated as they
start to read the subtle cues and guess that something is seriously
wrong, no matter how successful the parents think they have been at
hiding their feelings [11]. Children as young as five years of age can
question their own mortality in the face of serious illness. By late
adolescence all will contemplate this question [12]. Older children will
undoubtedly sense the difference in the attitudes of those around them
and may ask direct questions about whether they are going to die,
especially if parents previously gave them permission to ask questions.

It has been established that children, over the age of six who are told about a diagnosis of cancer, will experience less anxiety than those who are not told [13, 14]. Even very young children pick up on the anxiety being experienced by those around them and this can produce increased fearfulness. However, anxiety that is explained or contextualized is always easier to bear than anxiety rooted in ignorance [10].

Children need to know that it is all right for them to be anxious or scared, and that the best way to handle their feelings is to talk to those whom they trust [11]. In psychodynamic terms, anxiety is expected to be present as long as fears or feelings remain subconscious. Anxiety, which serves as an indicator of unconscious feelings or fears leaking into consciousness, may diminish when parents and caregivers provide information, understand children's fears, and help them articulate their feelings.

Secrets of this magnitude are difficult to keep, and they can cause divisiveness in the family structure [15, 8]. The risks of deception are great; trust is threatened, eroded, or destroyed by its discovery. Parents and caregivers who withhold the truth are not always good actors.

If children perceive an information gap, curiosity or emotional need may drive them to fill it—by speaking with other children, asking questions of available adults, drawing from their own life experiences, or using their imaginations. "No news" is often interpreted as withheld "bad news." Since children's imaginations can be more ruthless than any reality, being apprised of the truth may be vital to their psychological well-being.

Children who are capable and competent will usually be aware that they are facing a grave situation in which death is imminent. Caregivers encounter dying children who attempt to protect their parents by concealing their fears and not expressing their concerns about death. This places an enormous burden on children who may feel guilty for wanting to talk openly and thus risk hurting the people they love. This guilt increases exponentially as parents either hide their own feelings or openly demonstrate their grief and sadness. If children cannot discuss their concerns with their parents, they may experience more intense feelings of anxiety, stress, suffering, and depression.

For those children who have already determined that they are dying, the charade that shadows them can be onerous and isolating. This may engender feelings of guilt and subsequent stress in family members who survive them. Parents may find themselves wondering if their children might have given them a special farewell message had they been more open.

There is a tendency to downplay children's resilience and strengths while focusing on their vulnerabilities and functional limitations. Children who do not want to know whether they are dying will demonstrate their wishes through their behavior. For these children denial is a powerful tool; to fracture the protection it offers would be harmful. But, more commonly, after information is provided, children may move in and out of denial to protect themselves until they are ready to fully assimilate the proffered messages.

A study of children over three years of age with end-stage cancer revealed that when frank disclosure of the stage of the cancer was offered, the majority of children chose to know and made many of their own decisions regarding medical interventions [16].

Children as young as nine have clearly stated that they would want to know if they had a terminal illness. Their reasons were straightforward. They had objectives in life, and if they knew time was shorter than hoped, they would want to satisfy their most important and pressing goals while they still felt well enough [17, 18].

Most adolescents want to know the truth about their health care and to participate in decision-making. Some adolescents may wish to prepare advance directives while they are still able [19].

Ironically, children who have suffered through a long treatment process and are facing death may be more competent to participate in medical decision-making than their peers. Some enhancement of child competence may be the result of a decreased range of choices: for example, there may be fewer chances of making a mistake when life options are limited, i.e., striving to be an astronaut is not realistic, but dying at home is. In some situations parents do not know which of many treatment options is best; in such circumstances their children's expressed preferences can be the factors that determine action. These children need accurate, adequate information to help them make suitable end of life choices for themselves.

All children should be given the opportunity to express their concerns and wishes about the dying process and the site of death. Those children who prefer to die at home cannot have their wishes known or honored without honest and truthful discussion.

Control, autonomy, and a sense of belonging are important for dying children [18]. Secrecy and deceit rob them of such feelings and interfere with their compliance during palliative care.

Withholding information may interfere with a child's right to die. By not giving children the permission to die, we are forcing them to endure life and further pain and suffering, for the sake of their parents or caregivers.

The risk of suicide following the disclosure of bad news appears to be quite low, when adolescent cancer patients are considered [20]. Whatever the reality, it is important to point out that suicide may be a very rational act in response to anticipated pain, suffering, and death. It should also be mentioned that a few very negative counter-examples (e.g., teenagers tragically killing themselves when their prospects for remission were very good) actually may be insufficient evidence against a policy or practice.

ABOUT HEALTH PROFESSIONALS

"The transmission of information is related to characteristics of patients (sex, education, social class, prognosis), doctors (social class, background, income, and perception of patient's desire for information), and the clinical situation (number of patients seen)" [21, p. 2441]. It is also related to the age of both doctors and patients, and to the physician's experience within a given specialty [2].

Much of the ethics literature examines the "doctor-patient" relationship to the exclusion of the roles of other health professionals. Though teams are generally lead by doctors and final responsibility for treatment rests with doctors, it must be emphasized that the giving of information to patients is not primarily a medical or scientific decision. Rather, it is a moral decision, and in moral matters no one enjoys primacy by virtue of role or title. Health professionals are moral equals [22] and accordingly bear common burdens of moral responsibility. Each person involved in a child's care has their own perspective and insights that, if shared at the right moments, might be helpful [4].

Health professionals can have problems talking with dying children: they may feel pressure to maintain a stoic facade or the illusion of coping well; they may feel anger or frustration over professional and patient demands; they may experience inappropriate guilt over therapeutic failure; they may adopt paternalistic postures as a result of overidentification with a child or because of a need to control; they may use complex denial in difficult circumstances, and inappropriately attempt to prolong treatment; and they may hide behind euphemisms [3] or psychological walls. Also, there are health professionals who reveal too much information in order to relieve their own anxiety [3] or to protect themselves from potential litigation.

Unfortunately, "clinical objectivity" is often a less than stable quality. Whether one tells the truth depends less on the distinct personality and circumstances of the patient than on the particular values, biases, and fears of the professionals [23, 5]. Putting yourself "in your patients' shoes" is the best way not to understand what they feel; let them speak for themselves [5].

Health care workers should not forget that they are self-selected for their particular type of work, they talk about disease constantly, and the clinical terminology that is second nature to them can be very alien and frightening for others [8].

SOME RELEVANT ETHICS PRINCIPLES

It is a common practice in ethics debates to appeal to principles in support of one's claims. A principle is a general law, doctrine, or assumption that is basic to other truths. An idea or statement is elevated to the status of a principle when it is taken to be self-evidently valid or true, when there is solid evidence in support of it, or when an apparent consensus has emerged around its relative worth and importance. Unfortunately, even when there is agreement on which principles are relevant to a given issue, there may be significant disagreement over priority of place or application [24, 25]. With this proviso in mind, it is worthwhile to consider the following four principles that bear significantly on the sometimes elusive and fragile presentation of truth to a child: beneficence, best interests, nonmaleficence, and autonomy.

1. Beneficence

Beneficence is the doing of good, the treatment of disease and injury, or the alleviation of suffering [26]. It is this principle that guides the actions of both health professionals and parents as they provide care for children.

What is the "good" that can be done for children that are facing death? The answer hinges on the values espoused by participants in the life drama. These values are based on age, previous experience, culture, role, professional training, and other factors.

We make unfounded assumptions about each other's values all of the time. Unless these are spelled out, they can complicate discussions in unexpected ways.

The determination of the "good" is also contingent on participants being honest with themselves and forthright with each other. How do they interpret or bring meaning to suffering, pain, spirituality, and mortality? What do they believe to be the best interests or best quality of life for children and families? Which of their values coincide and which are disparate? Do they respect each other's perspectives and how do they decide whose values shall ultimately determine choices for action? What truths must be expressed by whom to achieve the best outcome?

The physician, for example, may believe that in the interest of research the child should continue therapeutically questionable treatment for as long as possible. The parents, on the other hand, may believe that the better choice is to protect their child from painful procedures for whatever time remains. The child may want the treatment to continue, and therefore, is angry over the parents' decision to stop it. Until all the protagonists openly and honestly express their own beliefs, fears, and values, mutual understanding cannot be reached and relationships may be weakened. This is not to say that children need to be cognizant of the intricacies of the discussions which occur between parents and professionals, or that parents should relate the detailed peregrination which helped them reach their decision. It is enough that there be a sufficient level of honest behaviour and self-revelation to break any communication log-jam.

2. Best Interests

Everyone would agree that it is in the best interests of every child to be well, active, happy, and able to anticipate a long lifespan. When these possibilities are extinguished we need to consider which goals should take their place. We also need to tailor these goals to the unique life context in which their realization will be attempted. Remember that the child's best interests will change over the course of the illness, especially as death approaches. Parents must learn to accept the fluidity of the concept of "best interests" and adjust their thinking accordingly.

From the moment of diagnosis, the child's role in the family will evolve within the changing dynamics. The best interests of the child must be paramount even when they are not immediately recognized by the child. For example, no child wants to be subjected to painful, invasive procedures. Parents need to develop negotiating skills that will help their child cooperate during treatment. This is not easy for parents because they instinctively need to protect their child from harm and suffering at all times. Unfortunately, they are not always able to because the necessity of treatment for life-threatening illness supplants the parent's role as protector. Open dialogue is necessary to safeguard the trust that underpins the parent/child relationship.

There may be times when there is disparity between the respective perceptions of professionals and parents concerning what is in the best interests of the child. These perceptions will vary with the stage of illness and the aggressiveness of the treatment, but such disparity is always a signal that honest discussion is required for resolution.

3. Nonmaleficence, or "Do No Harm"

Primum non nocere is a recognized cornerstone of medical practice. This principle [26] must be interpreted properly. It cannot be taken as an exhortation to never harm; physicians hurt patients all the time with painful examinations, tests, procedures, or treatments. Properly understood, the principle means that physicians should strive to ultimately achieve a positive balance of benefit over harm [27]. The older proscription, "So far as possible, do no harm," is better [24].

Bluntly stated, to lie is to harm (for all the reasons identified in this chapter). But telling the truth can hurt too. However, if done well it can and should hurt less. Attempts must be made to limit the existential anguish that may accompany the series of disclosures that are necessary from diagnosis through to death. The right words, at the right time, with the best continuing support possible are the ideal to which parents should aim.

4. Autonomy, The Right to Decide

While truthtelling has not always been perceived within ethical domains as an absolute obligation, most professionals now agree that there is "some duty of veracity and that it derives from the respect we owe to autonomous persons" [26, p. 371].

Miller examines the principle of autonomy from the following four perspectives: free action, authenticity, effective deliberation, and moral reflection [28].

Autonomy as free action implies that children who are facing death and wish to continue with treatment should be able to do so freely. On the same count, children who wish to have treatment withheld may do so freely. The construct of free action implies that honest dialogue has to occur prior to any decision. Several factors function here. The first is that children must be old enough to comprehend their actions and that they need to be adequately informed in order to make a decision. The second factor is that once children have made their decisions these must be respected (even if not supported or acted upon) by both professionals and parents.

Autonomy as authenticity means that the actions chosen by children are consistent with their attitudes and values. Such consistency is equated with personal integrity, and is taken as evidence of a relative degree of maturity. Here again, the construct of trust is implicit for children, parents, and professionals. Adequate information from other sources and a personal knowledge base are necessary in order for children to bring values to bear at critical decision junctures.

Autonomy as effective deliberation means that children and families who must make the decisions are aware of the consequences and alternatives, have evaluated these, and have reached their decisions appropriately. This also means that prior to the time that parents tell their children about their impending deaths, they have had open and honest dialogue with the professionals about the following concerns: the impact on the child, their fears that these children may lose hope or be angry, and how to provide all the support that their children will require. Effective deliberation implies careful thinking prior to any action being taken. There is no room for impulsiveness.

Autonomy as moral reflection means, in the first instance, that parents have evaluated and accepted the moral values that they have used to guide them to the decision to inform their children. It also means that the values they believe their children hold have been a critical part of that assessment. In the second instance, it means that children's responses to the information are framed in a manner consistent with their own moral values.

INVOLVEMENT IN THE CONSENT PROCESS

Currently, there is much discussion concerning the role of children in the process of consent. In some treatment centers, children as young as seven years of age are deemed competent to sign their own consent for treatment. In other jurisdictions, the children must reach the age of sixteen or seventeen before they are permitted to sign consents. At other centers, parents and children co-sign the consent for treatment. The purpose of this chapter is not to extend the debate about consent, but rather to emphasize that if children or adolescents are permitted to sign consents they should be informed appropriately for their age of the intent of the documents, and should not be expected to carry the full burden of decision-making as the treatment progresses.

It is morally reprehensible not to expect children, in an age appropriate manner, to participate in decision-making about aspects of their treatment, including the refusal of treatment. Equally, it is morally reprehensible to suppose, even for an instant, that children would bear the full responsibility for doing so.

QUALITY OF LIFE AS THE TRUTH UNFOLDS

Throughout the child's illness, the treatment received is intended to return the child to better health and therefore enhance quality of life.

In pediatric health care, it sometimes happens that the principle of the quality of life may be overshadowed by the principle of the sanctity of life. In this instance, the child's treatment is driven by the goal of survival and cure above all else. There is a cost, both emotionally and physically, to this approach. Although these two principles, quality of life and sanctity of life, seem complementary, they may, in fact, conflict and result in compromising the child's quality of life. The truth in these instances may also be compromised.

The desired and realistic quality of life for children needs to be articulated. For some children the control of symptoms and the absence of aggressive therapies will bring a maximal level of comfort and inner peace.

Parents know their children well and have an intuitive sense concerning their preferences. These same parents may be hesitant to discuss their feelings with health professionals. There have been situations in which parents did not realize that, when their child's death was imminent, they had the right to order the cessation of procedures and aggressive treatments.

It is incumbent upon professionals to initiate dialogue with parents. If conversation is not open and honest then children cannot be told the truth. Enveloping children in unrealistic hope for cure will inhibit them from communicating their concerns, raising questions about spirituality and death, and expressing love and concern for their parents. Children treated in this manner will die, in all likelihood knowing that they are dying, feeling alone, and not benefitting from appropriate psychosocial support.

FUTILITY: WHEN TREATMENT IS NO LONGER CURATIVE

A critical point will come in the continuum from diagnosis to death when treatment no longer provides sufficient benefit, and cure is believed to be impossible or to require too high a price to be achieved. Truthtelling at this time represents a multi-faceted composition which has to be carefully orchestrated by all the players. This need for a shift to a palliative focus is one of the most emotional decision points. Parents and professionals experience great difficulty replacing their hope for a cure with the hope for a peaceful death. Open dialogue is critical.

Professionals, by virtue of their access to and interpretation of medical information and despite the fact that they tend to treat diseases aggressively, may achieve this realization prior to parents. In this disparate state it may be incumbent upon professionals to continue treatment until parents have reached the point of acceptance with a clear realization that their child will not survive. However, it is critical that professionals not mislead and prolong treatment beyond, either the point of negligible therapeutic benefit, or the time they believe that parents and children have had enough.

Often the children begin to clearly articulate that treatment has become unbearable, or that the potential benefits do not justify the current means. Sometimes parents cannot accept the fact that treatment no longer offers any hope of cure. How can children question their mortality with parents who cannot accept that reality? A child's environment may become poisoned by pretence until such time that parents are ready for the next difficult steps.

SUFFERING AND THE PLACE
OF RELIGIOSITY

It behooves each caregiver to take the time necessary to understand parents' beliefs. In many instances these beliefs will be mirrored by children. Suffering and pain have an important place and meaning even in the religious belief systems of children.

No doubt the reader has an appreciation of how the variety of religious traditions and beliefs can produce many variations in truth-telling, as well as potential complications for families and caregivers. The information that is exchanged will be couched within frameworks of religious interpretation. For some the death of a child may be accepted more readily because of their belief in the manifest will of God. For others death may be a source of tremendous anguish because they believe a child is being punished for the "sins of the father." Some may believe that a child's suffering is an important means of reparation for sins. And still others will rage at the injustice of a world where the innocent suffer and die so young.

CULTURAL IMPLICATIONS AND
SENSITIVITY

We live in a world where millions of people from many cultures have made their homes in new countries. No longer can health professionals assume that parents and children will share cultural beliefs and values similar to their own. Yet frequently, treatment proceeds without a comprehensive cultural assessment of the family. Health professionals conscientiously conduct excellent physical, social, and psychological assessments, but rarely is the time taken to conduct a cultural assessment. It is likely that the cultural values of the country of origin are primarily responsible for moulding health and illness behaviors, caring and curative practices, and beliefs about death.

Truthtelling practices vary from culture to culture [29, 30, 2]. For example, in Japan patients will not be told that they have cancer because it is perceived as cruel to reveal such information [31]. Consequently, chemotherapeutic agents may be selected, not because they are most efficacious but, because they are least likely to have the tell-tale side-effects that point to a diagnosis of cancer.

Immigrants who have lived in their adopted country for a long time, or younger generations within a particular ethnic group, may adhere to other than their traditional health practices and beliefs. One cannot make assumptions but must ask each patient about respective beliefs.

Cultural variation may make the truth, which is acceptable to both parents and professionals, more elusive. When one considers that children who are at the center of the cultural debate may not share the same values as either their parents or the professionals, the need for a very careful cultural assessment is accentuated.

WHAT IF PARENTS NEED
TO DECEIVE?

The patterns of familial communication that were established before the intrusion of disease will be the same ones that serve families during the illness experiences. If openness and honesty prevailed before, then this pattern is likely to continue [13]. If communication patterns were closed, cautious, paternalistic, or protective then there may be a greater likelihood for attempted deception.

What may be new to the existing family dynamics is the ability of sick children to sometimes support and protect their parents by not talking about the possibility of death [18]. Parents may need to be taught how to detect and modify such behavior, or how to let down their own "walls." Parents should not be permitted to abrogate their responsibilities.

If children question staff members about their death rather than asking their parents, a "dance of secrecy" [17] may evolve which inevitably destroys trust and relationships.

If parents want to deceive should a doctor ignore their wishes and still reveal information to the child? If the physician chooses to tell, then two unfortunate things have happened. The physician has behaved paternalistically toward the parents and undermined the relationship with them [1], and the family structure has been threatened at a critical juncture [32]. Children almost always need to keep trusting their parents more than they need some information [8].

The obvious response to parents who wish to attempt deceit is that they are most likely doomed to fail. But they believe that the worry-free period that their child may enjoy is an important gift, even if illness ultimately intrudes and betrays the lie.

In the final analysis, parents generally know their children and themselves best, and their wisdom should be respected [15]. Remember that their choice to deceive is most often an act of love [33]. Encourage them to tell the truth if and when they feel the time is right, but do not cajole or pressure them. Parents' well-being will always have an impact on their children's well-being [8].

If a child knows the truth but the parent denies this, then the parent's interpretation should be respected. But the professional should gently offer evidence which suggests that the child may know more than the parent believes, and leave the door open to exploration of the matter [15, 18].

HIV/AIDS: A SPECIAL CHALLENGE

Compared to the domain of childhood cancer, we have relatively little research or experience to guide us in our disclosure decisions related to pediatric HIV or AIDS. We can assume that strong emotions, fears, and misconceptions are more likely to complicate exchanges of information.

The arguments made previously in support of pediatric truthtelling also apply to this population, however the potential for a very long illness-free period after initial infection (5 years or more [34]) would seem to count against a critical need for early disclosure. Unless, of course, a child is old enough to be sexually active [8].

Many of the arguments that support telling the truth presuppose relative accuracy of diagnosis, a fully competent patient, and a predictable natural history for the disease. These last two items may be absent with HIV infection or AIDS [34].

The fact that many of the children who are HIV positive also have an infected parent (over 70% [34]), a parent who has died, or live with foster parents means that stable and supportive family dynamics may be lacking. Parents may be struggling with their own burden, and coping through denial or by establishing discussion taboos. They may not want a child to figure out the parental source of infection (e.g., drug use, sexual activity) [8].

Foster parents may choose to conceal or disclose a diagnosis for the wrong reasons: they may wish to protect the child from a "bad" past, or they may wish to discredit natural parents and gain the child's favor. Accordingly, motivation should be explored in these family units [8].

The omnipresent social stigma may cause parents to believe that the fewer people who know their personal circumstances, the better [8]. Given the threat of persecution or discrimination, knowledge of diagnosis might also necessitate the unpleasant involvement of the patient in a protective web of secrecy and complicity [15].

An important unanswered question is whether the stress of knowing the diagnosis, or subsequently developing depression, will produce added immune suppression and actually lead to more frequent illnesses or earlier death [8, 34].

HOW TO TELL

Truthtelling remains the ideal, but it requires good judgement concerning pacing and content. How to tell the truth presents a challenge in negotiation, effective and meaningful dialogue, contracting, mutual respect, and provision of support and resources for families and health care providers.

Parents have a responsibility to be fully informed about the treatment and procedures required by their children. They should be encouraged to ask questions. Parents who are not adequately informed are often unable to be open and truthful with their children. It is difficult to tell the truth if one does not understand it. The onus is definitely on professionals to explain and repeat information as often as necessary until parents are comfortable with their knowledge. It is usually the parents who will first hear the questions posed by their children concerning the illness, hospitalization, pain and suffering, treatments, new medications, or even the lack of treatment. However, parents should not be expected to bear the full burden of telling their children about a potentially frightening diagnosis such as cancer, or that cure is no longer possible. The various members of the health care team who were present when parents were first given bad news, and who have supported them in an ongoing way, are the same people who can advise them on how to proceed. If the parents wish, these people can be present when the child is given bad news.

How the truth has been told in past, less-threatening, life situations will strongly influence the present. Together parents and professionals can discuss and decide upon the best way to talk with children. In these preliminary discussions it is important that the reactions of children be anticipated and appropriate professional support be available when they are told the truth.

Some children will respond with questions, anger, fear, or tears. Others will have had an intuition about their impending death and may express a sense of relief because their fears have finally been confirmed, and the charade that has been played around them is over.

Truth is told within frameworks of interpretation. Social, cultural, and spiritual values can differ greatly, even between individuals within the same family. Each participant in an exchange brings semantic variability and phenomenological peculiarities to the process. Children understand words differently than adults, they are not laden with the same baggage, and the impact of words will vary on them. Most significantly, they are unlikely to be bowled over by the full range of meaning and implication of words like "cancer" or "AIDS" [8].

Our truths to dying children are often couched in euphemisms. Euphemisms make health professionals and parents feel more secure, but they often cloud matters further. There is no single recipe for what to say and how to say it, but parents are the best judge of the type of language and non-verbal support that will be suitable for their children. Exactly how to tell, and the precise content (or disclosure limits) must be agreed upon by the health professionals and also by the parents. This consistency is "especially important in the pediatric case as the patient might be less able to reconcile minor differences in opinion, and various versions of the 'truth' " [32, p. 196].

Children's decisions can be shaped, supported, or undermined by the information that they are offered, and by the affect they detect in others.

Children's mental state, intelligence, maturity, attitude, questions, and rate of assimilation all help determine how much to tell and when [32]. Additional factors to consider are parental readiness and support.

Children obviously differ in their concepts of death. Roughly by ages five to seven, magical thinking begins to diminish and death begins to be recognized as a more permanent biological and social reality. Beyond age seven, children are capable of more logical thought [14]. By ages eleven or twelve they begin to develop a physiological understanding of illness [16]. For teenagers, death becomes more conceptually abstract and personally real.

Most likely, a very young child will not require a detailed explanation concerning his or her death. This child will respond to the increased comfort from the absence of invasive and painful treatments. For children of all ages the words one uses to talk about death must reflect compassion, love, and support.

Sometimes information flow should be guided by the questions that are asked rather than by information offered or assumed to be relevant by caregivers. However, caregivers must not lose sight of the fact that patients/parents may have complete trust that they will always be told what they need to know, without having to seek it out. Or conversely, they should be sensitive to the possibility that some patients/parents may not ask questions because they fear that caregivers may view this as an expression of mistrust [23].

Much of the literature about chronically ill children has shown that children do not usually ask important questions unless they already have some idea of the answer [15].

The following list identifies some key points when providing information to children:

1. Realize that children cannot be protected from all harm.
2. Recognize that children's imaginings may be much more harmful than the truth.
3. Tell the truth, but gently, and in degrees [35].
4. Consider whether children are able to bear, understand, or use the information you offer [4].
5. Bad news must always be framed within a message of continuing support and care [23].
6. Information and language must be appropriate to children's conceptual growth.
7. Be open, empathetic, direct, and unhurried.
8. Give time, opportunity, and encouragement to ask questions [23].
9. Let the questions be expressed through words, art, or play [15].
10. Let children control the pace; information must be wanted [4].
11. Be prepared to answer, or find answers, to the questions that the information you are presently offering may generate [3].
12. Answer just the questions that children ask without providing additional information or interpretation.
13. Give yourself permission to reopen a discussion or come back with an answer at a later time.
14. Be available in an ongoing way and provide opportunities for repetition or clarification.
15. Recognize that mutual pretence and denial have their place in the process of disclosure and need to be respected when they are useful.
16. Broach new topics by asking what children think or have already been told.
17. Correct misinformation.
18. Try to restrict difficult discussions to calm, safe moments or settings where intrusions and intruders are limited.
19. Recognize that children may play people off against each other in an attempt to elicit more information and confirm or repudiate suspicions.

20. Attempt to ensure consistency of disclosure-related affect across parental, sibling, relative, friend, and caregiver boundaries.
21. The process of information giving is not complete until all facts, possible consequences, and options for action have been specified to the degree desired by parents or children [3].
22. The right decision can feel like the wrong one; sometimes helping hurts and can produce cognitive dissonance.
23. At some time, every parent may need to be taught how, when, and what to communicate.

CONCLUSION

The truths that people exchange are subjective in nature, value laden, and shaped by social, cultural, religious, and professional perspectives of both the "giver" and the "beholder."

It is hoped that situations in which dying children are deceived are few, but where and when this happens the reasons and desired outcome must be carefully evaluated. The theoretical thrust of this chapter is intended to present a challenge to those who choose deception. The pragmatic thrust of this chapter recognizes that parents will lie for reasons of love and protection, but that such motivation may obscure the course of action that is truly in their children's best interest.

The weight of argument and experience tip the scales in favor of being truthful at all times and telling the truth when the time is judged to be right. It is the duty of parents to protect their children through gentle, well-timed disclosure. There may be exceptional cases when truthtelling should be delayed indefinitely, but what constitutes the exceptional must remain a subjective judgment by those who must assume this responsibility: the individual health professionals and parents working together.

There are stages in telling the truth to children who are facing death. The first is the identification of the values espoused by professionals, parents, and children; the second is recognition of the futility of further treatment and the acceptance of the inescapable outcome; the third is the provision of medical and psychosocial assistance required by parents and children from the professionals in order to determine what the truth actually is, and how to provide it on an ongoing basis; and the fourth stage is the identification and provision of the support and resources that families require once the truth about imminent death has been integrated into children's realities. Each of these stages is emotionally and physically stressful and fatiguing, and requires a trusting and open relationship among professionals, parents, and children.

We would do well to remember that trust, rooted in honesty, is the foundation for medical culture; it is fundamental to relationships, healing, and attempts to relieve suffering.

REFERENCES

1. M. S. Pernick, Childhood Death and Medical Ethics: An Historical Perspective on Truthtelling in Pediatrics, in *Difficult Decisions in Medical Ethics*, D. Ganos, R. E. Lipson, G. Warren, and B. J. Weil (eds.), Alan R. Liss Inc., New York, 1983.
2. D. J. Klenow and G. A. Youngs Jr., Changes in Doctor/Patient Communication of a Terminal Prognosis: A Selective Review and Critique, *Death Studies, 11*, pp. 263-277, 1987.
3. E. J. Cassell, Telling the Truth to the Dying Patient, in *Cancer, Stress, and Death*, J. Taché, H. Selye, and S. B. Day (eds.), Plenum Medical Book Company, New York, 1979.
4. S. A. Gadow, Truthtelling Revisited: Two Approaches to the Disclosure Dilemma, in *Ethical and Moral Dimensions of Care*, M. M. Leininger (ed.), Wayne State University Press, Detroit, Michigan, 1990.
5. L. Goldie, The Ethics of Telling the Patient, *Journal of Medical Ethics, 8*, pp. 128-133, 1982.
6. D. Bakhurst, On Lying and Deceiving, *Journal of Medical Ethics, 18*, pp. 63-66, 1992.
7. M. Sheldon, Truth Telling in Medicine, *Journal of the American Medical Association, 247*:5, pp. 651-654, 1982.
8. M. Lipson, What Do You Say to a Child With AIDS, *Hastings Center Report, 23*:2, pp. 6-12, 1993.
9. R. Buckman, *I Don't Know What to Say*, Key Porter Books, Toronto, Ontario, 1988.
10. D. B. Crom and C. B. Pratt, Stress, Cancer, Death—A Pediatric Perspective, in *Cancer, Stress, And Death* (2nd Edition), S. B. Day (ed.), Plenum Medical Book Company, New York, 1986.
11. D. J. Bearison, *"They Never Want to Tell You": Children talk about Cancer*, Harvard University Press, London, England, 1991.
12. J. Schowalter, The Child's Reaction to his own Terminal Illness, in *Loss and Grief: Psychological Management in Medical Practice*, Columbia University Press, New York, 1970.
13. D. W. Adams and E. J. Deveau, *Coping With Childhood Cancer: Where Do We Go From Here* (Revised Edition), Kinbridge Publications, Hamilton, Ontario, Canada, 1988.
14. M. K. Foley, Children with Cancer: Ethical Dilemmas, *Seminars in Oncology Nursing, 5*:2, pp. 109-113, 1989.
15. *Pediatric AIDS Foster Care Network Bulletin, 4*:1, pp. 3-6, 1992.

16. R. Nitschke, et al., Therapeutic Choices Made by Patients with End-stage Cancer, *The Journal of Pediatrics, 101*:3, pp. 471-476, 1982, and letters in *103*:1, pp. 167-169, 1983.
17. Paediatric Ethics Discussion Series, *". . . And Nothing but the Truth . . ."* (*Exploring the Information-Disclosure Dilemma*), Video, The Department of Bioethics, The Hospital for Sick Children, Toronto, Ontario, 1993
18. K. J. Pazola and A. K. Gerberg, Privileged Communication—Talking with a Dying Adolescent, *MCN, 15*, pp. 16-21, Jan-Feb., 1990.
19. R. G. Justin, Adult and Adolescent Attitudes Toward Death, *Adolescence, 28*:90, pp. 429-435, 1988.
20. J. Perrone, Adolescents with Cancer: Are They at Risk for Suicide?, *Pediatric Nursing, 19*:1, pp. 22-25, 1993.
21. H. Waitzkin, Doctor-Patient Communication: Clinical Implications of Social Scientific Research, *Journal of the American Medical Association, 252*:17, pp. 2441-2446, 1984.
22. E. Harris, et al., Nothing but the Truth?, *American Journal of Nursing, 83*:1, pp. 121-122, 1983.
23. I. Lichter, The Right to Bad News, in *Ethical Dilemmas in Cancer Care*, B. A. Stoll (ed.), The MacMillan Press Ltd., London, England, 1989.
24. R. Gillon, Telling the Truth and Medical Ethics, *British Medical Journal, 291*:30, pp. 1556-1557, November 1985.
25. D. M. High, Truth Telling, Confidentiality, and the Dying Patient: New Dilemmas for the Nurse, *Nursing Forum, 24*:1, pp. 5-10, 1989.
26. T. L. Beauchamp and L. Walters, The Management of Medical Information, in *Contemporary Issues in Bioethics* (3rd Edition), Wadsworth Publishing Co., Belmont, California, 1989.
27. Editorial, On Telling Dying Patients the Truth, *Journal of Medical Ethics, 8*, pp. 115-116, 1982.
28. B. L. Miller, Autonomy and the Refusal of Lifesaving Treatment, in *Moral Problems in Medicine* (2nd Edition), S. Gorovitz, R. Macklin, A. L. Gammadion, J. M. O'Connor, and S. Sherwin, (eds.), Prentice-Hall Inc., Englewood Cliffs, New Jersey, 1983.
29. P. Dalla-Vorgia, et al., Attitudes of a Mediterranean Population to the Truth-telling Issue, *Journal of Medical Ethics, 18*, pp. 67-74, 1992.
30. G. L. Brotzman and D. J. Butler, Cross-Cultural Issues in the Disclosure of a Terminal Diagnosis, *The Journal of Family Practice, 32*:4, pp. 426-427, 1991.
31. E. Feldman, Medical Ethics the Japanese Way, *Hastings Center Report, 15*:5, pp. 21-24, 1985.
32. G. Warren, Discussion Summary: Truth Telling in Pediatrics, in *Difficult Decisions in Medical Ethics*, D. Ganos, R. E. Lipson, G. Warren, and B. J. Weil (eds.), Alan R. Liss Inc., New York, 1983.
33. P. Maguire and A. Faulkner, Communicate with Cancer Patients: 2. Handling Uncertainty, Collusion, and Denial, *British Medical Journal, 297*:6654, pp. 972-974, 1988.

34. R. A. Olson, et al., Pediatric AIDS/HIV Infection: An Emerging Challenge to Pediatric Psychology, *Journal of Pediatric Psychology, 14*:1, pp. 1-21, 1989.
35. P. A. O'Connor, Truth Telling in Pediatrics—In Degrees, in *Difficult Decisions in Medical Ethics*, D. Ganos, R. E. Lipson, G. Warren, and B. J. Weil (eds.), Alan R. Liss Inc., New York, 1983.

Bibliography

Bok, S., Lies to the Sick and Dying, in *Medical Ethics* (2nd Edition), T. A. Mappes and J. S. Zembaty, (eds.), McGraw Hill Book Co., New York, 1986.
Rushton, C. H. et al., End of Life Care for Infants with AIDS: Ethical And Legal Issues, *Pediatric Nursing, 19*:1, pp. 79-83, 1993.
Warner, E., Should You Tell Your Patients the Truth?, *Canadian Medical Association Journal, 129*, pp. 278-280, August 1, 1983.

CHAPTER 15

The Influence of Spirituality on Dying Children's Perceptions of Death

L. L. (Barrie) deVeber

The philosophy of this chapter contends that spiritual care is a vital part of an holistic approach to caring for dying children and their families. This is particularly true in palliative (hospice) care where spiritual concerns are even more prominent than in other areas of medical care. Children are generally more open and less inhibited than adults when discussing various matters in life, including spirituality. This means that dying children are often more willing to examine spirituality and health care workers are challenged to pay particular attention to their spiritual needs and concerns.

Unfortunately, spiritual care is often overlooked because it is incorrectly equated with the beliefs and practices of formal religion and is not a priority of a significant number of health care providers and, to a lesser degree, of patients and families.

The first part of this chapter defines spirituality as distinct from religion; separates spiritual care from other forms of spirituality; assesses whether spirituality is necessary; determines whether children are spiritual; and delineates how religious convictions or beliefs affect spirituality. It is only when we understand the meaning and importance of spirituality that we can appreciate its influence on the child's perception of death and its application to clinical pediatric health care settings.

The second part examines some practical knowledge and working truths about children's spirituality including the phenomenon of near death experiences through the presentation of case histories. Finally, the chapter closes with practical advice to caregivers for dealing with the issue of spirituality and some religious convictions and beliefs that practitioners face on a day-to-day basis.

THEORETICAL CONSIDERATIONS

Spirituality Defined

My wife, Iola, and I participated in the International Work Group on Death, Dying, and Bereavement (IWG) subcommittee on spiritual care. This committee was comprised of a variety of professionals from different countries who struggled with the question of spirituality and eventually arrived at the following definition:

> Spirituality is concerned with the transcendental, inspirational and existential way to live one's life as well as, in a fundamental and profound sense, with the person as a human being [1, p. 33].

The difficulty faced by this group may be partly attributed to the lack of education about, and focus on, spirituality in our educational institutions. The subcommittee found that health care providers educated in health sciences faculties of universities in the western world receive little or no encouragement to develop their own faith system or discuss the implications of spirituality in a wider sense. Not surprisingly, the subcommittee found no evidence of courses on spirituality in the curricula of medical and nursing schools with the exception of a few schools that have religious affiliations.

Twycross, a British expert on pain control and palliative care, speaking at an international conference, provided the following definition of spirituality:

> The spiritual component of a personality is the dimension or function that integrates all other aspects of personhood. This relates to a concern with the ultimate issues in life principles and is often seen as a search for meaning in a person's life (why me, why him). Not to be confused with religion or religious, which is the practical expression of spirituality through a framework of beliefs often actively pursued in rituals and other religious practices. Everyone has a spiritual component, but not everyone is religious [2].

Spirituality is Not Necessarily Religion

The distinction between religion and spirituality, and the suggestion that religion is a sufficient but not a necessary condition for spirituality prevails throughout the literature. Highfield, in support of the existence of spirituality as an independent entity, developed the following definition:

> The spiritual dimension of persons can be uniquely defined as the human capacity to transcend self which is phenomenologically reflected in three basic spiritual needs:
> a) the need for self acceptance, a trusting relationship with self based on a sense of meaning and purpose in life;
> b) the need for relationships with others and/or a supreme other (e.g. God) characterized by non-conditional love, trust, and forgiveness; and
> c) the need for hope, which is the need to imagine and participate in the enhancement of a positive future [3, p. 2].

She points out that all persons experience spiritual needs whether or not they are part of a formal religious organization. She suggests that, "In contrast to spiritual health, religion is defined as the individual and community values, beliefs and practices through which persons attempt to fulfil spiritual needs" [3, p. 2]. In this sense, religion is a means to achieving spiritual needs rather than being equated with spirituality. Religion is a way in which people express their spirituality, whereas spirituality is that which separates humans from other beings—it is that realm of being that is concerned with the profound and ultimate questions of existence.

Stiles, from studying eleven hospice nurses and twelve adult patients' families, believes that spirituality refers to a hidden but energizing dimension that provides insight and new understandings of human experience [4]. According to her, spirituality involves transforming and transcending moments of human experience and requires one to be open and receptive. Further, she suggests that to know the spiritual is to know oneself and to know others [4].

Stile's study began with general questions about the hospice experience of nurses in hopes that spiritual matters would eventually be forthcoming. She concludes that if nurses view the "daily caring for patients and families as opportunities for spiritual insight and growth" there will be more personal meaning in their work [4, p. 244]. She also suggests that if nurses embrace patients and families as "strangers who may illuminate their lives," their approach may offer new meaning and spiritual growth to the patient care experience [4, pp. 244-245]. This may also revitalize nurses' professional lives, reduce burnout, and prevent them from leaving the profession.

Developing a spiritual relationship in this context requires being fully available to patients and families as well as providing knowledge and skilled nursing care. Stile's suggests that nurses should have a broad and secular conception of spirituality in addition to a more specific religious interpretation [4].

Spiritual Care Compared with Psychosocial Support or Pastoral Care

Amenta believes that spiritual support differs from psychosocial support because it consists of more personal involvement with patients at the deepest level. It is "walking in the valley of the shadow of death" with the patient [5, p. 178]. It may involve sitting, crying, or grieving with patients and families and incorporates transcendence, hope, guilt, forgiveness, reconciliation, rituals, and prayer.

Amenta stresses, as did the IWG subcommittee, that religious and spiritual systems should never be imposed on a patient but should be strengthened wherever possible. Amenta also concludes that:

> Spiritual care does not identify and solve problems in quantitative terms or in the traditional clinical sense. Effective spiritual care heightens awareness and/or promotes understanding and opens up blocked spiritual pathways [5, p. 182].

Eaton, a hospital chaplain, suggests that although anyone can be a pastoral caregiver, particularly if they have a strong faith background, pastoral care workers tend to have more training in the dynamics of loss, the grief process, and crisis management. They are also more knowledgeable regarding local clerical resources. She describes the spiritual accompaniment of patients and families as a journey through "a passage of fears that must be faced honestly and bravely" [6, p. 93]. She also suggests that, "to delve into such questions with another is to tread on holy ground, to be allowed to see the fiery spirit that lights their hearts" [6, p. 93]. This is a very dramatic way of illustrating the positive aspects of being involved in spiritual care, an area that many health care workers avoid because they do not feel comfortable sharing their beliefs or values with patients and families, perhaps because it is not fashionable or considered to be professional.

Smyth and Bellemare also try to distinguish pastoral care from spiritual care by describing pastoral counseling as a process requiring professional training and focuses on the development of listening skills and sensitivity to patients' needs. They agree that the same person can, at any one time, be a spiritual supporter, pastoral counselor, and representative of the patient's own religion. These roles may also be assumed by different individuals [7].

Wald contrasts the structured comforting Christian (Anglican) tradition of the British hospice system emanating from the work of Cicely Saunders with the North American system which tries to adapt to all religious and non-religious traditions. She emphasizes the fact that caregivers who are not educated in theology are called upon to minister and that clergy ordained in one faith are required to minister to people of different faiths. She also believes that compassion is common to all spiritual care. To be compassionate requires a degree of maturity and a sense of values that may come from a religious source, and/or from natural wisdom and experience [8].

Since pastoral care workers and clergy cannot always be available to dying children and their families, health care workers should be prepared to enter into dialogues about spirituality.

Weissman provides an existential view of spiritual care and believes that spiritual and pastoral concerns are more important to friends or family than to the dying patient, who is focusing more on medical and psychosocial problems. Although this does not seem to be the prevailing opinion, his insights emphasize the fact that a patient's physical and psychosocial needs must be attended to before we can expect to have a meaningful spiritual dialogue [9].

The Need for Spiritual Care

The IWG subcommittee concluded that when defined broadly, spiritual care should be an essential component of care for dying patients and their families. However, spiritual care has not received much attention in either the general literature on health care or the more specialized literature on adult and pediatric palliative and hospice care [1]. On the other hand, most people working in hospice and palliative care programs informally recognize the importance of spiritual care.

A palliative care assessment committee at the Montreal Children's Hospital that included physicians, nurses, parents, and chaplains examined and documented the issues of pain and symptom control, holistic care (including spiritual care), grief, loss, and staff stress when children were admitted to hospital with life-threatening illnesses. Their sample focused on family care and included a large number of premature infants and children with congenital anomalies, malignant diseases, cystic fibrosis, and other illnesses [10].

The study noted significant differences between the attitudes of hospital staff and parents toward the role of religious faith in their lives. It revealed that 33 percent of the staff reported no formal religious attachment compared to 17 percent of the parents [10, p. 58].

In addition, 60 percent of the staff would not attend a patient's funeral, although 75 percent believed that attendance would be healthy for the family. It was concluded that:

> Pastoral care resources were generally inadequate in the hospital and one of the six general conclusions was that pastoral care resources for the dying child and family needed upgrading and sustained hospital support in order to develop a dynamic, integrated, and interfaith pastoral care team capable of tending to the transcendent/existential needs of the secular persons who do not adhere to a particular religious tradition [10, p. 141].

In a small study at the Children's Hospital of Western Ontario between 1980 and 1990, bereaved parents were asked about their spiritual needs based on the broad definitions previously described by the IWG subcommittee and Dr. Twycross. Of twenty-two respondents, twenty indicated that they had spiritual needs when their children were dying and sixteen of the twenty responded that these had been fulfilled. In fifteen cases, support was provided by a local minister or priest, the congregation, or their own families. Support was obtained from a hospital chaplain in only two cases. When these parents were asked if they believed that there was a need for increased availability of pastoral care or spiritual help from the hospital, regardless of whether or not the spiritual care was related to a religious faith, eighteen out of twenty-two responded positively. At the conclusion of the survey there was no chaplain assigned to the Children's Hospital, but now we have the services of a part-time chaplain. In the interim, parents were served by a number of volunteer clergy from the community providing they stated their religious preference on admission.

I believe that the following situation further illustrates the need for a chaplain, especially for families who do not have formal religious attachment:

> Julie was an eight-year-old girl who was dying following surgery for an abdominal neuroblastoma with severe complications. The parents had stated that they had no religious preference, did not belong to a church, and did not have a minister. I did not know the family well and was only covering for the weekend, but I did ask them if they wanted the services of a hospital chaplain. To my surprise, they both eagerly responded "yes." When the chaplain arrived, she spent many hours with this family and eventually helped them arrange the funeral service for their child. Although I do not know the content of the dialogue between the chaplain and

the parents, one can assume that it did not relate to formal religion and yet was obviously of great benefit.

Can Spirituality be Measured?

Highfield, in a comprehensive study of adults, used a Spiritual Health Inventory (SHI) to determine if assessment of the spiritual health of patients by the nurses was as accurate as the patients' assessments of themselves [3]. The spiritual self-report inventory for patients focused on having a purpose in life, being accepted, and being forgiven for past actions, thoughts, and feelings. The spirituality inventory for nurses was slightly different and looked for expressions of guilt. Both inventories asked which caregivers were preferred and which were most effective in assessing and meeting patients' spiritual needs. It is interesting that chaplains were ranked second by nurses, but only fifth by the patients and families. For patients, the family members ranked first. Physicians were either ranked first or fifth by nurses and second by patients. Psychiatrists and social workers were ranked sixth or seventh by both [3, pp. 6-7].

The basic finding in this study was the marked incongruence between the nurse and patient SHI scores, suggesting that the nurses had not accurately assessed the spiritual health of the patients. This inaccuracy may be attributed to several factors. Highfield theorizes that the nurses may have focused more on physical and psychiatric rather than spiritual problems; they may not have expected to have any role in the spiritual care of patients; or they may have overlooked or avoided the need for direct discussion about spiritual concerns despite patients' desires. The influence of the nurses' ethnic and spiritual backgrounds and a definite limitation on time for the discussion of spiritual matters were additional factors [3].

Highfield concludes that nurses should improve their ability to communicate about, and be sensitive to, patients' spiritual needs and points out that the spiritual health inventory could be used to record the spiritual distress of patients. Highfield pleads for more research in this area and, recently, literature on the topic is beginning to appear. Although these studies were on adult patients, they may be applicable to pediatric patients, families, and health care workers [3].

Are Children Spiritual?

Robert Coles, writer, professor of psychiatry and medical humanities, and Pulitzer Prize winner, has studied children around the world and recorded their reactions to racial crisis, migration, poverty, and various types of hardship including moral and political stress. His latest book, *The Spiritual Life of Children*, was stimulated by a discussion with one of his mentors, Hanna Freud, the daughter of Sigmund Freud, who suggested that if he reviewed his life's work he might realize that he had missed something of importance [11]. In response, Coles and his family reviewed his tape-recorded sessions and notes from thirty years of working with children. During the process, he began to realize that children had often wanted to discuss spiritual matters but their needs were missed due to his insensitivity. Consequently, he began to interview children from a wide range of countries and religious backgrounds regarding their spiritual needs and eventually wrote a book on the subject [11].

In his book, I could find only one discussion dealing with spirituality and dying children. In this vivid account, a child from a Jewish family was dying of leukemia. A strong Jewish faith helped both the child and her family manage her illness and final days [11, p. 273].

Much of the literature on spirituality denies that young children have a sense of the spiritual. However, I believe that when we look for the spiritual dimension in our children, we may be looking from an adult's perspective. I would agree with Coles that children do have spiritual concerns and it is often our ignorance and insensitivity that influences our failure to see it. Handzo suggests:

> For the most part, children will talk to us only if they feel they are fully accepted children of God with a faith system that may be different from that of most adults, but one that is no less important . . . They may not talk about faith in the same way as adults, but their insights can be quite complete [12, p. 17].

Judith Allen Shelley, in *The Spiritual Needs of Children*, points out that although experts say children do not understand abstract religious concepts until they reach the age of twelve, it is clear that younger children may also understand [13]. At a very young age, children see their parents as God-figures but their conception of God or the spiritual is not limited to this. She suggests that children use parents as a bridge to God or the spiritual and it is difficult for children to develop a trusting or healthy relationship with a supreme being if the adults who are their main role models are uncaring, untrustworthy, and hurtful [13]. The problem is not in determining whether or not children are spiritual, but whether or not they are given a chance to develop their spirituality.

Perhaps even more telling is the need that children have for spirituality. Dubik-Unruh, in discussing children dying with AIDS, states that:

Depending on the child's age and functional capacity spiritual as well as emotional supports must be in place. Children as well as adults have spiritual needs which must be respected [14, p. 15].

Shelley, in examining the needs of hospitalized children, comments that children want formal religious discussion, despite the fact that there may not be any family background or experience to support this type of inquiry. She suggests that spiritual care is necessary for children and that:

Spiritual care is not merely a nice option for nurses who have a few spare moments. It is essential for the child's total development and outlook on life [13, p. 16].

Shelley notes that Piaget's stages of cognitive development include religious and spiritual development, and she also makes reference to spiritual development in relation to Erickson's eight stages of man. She quotes Meyer, a psychiatrist, in supporting her conclusion that children need spirituality for their development. Meyer suggests that:

Psychological development will enable our children to live in society and earn a living but spiritual development will enable them to understand the meaning of life [13, p. 26].

In working with young children, it is important for caregivers to emphasize the existence of a loving God, as opposed to a punitive God. Otherwise, children may feel that God will demand punishment for some remembered or imagined wrong.

In her examination of the literature, Shelley recounts how Marlow believed that children are not spiritually neutral because they have a natural interest in God and an inborn sense of the divine which can be nurtured by the family and the community. Marlow's three basic requirements for spiritual development are:

1. unconditional love with positive reinforcement,
2. realistic discipline, making children responsible for their actions,
3. a dependable and truthful support system [13, p. 34].

In continuing, Shelley referring to Marlow, reports that school age children can describe their conception of God. Children begin to want more detailed factual knowledge about their faith and start to conceptualize conscience, sin, and forgiveness, as well as religious rules and observance [13, p. 40]. They develop an abstract conception of God as being a power greater than themselves or their parents, are less inclined to describe God physically, and assign God character traits or responsibility for actions such as making the flowers, grass, or weather. These conceptions and the concepts of heaven and hell are understood and described in literal terms. By ages eight or nine, children begin to relate to God as individuals and develop ways to pray.

From ages ten to twelve, children begin to understand what it means to be a spirit. By the end of the elementary school years, many children have accepted that God is a creator, law-giver, and friend, and realize there are rules to be followed in accordance with God. They begin to develop a conscience that will bother them if they disobey and question the validity of what they have been taught about their faith [13].

Responsibility for the child's spiritual development usually rests with the parent or parents. However, during a child's hospitalization, nurses and health practitioners may also share in this responsibility. The role of caregivers is to be mindful of spiritual requirements and to integrate them into their approach, particularly in pediatric palliative and hospice care.

Van Heukelem suggests that seeing spirituality as an innate or inborn sense of the divine is not adequate for properly assessing the spiritual needs of children and families [15]. By starting with the assumption that spirituality is intuitive we may miss the point. She suggests that a series of diagnostic steps should be used for assessing spiritual need including: data collection, a proper diagnosis, a plan for action, implementation, and evaluation of effectiveness. She suggests that in the hospital setting, we should take a practical approach. We should evaluate the support systems of children, and analyze their bedtime needs and concerns, reading materials, leisure activities, greeting cards from visitors, and visits from family and friends to determine whether spiritual influences are present [15].

Presumably Van Heukelem's concern is that if we assume that an intuitive spirituality is present, we may overlook the specific needs of individual children. In order to provide effective spiritual support, I would endorse Van Heukelem's approach as a means of augmenting and supporting each child's need for spiritual development.

Regardless of whether spirituality is intuitive or learned, caregivers who accept the importance of spirituality can assume roles as facilitators in the development of spirituality. The problem is to assess how we can best meet the child's spiritual needs.

I would adopt Reverend Dane Sommer's observation that:

> Regardless of their religious heritage or the faith background of their parents, all children are spiritual. Like everyone, their spirituality is natural, creative and an adaptive force that both raises and resolves issues of life and death [16, p. 3].

In my work as a pediatric hematologist and oncologist, I have found rewards in discussing spirituality with families of my own and other faiths. In addition to validating my personal beliefs, these discussions increase my awareness and understanding of others and add a new and meaningful dimension to caring for children and families. I have found that once dying children are party to these discussions, they will join in very quickly and openly by adding their own personal thoughts and stories to the dialogue.

The Role of Religion

I agree that distinguishing spirituality from religion is an important step in recognizing the distinct spiritual needs of children that exist independent of religion. However, there is also a need for caregivers to understand the importance of religious convictions and practices in working with dying children. By comparing and contrasting the Protestant, Roman Catholic, and Jewish traditions in approaching the subject of death with children in general, Grollman offers the type of useful information that is in tune with what caregivers require [17]. This is endorsed by Lester and Ward who advocate training for hospice workers to include religious philosophies, beliefs about the after-life, and ceremonies and rituals of various religions. In their approach they used a four member panel representing different religions to educate hospice workers [18].

In my practice, I have learned that religious beliefs and practices are often the best vehicles for addressing the spiritual needs of some children as they involve thoughts and terminology that are familiar to children and in tune with the beliefs of one or both parents. Insensitivity or embarrassment can be avoided by becoming well-versed in the nuances of various religions or taking the time to consult with religious authorities when in doubt. I also believe that it is always worthwhile to ask children or families to tell us about their beliefs.

The value of religious beliefs is validated for older children in particular, in Balk's work with bereaved youths. Balk suggests that they use their religious beliefs to help accept loss and that religion becomes increasingly important and helpful as bereavement progresses [19].

Martinson and Enos, in emphasizing how we should encourage children to ask questions, points out that we need to be aware of cultural differences, some of which are closely tied to religious beliefs. For instance, in Japan and some other eastern countries such as Taiwan, parents do not usually tell children they are dying [20].

In a study of communication with dying children, parents, with religious faith as a source of support, reported that discussions of death with their children were more helpful than in families without religious faith. In dealing with death, religious faith was generally helpful or somewhat helpful in thirty-four of forty cases [21].

In closing this section, I must reiterate that little attention is paid to spirituality or religion in the education of health caregivers. In addition, as some Christian medical students that I counseled recently pointed out, many teachers in medical schools are openly critical of, and hostile to formal religion or any discussions about spirituality. Perhaps, because of these influences, I have seen deeply religious health caregivers hesitate to share beliefs, even with families of the same faith. I have heard them say, "That's not professional," or "Religion is a private matter." This is most unfortunate as these caregivers have much to offer.

NEAR DEATH EXPERIENCES AND SPIRITUAL CARE

The experiences of children who suffered cardiac arrest and were revived, provide useful information to help us understand whether or not children are concerned about spiritual matters. I believe that these experiences are often spiritual in nature and caregivers should be willing to elicit information and discuss spirituality as part of their care of gravely ill or dying children. Unfortunately, near death experiences are often either misunderstood or dismissed by caregivers.

Morse and his associates initially described near death experiences of children in a journal article in 1986 [22]. This led to funding for further research and subsequent publication of the book *Closer to the Light* [23]. This research, based mainly on intensive care unit experiences, compared 121 children who had been extremely ill but had not actually arrested with twelve children who had arrested and described near death experiences. Morse concluded that children had to be on "the brink of death" before they could experience the visions of the afterlife [23, p. 47]. His findings rule out theories that near death experiences result from medications, sleep deprivation, bad dreams, or subconscious awareness during surgery [23, p. 47].

In drawing his conclusions, Morse worked closely with eminent neuroscientists who, based on the earlier unreported work of Wilder Penfield, localized near death experiences to the right sylvian fissure connected with the right hippocampal lobe [23]. This conclusion leads Morse into a discussion of the soul and possible explanation of the intense light that is included in all near death experiences.

In his findings, Morse suggests that for children, as well as for adults, near death experiences are probably quite common. However, children seldom want to describe their experiences to anyone. They must be handled with sensitivity in order to help them share their thoughts and feelings as they legitimately worry about being ridiculed. One difference between adults and children is that children do not usually experience a life review. However, children in his study, as well as adults he contacted who had experienced near death experiences in childhood, were all inspired to change their lives. For many this was a very spiritual and religious experience [23].

Morse concludes that we have a lot to learn from children and their experiences and he quotes from Black Elk, a Native American spiritual leader who suggests that, "Grown men may learn from little children for the hearts of little children are pure and therefore the great spirit may show them many things which older people miss" [23, p. 131]. This parallels the Christian tradition where Jesus encourages the children to come to him because they are special and belong to the Kingdom of Heaven [24].

Some lessons from children who have had near death experiences reported by Morse include: "Love your neighbour and cherish life," "Do unto others as you would have them do unto you," "Clean up your own mess," "Be the best you can be," "Contribute to society," "Be nice, kind and loving" [23, p. 191].

Whenever caregivers learn of children's near death experiences, they should encourage them to talk about them. Children need to know that these are valid experiences and that they should not feel frightened. Talking about what has happened may also help children to be less fearful of the prospect of dying and may make the situation easier to face by all concerned.

Case Studies

Since I started my medical practice in pediatric oncology in 1961, I have had over 500 children die under my care. As I reflect back, during the 1960s when most children with cancer died, there was no psychological support available from social workers, psychologists, or clergy. In those days, when I did have free time, I had only minimal involvement in spiritual discussions with my patients. As with Coles, I do not think that I was tuned in to their spiritual needs or discussions about death, and yet most of them died in the hospital where I would have had the opportunity to talk with them. I believe that it took some time for me to overcome the death denial that prevents most physicians from engaging in such discussions. In those days, knowledge about the social, emotional, and spiritual needs of children was very limited and attention to their medical needs was the highest priority. During the 1970s, as the prognosis began to improve for children with cancer and there were fewer deaths, we began to promote death at home in keeping with the pioneering work of Martinson and Enos [20]. As this trend continued, there were fewer and fewer opportunities to talk with children about death or spirituality. During this time we also began to build teams consisting of social workers, psychologists, child life specialists, art therapists, and clergy, to help children and families deal with psychosocial concerns. As the survival rate continued to improve along with the intensity of treatment, my discussions with families were increasingly limited to medical facts and issues. Thus, my actual experience in talking to dying children is surprisingly limited and as a result, in the following case histories, I sometimes had to rely on the memories of the parents rather than on my memory of a child's actual words.

The lesson I have learned is that if we consider spiritual care of pediatric patients to be a necessary part of total patient care, then we should make time for such discussions. However, this is often easier said than done in the hospital setting where relaxed visiting rules mean that children are rarely without a visitor. In addition, once children are declared terminally ill and in need of palliative care, access is further reduced as they tend to be cared for at home and spend little time in the hospital. Finally, to enter into a discussion with a dying child about spirituality requires a special relationship with the child along with time and patience. Thus, it is more likely that a sensitive nurse, social worker, psychologist, child life specialist, art therapist, or clergy person will be carrying out this dialogue with terminally ill children. In this respect, I envy Komp's unique experience with dying children, especially in the context of a home care program that she was directing. This served as the basis for her wonderful books, A *Window to Heaven* and A *Child Shall Lead Them*, in which she describes how her Christian faith had been "derailed" during medical school and revived through her contact with dying children [25, 26].

The following case examples illustrate the spirituality of a small number of children from my practice.

Sara

Sara died at the age of fourteen after relapsing following a bone marrow transplant. Her mother was Hindu, although she was brought up in a Catholic convent and was well aware of Christian teachings. She wanted her daughter to have some knowledge about both of these religions. Her father was raised in the Hindu religion and wanted his daughter to have as much knowledge of Hindu as possible.

Sara did not verbalize any concrete ideas about her impending death, although she completed some wonderful paintings and drawings which expressed her spiritual concerns. Despite her illness and the treatment she had been a happy, cheerful child until the time following her relapse and final visit to the transplantation clinic. There, she was told that she had no hope of receiving a second transplant or being cured. On her return home, she became very depressed and one evening her mother heard her in her room crying out, "Why me? Why me?" It was as if she was talking to someone with greater power and authority. Her only other reference to her spiritual beliefs came when she stated that she believed after her death she would see her grandfather again.

Alex

When Alex was nine years old, he relapsed following a bone marrow transplant and was deemed incurable. His mother, Darlene, a single parent, had not been associated with a church or religion and had not taught him anything about formal religion. However, when he became terminally ill, he was curious about Jesus, and his mother sent for a pastor of a church that she had been associated with as a child. The pastor spent several sessions with Alex. Following each session, Alex remarked how much better he felt. He also said that he was no longer afraid to die because they talked about life in heaven. At other times, Alex was very reticent to discuss his dying and preferred to talk about everyday living. Nevertheless, he welcomed the attention of the mother of another seriously ill child who was a devout Roman Catholic. When she prayed with him and said the rosary, Alex stated that the experience was very reassuring.

Michael

Michael was seventeen years old and in the terminal stages of acute myelogenous leukemia. He had a very low platelet count and was not really fit to travel. However, his last burning wish was to go to a friend's cabin on Manitoulin Island and catch a pike in the open water, a new experience for him. In spite of protests from members of the medical and nursing staff, I arranged for him to go on this trip. A helicopter was standing by at the nearest medical center in case he should start to hemorrhage or encounter other complications. It was not needed. On the bookshelf in my office is a picture of Michael with a pike in one hand and a glass of beer in the other. He has a big smile on his face. He died the next day. Although his family were devout Christians and he had attended religious services, his fishing trip was, in a sense, a spiritual experience for him at that time in his life. This case emphasizes that it is important to be sensitive and open to this type of spirituality.

Carol

Carol was seven years old and dying from acute leukemia when I visited her at home. After some discussion in the presence of her mother, I was reassured that all was going well. I was told she had accepted her death and believed she would go to heaven. As I was about to leave, Carol asked to see me alone. With some hesitation she asked, "Will I get to heaven?" In retrospect, I wish I had explored this matter more with her but, at the time, all I could do was to tell her I was sure that she would be accepted into heaven.

Peter

Peter was a seven-year-old boy who was dying at home from disseminated lymphoma. He told his mother that he knew he was going to heaven because he knew it would be a better place. His main concern was that it would take a long time before he would see his parents there and he would miss them. He also wondered if there was "anyone else in heaven besides kids." He asked for prayers from visitors for himself and his family. When the minister came to visit and wanted to leave very quickly, Peter asked him to come back because he wanted to talk to him about Jesus. It was fortunate that Peter made his spiritual needs known very clearly as sometimes clergy, like other caregivers, avoid such discussions due to their own discomfort.

Bob

Bob, age thirteen years, became comatose due to a large brain tumor that complicated treatment for acute leukemia. Although the neurology service was anxious to investigate the tumor and begin treatment, his parents who were Mennonites, knew that he was incurable and decided to take him home to die. He awakened from his coma Friday night and remained awake until Saturday morning when his parents talked to him about dying, going to heaven, and meeting his grandmother and two other patients that he knew who had already died. Bob, who was a young lad of very few words, responded, "I have got more friends than that up there." Shortly after, he became comatose and died. His parents wished they had asked him for more details. In retrospect, given his history, it is possible that he had a near death experience and had seen some other people in addition to his grandmother and the two other patients.

Diane

Diane was eight years old and dying of Ewing's sarcoma when her parents called me to her home because they were concerned about her fear and agitation. Diane and her family believed in heaven, and she had apparently been resigned to dying and going to heaven. Diane asked to see me alone and then asked me what it was like to die. It was apparent that her fear and agitation arose from this question, possibly reinforced by frequent media presentations of violent death. I tried to reassure her that I had seen many children die and that it had always been a peaceful experience. However, I also discussed my knowledge of near death experiences and this seemed to reassure her. Although these experiences have been questioned as to whether they are a true vision of heaven, or some other hallucinatory phenomenon, I believe that they provide a message that dying is peaceful and, as a result, I had no problem in conveying my belief to Diane.

Rose

Rose, age ten years, had been frequently asking me if we had found a bone marrow transplant donor for her. This was her only hope of cure after her fourth relapse of acute lymphoblastic leukaemia. After I finally told her that we really did not believe this would happen, she told me about her dream from the week before. She said, "An angel came to me and told me I would die soon and go to heaven and that after this happened, my little brother would behave badly." Apparently, Rose had not told anyone else about this dream. I continued our dialogue by asking her if she believed that dreams came true. She said, "What do you think?" and I said, "Yes, sometimes they do." She cried, I hugged her, and then left. Soon after, I wished I had spent more time with Rose and wondered if I had left because I was uncomfortable with her being upset. Previous to this, her father and step-mother had told me that they did not believe that Rose knew how sick she really was (with which I politely disagreed) and this probably led me to talk with her. I mentioned the dream to her parents and they were both quite surprised. Talking with her about this dream subsequently led to a more comfortable relationship between Rose and her parents.

I initially found these, and other encounters with dying children to be difficult because I was very unsure of how to deal with their direct questions. However, once I overcame my professional inhibitions, I found that providing simple honest answers and being unafraid to express ignorance made the encounters much less difficult.

A PRACTICAL GUIDE TO DISCUSSING SPIRITUAL ISSUES WITH DYING CHILDREN

From a combination of my experience and the literature, I believe that there are two basic questions to pursue with dying children that should be asked in terms they can easily understand: 1) How they describe God; and 2) Whether they believe that God acts in a meaningful way for them. An important principle would be to let the child set the agenda. For instance, if you engage in prayer with terminally ill children, ask them what you should pray about, listen to them carefully, and follow your intuition with respect to how you respond. What have they told you about their beliefs? Can you tailor your response to their thinking?

Entering into a dialogue with young children about spirituality or religion can be difficult because they tend to mix logical and concrete thinking with fantasy. By school age, they frequently have an unending array of specific questions and will point to and notice any inconsistencies in your story. But even school age children, due to their active fantasy life, may accept stories, analogies, and other religious parables at face value. For instance, as Prescott-Erickson relates, because of a Bible story, one child was afraid of being buried alive as God's punishment for some wrong-doings she had done. In dealing with such concerns, especially when children are dying, Prescott-Erickson suggests that puppets, dolls, and art therapy be used to encourage children to express their thoughts and deal with their anxieties. She stresses that it is important to allow children to feel comfortable with God and believe they are forgiven for those things that they feel guilty about [27].

In the Christian tradition, children may have difficulty understanding that the God they have been taught about would allow this to happen to them and think that they are being punished [25]. Dane Sommer suggests that the concept of a loving God is the least confusing to children when describing how God functions. For Sommer, a God that will help them through this period of distress and be ready to receive them in heaven is more acceptable than the concept of the all powerful God who might have caused this problem and has the means to rectify it [28].

Prescott-Erickson suggests that when dealing with spiritual concerns, caregivers should:

1. Explain who they are and why they have scheduled the visit, linking their purpose to spiritual concerns and needs.
2. Arrange an individual appointment with the child, somewhere where the child is comfortable.
3. Guide the conversation, based on the child's responses and questions, and keep the answers simple. Honesty and directness are as important as making regular follow-up visits [27, pp. 111-112].

In her work, Prescott-Erickson has encountered questions or comments such as: "Does God kill good people?" "I was a bad girl, God is making me die," and "What is heaven like?" She points out that for those of the Christian tradition there are many bible stories concerning Jesus and children and these can be used to comfort children. However, you must also be able to admit that you do not have all the answers to difficult questions. You have to be honest and reassuring at the same time [27, p. 113].

For children without a specific faith, the classic butterfly analogy used by Elisabeth Kübler-Ross is helpful. A child describes this analogy as follows:

> The caterpillar gets in a cocoon and goes into a deep sleep and wakes up beautiful and able to fly. That's what will happen when I die . . . I'll wake up and be able to fly in heaven and I won't hurt no more [27, p. 105].

It is important to remember that "all people are spiritual, and all people have spiritual needs," regardless of their age or faith background [28, p. 225]. Children, like adults, in the face of an impending death will experience a spiritual crisis. Although the language, the responses, and the ability to describe this experience will not be as sophisticated as those of adults, it is no less real. The caregiver must respond to the spiritual needs of dying children by assessing the particular needs of each child and talking openly and honestly.

In closing, I offer the following comments on spirituality:

1. Spirituality must be defined broadly and incorporate the recognition that it may stand on its own or be closely linked with religious beliefs and practices.
2. Thus defined, spiritual care should be an integral part of care of dying children and their families, regardless of their religious affiliation.
3. Spirituality cannot only be defined, but can also be assessed, in respect to the concerns and needs of patients, caregivers, and families.
4. Spirituality and spiritual care are generally not taught or encouraged in the training of caregivers. Consequently, educators in health science faculties are challenged to change their approach to meet a valid need.
5. Dying children are particularly open to spiritual dialogue and there is a small but significant collection of literature available to assist caregivers in this area.
6. Dying children, families, and caregivers will all benefit from increased spiritual dialogue.
7. There is a need for further applied research on the spiritual dimensions of care in pediatric palliative care and hospice programs where the spiritual needs of children and their families are most intense.

ACKNOWLEDGMENT

I acknowledge the editing assistance of Michael Lacy and Iain Mackinnon, and the research assistance of Judy Wolfe and Elyse Pike.

REFERENCES

1. C. A. Corr, J. D. Morgan, and H. Wass (eds.), *International Work Group on Death, Dying, and Bereavement: Statements on Death, Dying, and Bereavement*, International Work Group on Death, Dying, and Bereavement, London, Canada, 1993.
2. R. Twycross, *How Whole is Our Care?*, address to the Seventh International Congress on Terminal Care, Montreal, Canada, 1988.
3. M. F. Highfield, Spiritual Health of Oncology Patients—Nurses and Patient Perspectives, *Cancer Nursing, 15*:1, pp. 1-8, 1992.
4. M. K. Stiles, The Shining Stranger—Nurse-Family Spiritual Relationship, *Cancer Nursing, 13*:4, pp. 235-245, 1990.
5. M. D. Amenta, Paediatric Hospice Care, in *What Helps*, B. Martin (ed.), Children's Hospital of Los Angeles, Los Angeles, 1989.

6. S. Eaton, Spiritual Care: The Software of Life, *Journal of Palliative Care,* *4*:1 & 2, pp. 91-93, 1988.
7. P. Smyth and D. Bellemare, Spirituality, Pastoral Care, and Religion: The Need for Clear Distinctions, *Journal of Palliative Care, 4*:1&2, pp. 86-88, 1988.
8. F. Wald, Spiritual or Pastoral Care: Two models, *Journal of Palliative Care, 4*:1&2, pp. 94-97, 1988.
9. A. Weissman, Ultimate Questions on Existential Vulnerability, *Journal of Palliative Care, 4*:1&2, pp. 89-90, 1988.
10. B. M. Mount and L. McHarg, *Montreal Children's Hospital Palliative Care Assessment Committee Report,* Montreal Children's Hospital, Montreal, Canada, 1987.
11. R. Coles, *The Spiritual Life of Children,* Houghton Mifflin Co., Boston, 1990.
12. G. F. Handzo, Talking About Faith with Children, *Journal of Christian Nursing,* pp. 17-20, Fall 1990.
13. J. A. Shelley (ed.), *The Spiritual Needs of Children,* Intervarsity Press, Downers Grove, Illinois, 1982.
14. S. Dubik-Unruh, Children of Chaos: Planning for the Emotional Survival of Dying Children of Dying Families, *Journal of Palliative Care, 5*:2, pp. 10-15, 1989.
15. J. Van Heukelem, Assessing the Spiritual Needs of Children and Their Families, in *The Spiritual Needs of Children,* J. A. Shelley (ed.), Intervarsity Press, Downers Grove, Illinois, pp. 87-93, 1982.
16. D. R. Sommer, How to Find God in a Children's Hospital, *Bioethics Forum,* pp. 3-8, Winter 1993.
17. E. Grollman (ed.), *Explaining Death to Children,* Beacon Press, Boston, 1967.
18. L. Lester and D. Ward, Youth Hospice Training, *Death Studies, 9,* pp. 353-363, 1985.
19. D. E. Balk, Sibling Death, Adolescent Bereavement, and Religion, *Death Studies, 15,* pp. 1-20, 1993.
20. I. M. Martinson and M. Enos, The Dying Child at Home, in *Hospice Approaches to Pediatric Care,* C. A. Corr and D. M. Corr (eds.), Springer Publishing Company, New York, 1985.
21. J. Graham-Pole, H. Wass, S. Eyberg, and L. Chu, Communicating with Dying Children and Their Siblings: Retrospective Analysis, *Death Studies, 13,* pp. 465-483, 1989.
22. M. Morse, D. Castillo, D. Venecia, et al., Childhood Near-Death Experiences, *American Journal of Diseases of Children, 140,* pp. 1110-1113, 1986.
23. M. Morse and P. Perry, *Closer to The Light: Learning from Near Death Experiences of Children,* Villard Books, New York, 1990.
24. The Holy Bible, Matthew, 19:14.
25. D. Komp, *A Window to Heaven,* Zondervan Publishing, Grand Rapids, Michigan, 1992.

26. D. Komp, *A Child Shall Lead Them*, Zondervan Publishing, Grand Rapids, Michigan, 1993.
27. B. J. Prescott-Erickson, The Terminally Ill Child, in *When Children Suffer: A Sourcebook for Ministry with Children in Crisis*, A. D. Lester (ed.), Westminster Press, Philadelphia, 1987.
28. D. R. Sommer, The Spiritual Needs of Dying Children, *Issues in Comprehensive Pediatric Nursing, 12*, pp. 225-233, 1989.

CHAPTER 16

Challenges in Developing a Children's Hospice

Betty Davies and Brenda Eng

Pediatric hospice care designates a program or approach to care that seeks to maximize the present quality of life by adapting principles of palliative care to children, their families, and to other concerned persons who are coping with serious or life-threatening illness, the imminent likelihood of dying, or the aftermath of death [1]. Across Canada, there are adult hospice units in about two dozen hospitals, and a few free-standing hospices. In the United States, there are many more. But Canuck Place, located in Vancouver, British Columbia, will be North America's first free-standing hospice specifically for children. The purpose of this chapter is to discuss the challenges that we have encountered to date in the development of Canuck Place. It is important, however, to emphasize that

> pediatric hospice programs cannot be developed through a cookbook approach. Faced with a special population needing special services and considering the resources currently available, each community, it is hoped, will be able to develop its own equally valid solution to the challenge of providing pediatric hospice care [2, p. 28].

BACKGROUND

The first free-standing children's hospice anywhere in the world was Helen House, founded in 1982 in Oxford, England. Helen House is the actualization of an idea which grew out of the tragic illness of one small child, Helen. In turn, Helen House inspired the development of

Canuck Place. In 1988, Brenda Eng, a pediatric nurse, spent four months at Helen House. Upon her return to Canada, she led a small steering committee which formed HUGS (Human Understanding, Growth and Sharing) Children's Hospice Society in 1990 and began working toward the establishment of a hospice in Vancouver.

When Canuck Place opens in 1995, it will provide a warm, welcoming, home-away-from-home atmosphere for eight children, from infancy to seventeen years. Two suites will be able to accommodate families of four who may come from any part of British Columbia.

The scope of the hospice program at Canuck Place, once it is fully developed, will encompass a broad spectrum of services. A basic premise of the hospice program is that home based care is the preferred option. In some circumstances however, periodic in-house care is appropriate. A further premise is that bereavement support is an integral part of all hospice programs. The hospice program therefore, will work with existing services and organizations to provide three components of care: respite, palliative and bereavement. Each component will include activities related to assessment and referral; delivery of care to children, families and others; education; and research.

Participating in the process of nurturing a dream to grow from an abstract idea to a concrete reality has been exciting and sometimes overwhelming. Numerous challenges have marked our path, and unknown challenges lie ahead. Based upon a survey of current Board members and our own experience, the following describes six major challenges we have faced to date, and how we dealt with them.

MAINTAINING THE VISION

What is vision? Essentially, vision is a mental image of a possible and desirable future state. This image or vision may be as vague as a dream or as precise as a goal. Vision helps us to position ourselves so that we might create and take advantage of opportunities [3]. Without vision, one does not know which direction to pursue.

Brenda had a vision of a place where terminally ill children might be cared for comfortably, with compassion, and away from the hustle and chaos of a hospital environment. She first described that vision in an early paper completed in graduate school. Betty had a dream of creating a place where grieving children might freely express their feelings and thoughts, and be assisted to integrate a traumatic experience into their developing lives. Our vision, our dreams are coming to fruition in the creation of Canuck Place. The momentum we gain from this experience sustains us when the going gets a little rough. The challenge, however, is clearly expressing the vision and maintaining it, sharing it with others so that they too benefit from its inspiring power.

One of the first challenges in sharing the vision was to justify the feasibility and the viability of a children's hospice in the province. We had to identify clearly that our perception of a gap in health care services was well founded. The existence of such a gap did not imply that the current services were inadequate, but rather that more could be done to optimize care for children with progressive life-threatening illness and their families.

The changing face of illness in recent years has been and continues to be a factor to consider in planning health care for children. For example, significant advances in technology and medicine have reduced mortality and morbidity from conditions of which children previously died. Consequently, the focus of care has expanded to include children with chronic illnesses in addition to those with acute illness. In an American study, chronically ill children, while comprising 2 percent of the nation's population, use 60 percent of all inpatient resources for children, including diagnostic services [4]. This small minority accounts for about 40 percent of all pediatric inpatient days in hospitals. Thus, while the total number may seem small, these children account for an inordinate amount of health care resources, and attention must be paid to adapting the current system to include care for such children [4].

Moreover, the chronic illnesses of childhood are physiologically diverse, variable in life expectancy, and different in treatment. Many of these illnesses involve a course of slow degeneration and premature death. Several major categories of childhood chronic illness occur more frequently than other diseases and result in childhood mortality: neoplasms and leukemias, respiratory diseases, congenital anomalies, disorders of the central nervous system, and a small but growing number of children with AIDS. Consequently, a model of living-dying care must be organized around values that encourage programs to meet a variety of needs among those in the living-dying interval and that recognizes diversity within the population of people who are dying. This, in itself, is a challenge for health care professionals since current methods of responding to the dying have developed from models of care for the sick that emphasized curing disease and restoring function. As a result, health care professionals have tended to focus on diagnosing, prolonging life and curing disease. It takes time to change focus, to realize that people who have illnesses that cannot be cured or whose ability to function will continue to deteriorate, need a model of care that emphasizes quality rather than length of life.

While it was generally recognized that the unmet needs of children living with life-threatening conditions demand attention, there continued to be debate as to the most beneficial approach, level and location of care. Of course, there is no right way to develop a pediatric hospice program. Each local situation—its needs, its resources, and the commitment of its people—determines the existence, dimensions, and quality of its own pediatric hospice care. Consequently, we chose to describe the situation in British Columbia as a way of documenting the need for a children's hospice program in this province. The needs assessment was based on statistical data pertaining to the numbers of children who die in the province from progressive life-threatening illnesses, interview data with health care professionals, interview and survey data from parents who represented potential users of the hospice program, and data from the literature [5]. The final report provided a logical argument in favor of the hospice program. Moreover, it provided a rational basis for a project that had heart-rending emotional appeal. The document serves to share the vision with Board members, the public, the professional community and potential and actual funding sources, including appropriate government departments.

The needs assessment also served as the foundation for the creation of a business plan [6]. This document encapsulates the overall plan for developing the hospice program, and thereby has also helped to maintain the vision. Both documents are critical in the ongoing development of the clinical program.

CREATING A TEAM

As said in other circumstances, "Coming together is a beginning, keeping together is progress, working together is success." This also fits with our experience. Working together is a collaborative process in which individuals listen to and respect one another, share similar values, and divide responsibilities.

In the beginning, the Steering Committee was comprised mostly of caregivers and parents who shared a common interest in optimizing the quality of care provided to children with life-threatening illness and their families. This group developed the initial mission statement and objectives for a children's hospice. Ground rules were established that focused on cooperation and decision-making by consensus. The structure was informal, with each member contributing to the tasks at hand.

The Steering Committee reached a point where the members realized that their idea would not be viable without funds and a location for the hospice. The expertise of someone knowledgeable in fundraising, public relations, and communications was necessary, someone who could translate the concept into language that potential donors could understand. Our immediate goal then changed direction, from focusing on program development to public relations and fundraising. We established a non-profit society, and disbanded the Steering Committee. Our first Board of Directors was created and included individuals who represented all the necessary components, that is, fundraising, communications, public relations, building management, and clinical aspects. The primary focus was to inform the public and the private sector of our project as a means to finding financial support. For a time, the process became somewhat autocratic as decisions needed to be made quickly and with attention to legal details. The Chair of the Board and those individuals with the required expertise made the necessary decisions with the Board's approval. The needs assessment and then the business plan were completed as background data for marketing and fundraising. Potential locations for a site were negotiated. Individuals with expertise in these various areas took on the responsibility of completing the tasks. Then, as the public became more informed about Canuck Place, and as funding became more established, attention turned once again to the details of ongoing program development. Some individuals argue that it is unwise to develop a program if funding is not in place; others argue that a clearly developed program is essential for securing funding. We have found truth in both arguments—the challenge is to maintain a balance between focusing on fundraising and on program development so that both aspects receive the attention they deserve.

As the project progressed from the simple to the complex, we found it to be a process well characterized by Styles' premise that factors entering into successful collaborative efforts are pyramidal or hierarchical [7]. Basic elements must be met before other aspects can develop securely and soundly, and each phase of the process involves returning to the base and reassessing the elements.

At the base of the pyramid are individuals who share a common interest and possess a fundamental compatibility. Ideally, these persons represent the participating units, but out of necessity, must be in positions of greatest influence. Recruiting the appropriate individuals for each phase of the project is crucial to success. Second, a sense of specific purpose is critical. Aimlessness and empty processes are frustrating and futile and perhaps ultimately destructive. With each phase, a new focus was clarified and new tasks were identified. A set of principles or ground rules for the collaborative relationship, whether spoken or unspoken, is essential regarding such matters as values, expectations, and communications. We began with a small group in which communication was easily maintained through brief telephone conversations and handwritten memos between meetings. Consensus was easily achieved. As the project grew, communication among a larger number of people and between various committees and other groups became more challenging. And, last, structure with its roles and relationships, has its place in the building of a collaborative endeavor. Again, with increasing complexity, the structure has changed. Approximately four years after the initial meeting of the Steering Committee, we hired an Executive Director to manage the affairs of Canuck Place, and other staff to assist in developing various components of the hospice program.

People

Recruiting people must be done with care to increase the probability of a successful experience. The "4 C's" of collaborative work can be applied to finding the right team of people to create the hospice: contribution, communication, commitment, and compatibility.

Contribution

Board members and staff have been selected for the unique nature of their contributions: they possess a particular skill necessary to the work of the Board; they have had valuable experience relevant to fulfilling the vision; or, they may be knowledgeable about the workings of particular structures or other agencies. Each individual brings something unique to the Board and to the whole organization. The challenge is to respect individual contributions and to use various strengths constructively, which in turn creates a sense of community and collaboration. It is helpful to clarify the role of all Board members and their status on the Board as individuals, or as representatives of particular agencies or organizations. The aim is to develop a working board, not a "name" board. This presents another challenge: to identify potential Board members who have the expertise required for the various tasks which need to be completed.

One specific challenge has been to adequately inform those Board members, who have had limited or no direct experience in hospice care, about the hospice concept. Their commitment to the project has gradually and enthusiastically developed through their participation. It is essential that individuals are able to somehow mesh personal goals with the project's goals. A related challenge is to recognize that each person has different skills and contributions to make during certain phases in developing the concept.

Communication

Communication is important to identify if there is "goodness of fit" in both personality and communication styles among Board members and staff. At minimum, it is important that team members be able to tolerate one another well enough to work together.

Commitment

Finding individuals who will maintain their commitment to the project may be a challenge. Commitment includes time, energy, and resources. Groups work better if all members have relatively the same level of commitment and if they give the project the same level of priority in their lives. To tactfully manage situations where an individual lacks the requisite commitment, requires a safety net, an established procedure for moving such individuals off the Board or from a staff position. Sometimes however, commitment is affected by factors outside of the group members' control and such situations need to be tolerated. In addition, it is important not to expect all individuals to make a life-long commitment to the project.

Compatibility

Compatibility by no means implies that all members should be alike, but rather, that the members of the team should fit together to make an effective, functioning whole. Compatibility means that members find ways to recognize and appreciate one another's similarities and differences as well as ways to make members' differences an asset to the team. Compatibility also means finding ways to harmonize very different styles, so that team members maintain respect for one another and bring out the best, rather than the worst, in each other. A working team may have a member who sees the big picture; one who thinks up ideas like a bubbling cauldron; another who plays the devil's advocate whenever a new idea is shared; someone who says, "Let's stop and think about this for a moment"; and yet another who insists, "Charge ahead!" Such a mixture can lead to a challenging and exciting experience in collaborating to develop a hospice. It must also be remembered that the people who develop the concept may not be the people who maintain the system. Some creative and innovative persons may be more interested in developing the ideas than in the day-to-day management. Others may not be as creative, but have excellent organizational skills which are necessary to the smooth ongoing functioning of the program.

Purposes

The overall purpose of Canuck Place has been addressed in the earlier discussion of the first challenge, maintaining the vision. Each phase of development has had its own purpose. For example, the Steering Committee clearly identified its purpose in laying the groundwork for the project; the purpose of the subsequent phase was to identify one or more individuals who could assist with fundraising and public relations. Completing the needs assessment and the business plan were clear purposes at different stages. Currently, the purpose focuses on the building renovations. Other purposes, such as fundraising, public relations, and program development are less phase-specific, and are of an ongoing nature. It is important to clarify the priorities of each purpose, and to clearly state expectations for all members of the team in order to support high quality participation.

Decision-Making

Hospice, as a philosophy and an approach, requires interdisciplinary teamwork that implies the coming together of individuals of various disciplines, personalities, insecurities, strengths, and abilities. When we began, decisions were made through shared discussion and consensus by the members of the Steering Committee. As we progressed to having a Board, we have had to face challenges related to our increasing size and complexity. For example, a decision which has long-term implications for the future of the hospice requires a process by which there is consensual agreement. In contrast, decisions that have more practical and immediate implications can be made by an appointed sub-group. The challenge is to decide which decisions require which method of decision-making.

Challenges related to leadership have been critical. Various types of leadership are required at different points in time. For example, to take the group from a volunteer organization to a funded organization, it was necessary to provide leadership in the form of a chief executive officer. However, such a position could not be filled until funds were in place. Clinical leadership was also required to accurately portray the ultimate purpose of the facility in terms of the children and the families who will receive care.

The ability of group members to arrive at a consensus was tested early in the collaborative process, and continues to be tested in each new phase of development. Board and staff retreats, facilitated by an outside consultant, have served to equalize information and formulate goals. Consensus, like compatibility, is a never-ending process of communication, compromise, and negotiation.

Credit in collaborative endeavors can be a complicated issue. In successfully meeting the challenge of creating a collaborative team, we must acknowledge that the development of Canuck Place to date is the product of the generous efforts of many individuals. For example, the hours donated by our fundraiser are too many to count, the time donated by our lawyer have saved us thousands of dollars. The same holds true for the engineer who chairs our building committee and the chartered accountant who is our treasurer. Many of our Board members contribute countless hours, over and above their regular work weeks. Their contributions in terms of time, effort, and dollars saved for the hospice, must be acknowledged. In addition, we are challenged to find creative and appropriate ways to recognize and acknowledge the contributions of our financial partners and other donors. Without their support, the hospice vision would not be realized in the same way.

Structure

The structure has evolved as the concept developed, and continues to do so. The ongoing challenge is to form the best structure for getting the work done. For example, when we first created the HUGS Hospice Society and its Board, numerous tasks were identified and assigned to various committees . . . a total of eighteen different committees! Not only was communication among all the committees a problem, but some individuals were being spread too thin across too many committees. Now, we have four major committees: Finance, Fundraising and Public Relations, Building, and Hospice Care. Each is chaired by a Board member. One advantage of these smaller committees is that there is a committed working group to accomplish the tasks. Using a small number of people, however, can limit the input from all appropriate sources. Consequently, another challenge is to find ways of soliciting that input. For example, the hospice care committee values the input of consumers, volunteers, and health educators whose students might be placed in Canuck Place. The consumer perspective might be represented if a parent were on the committee. However, the contribution of that one parent will be influenced by the extent of his/her experience. A focus group comprised of several parents would be more representative of the various views of consumers. The current structure is more efficient, although a continuing challenge is to maintain communication among the committees and other Board members.

Another challenge stems from changing the structure from volunteer to staff positions. For example, we needed to identify which aspects of various positions would continue on a volunteer basis, and which ones would be part of paid positions so that fair and satisfactory contracts could be established. As we continue to evolve and Canuck Place opens, our structure will continue to change and we will encounter new challenges in this regard.

The process of structuring a collaborative team requires the understanding that all persons come to the project with their own personal agendas and their own problems. Facing the challenge involves accepting all of these factors, and appreciating that individuals are prepared in different ways to be stretched to reach beyond their known capacities. It includes maintaining the belief that "all will work out for the best." It is finding the balance between the excitement of pioneering, the satisfaction of doing something for the first time, and the fear that it may not work.

TELLING THE STORY

To tell the story—to continually reinforce public and professional awareness—is another major challenge. Part of this challenge was to identify the kinds of background information required by various groups, i.e., government, major corporate sponsors, and professionals. Some individuals and groups demanded statistical information and documented evidence of the need; a needs assessment provided information for this purpose. Others required a more detailed plan of operation; a business plan met their needs. As Canuck Place becomes a functioning program, we must meet the challenge of "coming through" with what the public expects and believes we are to be within the realities of the resources and time available.

Another component of telling the story involves developing a marketing plan for various public forums. For example, strategies must be developed to relate, not only to the donating public, but also to the health care and professional public. There is the potential that being "the new kid on the block" in the health care arena will be threatening to existing health care providers and agencies. How, then, do we introduce the concept in a manner that will invite cooperation and encourage the building of bridges, rather than competition and antagonism? Ongoing challenges are to present our mission clearly, not dogmatically; avoid becoming "all things to all people;" and refrain from the "rescuer" role which tries to fill all the identified gaps in the system.

The success that we have had in the area of fundraising and public awareness may provide a challenge in relating to the professional community. As yet, we have no track record in terms of services offered and still, we have been successful in fundraising. We have made a serious attempt to include representatives from various groups who provide care to children and their families. We have a multidisciplinary Professional Advisory Committee which consists of members who are primarily involved in the care of children, both in the local children's hospital and within the community. In addition, several representatives (operational and medical) from the local children's hospital sit on our Board, serving primary functions of communication and liaison. In addition, we have made presentations to the larger professional community at local health conferences, and national and international palliative care and pediatric conferences. Feature articles have been written in local nursing journals and two papers have been published [8, 9]. We have presented to nursing students, local pediatric practice groups, and are beginning to present to physician groups. As the opening draws closer, we are focusing more attention on specific ways of relating to others in the professional community with regard to the care of children with progressive life-threatening illness.

A provincial daily newspaper, The Vancouver Sun, has been a principal force in telling the story of Canuck Place. Their role has been manifold: (a) to differentiate from the services provided by Ronald McDonald House; (b) to educate the general public about children's hospice care—its philosophy, components, and program services; and (c) to raise funds from its readership.

The story is also being told through video, radio interviews, community newspapers, and employee groups which are fundraising for Canuck Place within their own companies. Individuals who provide fundraising, public relations, and clinical leadership for the project play a critical role in telling the story because they are key spokespersons for many interrelated purposes. For a time, the captain of the Canucks Hockey Club was appointed honorary spokesperson for the Canuck Foundation. This avenue of spokesmanship attracts another public audience and represents a different aspect of commitment to Canuck Place. Another way of telling the story has been through selectively and sensitively describing the realities of death in childhood by sharing the stories of some children and their families. A continuing challenge here is to tell the stories so as to educate the public, while respecting families' rights to privacy.

SEEKING AND MAINTAINING FINANCIAL SUPPORT

Funding is often the most worrisome challenge for any new venture such as ours. One aspect of the challenge centers around the fact that it is more difficult to obtain funding for long-term operating, than it is to get funds for the bricks and mortar. Both aspects of fundraising must be tackled. Our success derives from the strong leadership of an individual who understands the business, corporate, fundraising, and marketing worlds, and who is able to translate the original concept into language that appeals to potential public donors. He knows how to put the right pieces of the puzzle together in terms of resources—money, people, and time. This leadership, in combination with Brenda's representation of the clinical components, paved the way for a partnership with the owners of the Vancouver Canucks. Through their community service arm, known as the Canuck Foundation, they have become a leading force and subsequently, the principal benefactor for capital and operating fund campaigns for Canuck Place.

The process of fundraising has been one of introducing donors to a concept of caring for children and their families, and inviting them to participate. Donors are sought for their stability and character in the community and for the possibility of having provincial impact because of the province-wide nature of services through Canuck Place. Such donors represent the potential for fundraising for Canuck Place and also have the capacity to raise funds for individual children and their families from their own communities. Donors are invited to participate based on what they do best. For example, the newspaper could inform and educate the public, a funeral home corporation could support the bereavement program, and a major realty firm could sell deeds of "real estate" for the children's garden at Canuck Place.

The fundraising approach has been one of building "relationships for tomorrow" by seeking funds for initial capital as well as ongoing operations. Its aim is to create partnerships rather than seek one-time donors because the challenge is to establish a system of funding that will maintain us once the current window of opportunity has closed. Once financial support is obtained a resultant challenge is to maintain good relationships with our donors and to develop appropriate programs of donor recognition.

BUILDING THE FACILITY: GIVING HOSPICE A HOME

Finding a suitable location for Canuck Place has been a multifaceted challenge. Several criteria were developed for the site: proximity to a major pediatric acute care facility, accessibility by several modes of transportation, proximity to other services so that children and their parents might engage in outside activities, and, at the same time, find a place that provides a peaceful milieu. We examined the pros and cons of constructing a purpose-built facility versus renovating an existing building. The cost of each approach was similar, therefore, the challenge was to consider several sites in order to find the optimal one.

First, we considered the possibility of sharing a site with a local church. The proposed plan was for the hospice to lease the land owned by the church, and to be responsible for the building of the facility to meet the needs of both parties. The church would then lease space from us. Discussion ensued centering on issues of mixed-user space and protecting the interests and the privacy of the groups involved. The challenge then became one of clarifying our own values and assumptions integral to providing hospice care for children; as a result, we stepped away from the arrangement.

A second consideration was to work with an existing major health care institution to explore the feasibility of building on their existing land. Even though the sharing of resources seemed like a practical idea for both parties, issues surfaced around how we might become a "dumping ground" for patients who might not meet hospice criteria and how we would deal with a slow-moving hospital board of directors. Again, we were forced to re-examine our own goals and our vision.

While we were in negotiation with this facility, we launched a public announcement in the local provincial newspaper about the partnership between HUGS Children's Hospice Society, Canuck Foundation, and the Vancouver Sun to build the hospice. At the same time, a consultant working for the city was considering potential uses for a turn of the century heritage home which had been donated to the City of Vancouver by Mrs. Elizabeth Wlosinski. The mansion is set in 1.1 acres of established grounds in a quiet residential neighborhood, only a few blocks from the children's hospital. Subsequent interactions led to our leasing the site for the hospice, known now as Canuck Place at Glen Brae.

Having obtained a "perfect" site, the situation was not without its own problems which were related to the legalities of the lease, and gaining the support of some surrounding neighbors. While it was not a major challenge in our experience, neighborhood support can be an insurmountable problem because of the potential deep-rooted anxieties and fears surrounding death, particularly of children. Meeting this challenge was facilitated by the history of the local Ronald MacDonald House which, ten years ago, had become established in the same neighborhood. Since that time, Ronald MacDonald House had become a "good" neighbor having made many contributions to the community. The previous use of Glen Brae was another advantage: for over forty years, this heritage mansion served as a private hospital, thereby, familiarizing the neighborhood with the concept of a care facility.

There have been several challenges associated with the physical building. Obtaining the necessary building and development permits has been somewhat complicated by the fact that we are renovating a heritage site, emphasizing the political nature of working with city and provincial governments at both the bureaucrat and politician levels. Having an experienced engineer as Chair of the building committee, and other Board members who are familiar with the workings of City Hall has been instrumental in the process.

Extensive restorative and renovative work were required to Glen Brae, all within the spirit of respecting the mansion's heritage while creating a warm, friendly, child-oriented environment. As a four-story building, in contrast to the one-level purpose-built children's hospices in England, it has required architectural creativity. One major addition at the back of the house involved installation of an elevator to transport children in beds or wheelchairs from any floor directly into the garden.

Working out satisfactory utilization of the space among the three components of the hospice program has been an additional challenge. There is a natural flow between the respite and palliative care components, but the bereavement program has a mixed user group. As a result, we have had to work at clarifying how to balance the use of this space within the picture of the whole program. The multipurpose space, for example, is designed for a variety of events, including staff and volunteer training, bereavement groups, and other meetings.

DEVELOPING THE CLINICAL PROGRAM

The overall challenge in developing the clinical program is to translate the vision of care into service delivery which serves children with progressive life-threatening illness and their families from anywhere in the province; is family oriented; captures the home away from home philosophy; complements existing services; and fosters a collaborative approach to care which maximizes quality of life. It is this challenge that is our current focus as we more specifically define the various aspects of the program.

As the program is implemented, additional challenges will relate to hiring staff, recruiting volunteers, and developing training programs. In addition to the appropriate qualifications, we will seek people whose attributes make for optimal hospice staff: a high tolerance for ambiguity, flexibility, and an appreciation for individual differences; good external support networks and a realistic awareness of personal limits; joie de vivre and a sense of humor; an open communication style, an ability to listen and a tendency to value self-awareness as assets; empathy; and a willingness to continually learn. Another ill-defined personal characteristic that may affect one's ability to work with dying children is their comfort with death:

> Becoming a clinical practitioner who can move toward instead of away from children who are dying does not come easily. Rather, it requires a willingness to experience again and again the strong and varied feelings that come with human-to-human involvement during periods of crisis and change [10, p. 14].

A related challenge is the integration of volunteers at Canuck Place without imposing demands that can potentially take away the staff's energy which would otherwise be directed to the children and their families. There is a need for volunteers in a variety of capacities including positions at the Board level, assistance with special events and events related to fundraising, day-to-day functioning in service delivery, and participation in policy making. The challenge is to find the right "fit" between individuals, their talents, and the needs of the organization, as those needs evolve.

In developing the hospice, we have been challenged to find specific information about the evaluation of hospice programs for both adults and children. We are meeting this challenge by incorporating into our work, from the beginning, an evaluation component which will ensure that we are offering quality care within the limits of our finances and other resources. Moreover, we want to ensure that the hospice program is based on sound principles, and that the care delivered is research-based. Through research, we want to contribute to the general knowledge about caring for children with progressive, life-threatening illness and their families. Pursuing such research goals while maintaining an active service program will be an ongoing, but worthy, challenge.

Finally, there is the challenge of remembering that we can only do our best in terms of developing high quality programs. Once we open Canuck Place we will need to face the challenge of changing to better meet the needs of the children and families as those needs become evident.

CONCLUSION

Many challenges have accompanied the establishment of Canuck Place. The determination to meet these challenges has been facilitated by finding suitable levels of personal commitment, so that individuals do not become overly committed at the expense of their own health and well-being. It has come from recognizing that no one is immune to burn out, no matter how much one believes in the project. It has to do with knowing one's own vulnerabilities, strengths, and limitations. It also has to do with maintaining one's own boundaries. Mount suggests that the "primary task of adult life is to recognize, understand and accept our own personhood, our own feet of clay, our own woundedness" [11]. Fulfilling this task is an ongoing challenge.

Through it all, we have been sustained by remembering first, that children's hospice can make a difference. It facilitates the participation of parents in assuming the role of primary caregiver. It supports the inclusion of the patient and the family in the decision-making process to the best of the family's capability and commensurate with their desires. This comprehensive care can have a lasting impact on the lives of family members and friends, making it possible to find some solace and comfort mixed in with the grief [12]. Second, we are sustained by remembering the words of Cardinal Newman: "Nothing would be done at all if a man (or woman) waited until he could do it so well that no one could find fault with it."

REFERENCES

1. C. A. Corr and D. M. Corr, In our Opinion...What is Pediatric Hospice Care? *Children's Health Care, 17*:2, pp. 4-11, 1988.
2. D. Wilson, Developing a Hospice Program for Children, in *Hospice Approaches to Pediatric Care*, C. A. Corr and D. M. Corr (eds.), Springer Publishing Company, New York, pp. 5-30, 1985.
3. B. Davies, Clearing our Vision Through Research, *Canadian Nurses Journal, 86*:6, pp. 20-22, 1990.
4. Caring Institute of the Foundation for Hospice and Home Care, *The Crisis of Chronically Ill Children in America: Triumph of Technology—Failure of Public Policy*, Author, Washington, D.C., 1987.
5. B. Davies, *Assessment of Need for a Children's Hospice Facility in British Columbia*, HUGS Children's Hospice Society, Vancouver, B.C., June 1992.
6. Health Management Resource Group, *A Children's Hospice Program at Canuck Place: Business Plan*, HUGS Children's Hospice Society, Vancouver, B.C., April 1993.
7. M. Styles, Reflections on Collaboration and Unification, *Image: The Journal of Nursing Scholarship, XVI*:1, pp. 21-23, 1984.
8. B. Davies and B. Eng, Development of a Children's Hospice, in *Shaping the Future of Child Health: Challenges for Nurses*, H. Clarke and B. Davies (eds.), Vancouver, B.C., pp. 81-84, 1993.
9. B. Eng and B. Davies, Canuck Place: A Hospice for Children, *Canadian Oncology Nursing Journal, 2*:1, pp. 18-20, 1992.
10. M. M. Suarez and J. Q. Benoliel, Coping with Failure: The Case of Death in Childhood, *Issues in Comprehensive Pediatric Nursing, 1*:3, pp. 3-15, 1976.

11. B. M. Mount, Challenges in Palliative Care: Four Clinical Areas that Confront and Challenge Hospice Practitioners, *Journal of Hospice Care*, pp. 3-10, November/December 1985.
12. C. E. Koop, Foreword, *Hospice Care for Children*, A. Armstrong-Dailey and S. Z. Goltzer (eds.), Oxford University Press, New York, 1993.

CHAPTER 17

Using Story to Help Children Cope with Dying, Death and Bereavement Issues: An Annotated Resource

Donna R. O'Toole

INTRODUCTION

There is a now a large and growing body of literature that demonstrates how personal narrative and story can help children and adults facing the adversity of illness, loss, and grief. This chapter serves three distinct purposes. First, it serves as an adjunct to Chapter 2 by the same author in this volume of *Beyond the Innocence of Childhood*, which discusses how story and active imagination can be used to help seriously ill children and their families. Interested readers can use this information to enlarge their knowledge of materials that substantiate the healing power of narrative. While the twenty-nine annotated listings for professionals and parents are by no means an exhaustive list, they do represent definitive works in the field of narrative thought and practice.

The second use of this chapter is as an annotated guide for those looking for current and available storytelling and story reading materials. In this regard readers will find forty fiction books. Of course, it is not possible to provide an authoritarian discourse of books on any of the given topics below, since individual circumstances, point of view, and cultural influences are so vast. Nonetheless, the stories listed here will provide a rich and rewarding sampling of what literature has to offer. Diverse audiences will benefit from reading these books, including healthy children and adults who are not currently dealing with issues of illness, loss, or grief. Lastly, readers will find listings of names and addresses of six organizations that specialize in a wide variety of mail-order books, and audio and videotapes related to serious illness, dying, death, bereavement, and hope.

Those who wish to make full use of the richness of story are encouraged to contact their local and regional librarians and to search for opportunities to engage the counsel of the thousands of persons who are carrying out the oral traditions as professional and lay storytellers. Information on storytelling conferences and a directory of storytellers in the United States and Canada are listed at the end of this chapter.

THERAPEUTIC STORY RESOURCES FOR PROFESSIONALS AND CAREGIVING ADULTS

Annie Stories, D. Brett, Workman Publishing, New York, 1988—A clinical psychologist provides nine stories to be retold to help children cope with a variety of real-life emotions and anxieties: nightmares, going to the hospital, dealing with pain, coping with divorce, and coping with the death of a loved one.

Awakening the Hidden Storyteller, R. Moore, Shambhala, Boston, Massachusetts, 1991—A master storyteller, the author teaches how stories can be used to build traditions in families. Precise, step-by-step instructions are given throughout.

Biblio/Poetry Therapy, The Interactive Process: A Handbook, A. McCarty Hynes and M. Hynes-Berry, Westview Press, Boulder, Colorado and London, England, 1986—This handbook is designed to teach both professionals and lay persons how to use the whole spectrum of literature, from poetry to science fiction, to promote greater self-knowledge, to renew the spirit and, in general, to aid in the healing process.

The Call of Stories: Teaching and the Moral Imagination, R. Coles, Houghton Mifflin, Boston, Massachusetts, 1989—The author, a skilful psychiatrist, develops the thesis that humans are always able to relate to and learn from stories. In this book Coles makes clear his profound belief that, especially during periods of distress, stories abound in therapeutic value.

Cartoon Magic—How to Help Children Discover their Rainbows Within, R. Crowley and J. Mills, Brunner/Mazel, New York, 1989—An appealing book that offers parents, counselors, and

---

* Titles marked with an asterisk contain references and stories that are directly related to dying, death, and bereavement.

therapists innovative techniques for using cartoon characters and cartoon drawings to help children confront fears.

Creative Storytelling: Choosing, Inventing, and Sharing Tales for Children, J. McGuire, Yellow Moon Press, Cambridge, Massachusetts, 1985—An informative text that provides guidelines for sources and types of stories, how to match stories to age levels and interests, techniques for remembering and adapting stories, and how to utilize your own experiences to create new stories.

Freidman's Fables, E. Freidman, Guildford Press, New York, 1990—This book offers twenty-four fables that can be used to give the reader or listener distance from his or her own real life encounters. The stories offer new perspectives when dealing with adversity.

From Wonder to Wisdom, C. A. Smith, Penguin Books, New York, 1989—Drawing on the best in classic and contemporary literature for children, the author illustrates how a simple story can convey a deeply evocative message to help children persevere through challenging situations.

Homemade Books to Help Kids Cope, R. Ziegler, Brunner/Mazel, New York, 1992—An informative and highly useful guidebook that shows how anyone working with children can help them cope with difficulties through personal storytelling and bookmaking.

The Illness Narratives, Suffering, Healing and the Human Condition, A. Kleinman, Basic Books, New York, 1988—Based on twenty years of clinical experience studying and treating chronic illness, a Harvard psychiatrist and anthropologist argues that interpreting the illness narratives of clients is an art tragically neglected by modern medical training. The author makes a case for listening to illness narratives as a means to ameliorate suffering.

My Voice Will Go With You, The Teaching Tales of Milton H. Erickson, S. Rosen, W. W. Norton, New York, 1992—These are the collected and edited teaching tales used by a master clinician, Milton Erickson. How to increase the reader's learning commentary on the teaching tales is provided.

Narrative Means to Therapeutic Ends, M. White and D. Epston, W. W. Norton, New York, 1990—The thesis of this book is that people experience problems when the stories of their lives do not sufficiently represent their lived experience. Therapy then becomes a narrative process of storying or re-storying the lives and experiences of these people.

Personal Mythology—Using Ritual, Dreams, and Personal Imagination to Discover Your Inner Story, D. Feinstein and S. Krippner, Los Angeles, California, 1988—A practical guide that demonstrates how personal myths are developed and how they can be altered to enhance well-being in times of crisis and change.

Telling Your Own Stories, D. Davis, August House, Little Rock, Arkansas, 1993—This resource will help adults of all ages remember their stories and organize them for family or performance telling.

Storied Lives, G. C. Rosenwald and R. Ochberg (eds.), Yale University Press, New Haven, Connecticut, 1992—The authors tell us that personal stories are not merely a way of telling someone (or oneself) about one's life; they are a means by which identities are fashioned. What stories emphasize and omit, their stance as protagonists or victims—all shape what individuals can claim of their own lives.

*Stories of Sickness, H. Brody, Yale University Press, New Haven, Connecticut, 1987—A philosophical inquiry into the significance of storytelling or narrative for medical practice, philosophy of medicine, and medical ethics.

The Stories We Live By, Personal Myths and The Making of the Self, D. P. McAdams, William Morrow and Company, New York, 1993—The author, a psychologist whose research has led him outside the bounds of academic psychology, presents his innovative theory of human identity, i.e., the way in which we define ourselves is often an unconscious process of creating a heroic myth. A provocative and highly instructive text for all who are seriously interested in the influence of narrative on human development.

Storytelling: Folklore Sourcebook, N. J. Livo and S. A. Rietz, Libraries Unlimited, Englewood, Colorado, 1987—An excellent resource that provides bits and pieces of many categories of folklore to trigger their possible inclusion in stories we tell, write, and read, but especially tell.

Storytelling: Process and Practice, N. J. Livo and S. A. Rietz, Libraries Unlimited, Littleton, Colorado, 1986—This extensive volume presents vital information on the value, process, and presentation of the oral traditions.

*Storymaking in Bereavement, A. Gersie, Jessica Kingsley Publishers, London, England, 1991—An exceptional resource for those wishing to use storymaking and storytelling with bereaved individuals. The uses of stories in therapy are explained. Specifically, bereavement counseling through storymaking is addressed. The final section provides storymaking structures that can be used with particular stories in group work.

*Storytelling in Psychotherapy with Children, R. Gardner, J. Aronson, Inc., Northdale, New Jersey, 1993—A potpourri of practical

storytelling techniques is provided in a readable format by a seasoned child psychiatrist. As well as providing an in-depth look at his storytelling technique, the author illustrates the use of storytelling games and dramatizations.

Story Writing in a Nursing Home, A Patchwork of Memories, M. Tyler John, The Haworth Press, New York, 1991—An exceptional resource that outlines how story-writing has been developed and used as a therapeutic process in nursing centers.

Symbol, Story and Ceremony, Using Metaphor in Individual and Family Therapy, G. Combs and J. Freedman, W. W. Norton, New York, New York, 1990—Building on the work of Erickson, Bateson, and their followers, this book provides invaluable information on the construction and therapeutic use of symbols, stories, and ceremonies.

Therapeutic Metaphors for Children and the Child Within, J. Mills and R. Crowley, Brunner/Mazel, New York, 1986—The authors provide a thorough background of the history, nature, and dynamics of metaphor, demonstrating its rich heritage in both spiritual and psychological traditions. This book has a non-analytical orientation. There are extensive case examples that illustrate the therapeutic uses of artistic metaphors, cartooning, and storytelling.

Touch Magic, Fantasy, Fairies and Folklore in the Literature, J. Yolen, Putnam, New York, 1981—Yolen passionately details how children today are facing a serious loss of story, and therefore, are losing the imaginative capacity that assists them in learning and in dealing with human experience and suffering.

The Uses of Enchantment: The Meaning and Importance of Fairy Tales, B. Bettelheim and A. A. Knopf, New York, 1976—A classic in the field that outlines the importance and uses of fairy tales as a way to communicate culture and well-being.

What's Your Story? A Young Person's Guide to Writing Fiction, M. D. Bauer, Clarion Books, New York, 1992—An award winning novelist guides beginners through the creation of a short story, offering practical, reassuring advice every step of the way.

Writing For Your Life: Discovering the Story of Your Life's Journey, D. Metzer, Harper Collins, San Francisco, California, 1992—In this resource for writers and non-writers alike, Metzer helps us explore ourselves and our creativity through journals, autobiographies, stories, fairy tales, dreams, and myths.

You Don't Have to Die—One Family's Guide to Surviving Childhood Cancer, G. Gaes and C. Gaes, Villard Books, New York, 1992—This book tells the amazing story of one family's determination and action as they face the fears, concerns, and treatment of their young son after his diagnosis of cancer. The book is filled with practical suggestions that will be inspiring and indispensable to other parents facing similar challenges.

STORIES TO READ ALOUD AND TO TELL

The following stories are often presented in story-book form and appear to be for young children. However, most of these stories adapt well to the oral tradition of storytelling. When told, rather than read, they are useful to people of all ages. Other story sources can be found in folklore and ancient myth.

DEATH AS A PART OF LIFE AND DEATH AS TRANSITION AND TRANSFORMATION

Annie and the Old One, M. Miles, Little Brown and Company, Boston, Massachusetts, 1971—Annie learns from her Navajo grandmother that life and death are woven together like the rhythm of growth and decline in nature—that all life is, and always will be, a part of the earth.

The Dream Tree, S. Cosgrove, Price, Stern & Sloan, Los Angeles, California, 1974—The mystery of the transformation of one life form to another is told as a young caterpillar learns how a cocoon becomes a butterfly.

The Education of Little Tree, F. Carter, University of New Mexico Press, Albuquerque, New Mexico, 1976—The true-to-life story of a young Cherokee boy whose mother and father have both died. Little Tree goes to live in the mountains with his grandparents who nurture him and teach him the ways of nature. Little Tree faces many losses and finds a deep and abiding reverence for the cycles of life.

Gentle Closings, How to Say Goodbye to Someone You Love, T. Menten, Running Press, Philadelphia, Pennsylvania, 1991—These are the brief stories of people who have faced illness and death in their families. The vignettes are inspirational, down to earth, easy to read, and to retell.

The Golden Heart of Winter, M. Singer, Morrow Junior Books, William Morrow and Company, New York, 1991—Three sons of a black-smith are sent on a journey to find a thing of great value. The youngest son finds the golden heart of winter which holds the secret of the balance between life and death. Through perilous experiences the three sons learn how to honor both life and death.

Mrs. Huggins and her Hen Hanna, L. Dabcovick, E. P. Dutton, New York, 1985—When Mrs. Huggins' dear hen Hanna becomes sick and dies, Mrs. Huggins buries her and returns sorrowfully to her cottage. Her tears of grief are interrupted when she learns one of Hanna's eggs has hatched. A life cycle story with inter-generational teaching opportunities.

Love You Forever, R. Munsch, Firefly Press, Scarborough, Ontario, 1986—An inter-generational story about how love persists and transcends time, space, and even death. The story lends itself well to audience participation and repetition of the theme, "I'll love you forever, I'll like you for always."

The Man Who Wanted to Live Forever, retold by S. Hastings, Henry Holt, New York, 1988—A young boy who wishes to live forever finds a far away castle that promises him eternal life. After living to be several hundred years old he decides to visit the village of his youth. There he meets death who gently leads him away. Based on an Italian folktale, this story can also be found in story anthologies.

The Redheaded Woman, H. Eustis, Green Tiger Press, LaJolla, California, 1983—An allegorical tale that brings young Maude Applegate face to face with Mr. Death. From Mr. Death and his grandmother she learns the secrets that death carries and the important role death plays as a part of life. Maude comes to see death as a compassionate friend. She finds her own true nature and vitality by living side-by-side with death.

Savitri, retold by A. Shepard, Albert Whitman and Company, Morton Grove, Illinois, 1992—An ancient, well-known, and loved tale from India that was passed down in the oral tradition for centuries. Princess Savitri marries Satyavan, even though she knows he is destined to die in one year. When Satyavan is stricken, Savitri pursues death until she wins back her husband's life by her tenaciousness and wit. Years later, after Satyavan and Savitri have lived a long life they face death without fear or tears.

Nana Upstairs and Nana Downstairs, T. de Paola, Penguin, New York, 1973—An inter-generational tale of a young boy, his grandmother, and his great grandmother. The boy grows and his grandmothers die, but the boy feels their presence with him through his experiences with nature and through his loving memories.

STORIES AND BOOKS ABOUT SERIOUSLY ILL AND DYING CHILDREN

The Angel Who Forgot, E. Bartone, Green Tiger Press/Simon and Schuster, New York, 1986—A young boy is ill and calls for an angel to come to heal him. When the angel appears it is confused and has forgotten how to heal or bring comfort. Over time, the boy's mother learns that the angel lost his healing powers because he once lost his beloved horse. In his grief the angel threw all his memories away, and with his memories gone he no longer knows how to heal. The mother retrieves the memories, the angel regains his powers, and her child is healed.

Cell Wars, F. Balkwill, CarolRoda Books, Minneapolis, Minnesota, 1994—Young readers and their parents will find this an excellent way to help them visualize how cells in the body work to assist the body in healing. Colorful illustrations abound throughout the book.

Gentle Willow, J. C. Mills, Brunner/Mazel, New York, 1993—A story written for dying children to give them a comforting metaphor. Gentle Willow is not well, and nothing her friends do can make her better. The story presents a "transformational" way of experiencing emotions associated with dying and death.

In the Hospital, P. Alsop and B. Harley, Moose School Productions, Topanga, California, 1990—This audio tape and book provide lightheartedness and entertainment, while offering many ideas about how children can increase their ability to cope with their fears and with the rigors of treatment.

Little Tree, J. C. Mills, Brunner/Mazel, New York, 1992—In this healing story, a little tree loses some of her branches in a storm. She experiences the emotions of fear, self-blame, and worry so common to children facing serious medical problems. The tree wizards who treat her represent the spiritual, psychological, and medical approaches to treatment as well as the hope for recovery and a fruitful and happy, albeit changed, life.

No Longer Afraid, D. Sanford, Questar Publishers, Portland, Oregon, 1993—This is the true story of Jamie following her diagnosis with cancer. The story shows how Jamie develops the ability to face her fears. She learns that, although she is limited by her illness, she still has the power to make choices.

On the Wings of a Butterfly, M. Maple, Parenting Press, Seattle, Washington, 1992—Lisa, a child dying of cancer, finds comfort and support in her friendship with a caterpillar who is preparing for its transformation into a Monarch butterfly. The two share their fears and questions and embrace the unknown together.

Sadako and the Thousand Paper Cranes, E. Coerr, Putnam, New York, 1977—The story of a young Japanese child who maintains hope as she lives and dies with leukemia. Her courage inspired a monument in Hiroshima Peace Park that is visited each year by thousands of young children who remember Sadako as a symbol of peace.

Swan Sky, Tejima, Putnam, New York, 1988—This inspirational and metaphorical story is a translation of Ōhakuchō No Sora, originally published in Japan. Despite the devoted attentions of her family, a young swan becomes sick and dies. After her death the swan family are called by the winds to journey to their northern summer home. When they arrive they are greeted by a rising sun that spreads its wings of warmth across them. In the sun they see their loved one who has died and are comforted and blessed.

The Velveteen Rabbit, M. Williams, Doubleday, Garden City, New York, 1975—A young stuffed bunny becomes real only after he has had a lot of rough wear—he looses his fur and looks old and shabby. This bunny, who has been transformed by love, comes to see life in a whole new way. A story enjoyed by people of all ages.

STORIES AND BOOKS WRITTEN BY SERIOUSLY ILL OR BEREAVED CHILDREN

Another Look at the Rainbow, G. Murray and G. Jampolsky (eds.), Celestial Arts, Berkeley, California, 1982—Thirty-four children (ages 6 to 24 years) tell about their feelings and experiences as siblings of seriously ill children. Included are: their first reactions, how they dealt with fear, loneliness, jealousy, and guilt and how they faced the problem of death.

Children Facing Death, J. Loomis Romond, Abbey Press, St. Meinrad, Indiana, 1989—The author completed extensive interviews with eighteen children (ages 6 to 14) whose brother or sister had died. She then worked with the children in completing letters to help other children dealing with the death of a sibling. This book is the compilation of the children's letters. This resource provides a wealth of information and is instilled with hope.

How to Fight for Your Life, J. Krementz, Little Brown and Company, Boston, Massachusetts, 1989—A collection of deeply personal, inspiring stories and photographs of fourteen children, ages seven to sixteen, who are living with life-threatening illnesses.

I Will Sing Life, Voices From the Hole in the Wall Gang, L. Berger, D. Lithwick and Seven Campers, Little, Brown and Company, Boston, Massachusetts, 1992—Seven remarkable children, living with AIDS, sickle cell anaemia, cancer, and physical disabilities share their poems and stories and tell how and why they are able to "sing life" in spite of their various illnesses.

My Book for Kids with Cancer, J. Gaes, Melius and Peterson, Aberdeen, South Dakota, 1987—The true story of Jason Gaes, who at the age of six years was stricken with a rare and deadly form of cancer. Jason struggled and survived. He tells his story to help other kids know what treatments and feelings they will face and to offer hope and encouragement. Today, Jason is a young teenager who plans one day to be a pediatrician.

My Journey of Hope, S. J. Kova, Harper Collins, San Francisco, California, 1993—Eleven-year-old Sarah Jean Kova tells other children how to keep their spirits up after they have been diagnosed with cancer. Sarah talks about the possibility of death and how her belief in God helps her through her treatments and her fears.

When I Die, Will I Get Better? J. Breebaart and P. Breebaart, Bedrick, New York, 1993—This is the story that five-year-old Joeri made up after his brother died of a sudden illness. The book is illustrated by Joeri's father. The story features a host of animals who behave in very human ways. The ending, which finds Joeri and his friends at play in the field where Joe Rabbit is buried, is both poignant and hopeful, and may be a real boost to story listeners struggling with grief.

LOSS AND BEREAVEMENT

Aarvy Aardvark Finds Hope, D. O'Toole, Mountain Rainbow Publications, Burnsville, North Carolina, 1989—This is available as a book, teaching guide, and video and audiotape and is a useful resource as a teaching story for bereavement counselors, teachers, and children. The story uses animals to illustrate the grief process as well as the supportive helping process. Aarvy Aardvark has become an orphan and is so sad that he wishes he could die. He is helped by his imagination and by a wise Rabbit who is willing to be with Aarvy through his anger and pain. A strange turn of events helps Aarvy release his sadness and regain hope.

Badger's Parting Gifts, S. Varley, Mulberry Books, division of William Morrow, New York, 1984—Old Badger is dearly loved by the woodland creatures. But Badger is growing old and he tells his friends he will soon die. When Badger dies the other animals are overwhelmed with sadness. When they gather together to tell stories about the gifts that old Badger gave to each of them they realize that, though their loss is sad, these stories and gifts can still fill their hearts with gladness.

The Black Dog who went into the Woods, E. Thacher Hurd, Harper and Row, New York, 1980—After their old dog goes into the woods and dies, each family member has a special dream about Black Dog. As the full moon touches their faces they wake from their dream and whisper their good-byes to their beloved pet. In the morning the family members share their dreams with each other and tell how each said farewell to Black Dog.

Christmas Moon, D. Cazet, Bradbury Press, New York, 1988—A story about the impact of death on a very young child and the importance of tender memories and loving support by adults.

I Don't Care, M. Sharmat, Macmillan, New York, 1977—A story that illustrates how children can move through a response to loss. When Jonathan's blue balloon with a smiling face blows away he tries to deny that it had any real importance to him. When the reality of the loss hits he cries and cries. As he cries his loss works its way deeply into his heart. Jonathan realizes he can resume living because the memory brings comfort and warmth for him.

Nadia the Willful, S. Alexander, Random House, New York, 1983—A retellable and readable tale that illustrates the importance of remembering when grieving the loss of a loved one. Nadia has a special relationship with her older brother. When he dies, Nadia refuses to forget him, even though Nadia's father tells her she must never again speak her brother's name. Nadia refuses to obey her father. Gradually, her father learns that Nadia's refusal to forget is a wise choice, and he too comes to remember his son and speak his name.

The Tenth Good Thing about Barney, J. Viorst, Macmillan, New York, 1971—When a little girl's cat named Barney dies, the girl expresses her feelings and tries to remember ten good things about Barney. The story provides a logical explanation of death, shows the role of rituals for commemoration and demonstrates that even young children have different—and sometimes clashing beliefs about what happens after death. Also available as a video.

Through the Mickle Woods, V. Gregory, Little Brown and Company, Boston, Massachusetts, 1992—After his wife's death a grieving king is mysteriously led by a young boy to an old bear's cave. The bear tells the king three stories so that he will find the courage to go on living.

STORIES AND BOOKS ABOUT FEELINGS

Fear

Alexander and the Dragon, K. Holabird, Clarkson Potter, New York, 1988—Young Alexander has a dragon in his room and his parents do not believe him when he tells them. Alexander faces his fear (the dragon) and learns that when dragons are faced with bravery and determination their negative powers vanish.

St. George and the Dragon, retold by M. Hodges, Little Brown and Company, New York, 1984—The retelling of the dramatic battle between good and evil. George perseveres in fighting a fierce dragon in this timeless tale of a legendary hero who risks his life to rescue others. It is easy to draw the metaphor of the fears and fierceness that one faces in grief and in the losses associated with life-threatening illness.

Anger

Angry Arthur, H. Orum, E. P. Dutton, New York, 1982—When things do not go the way Arthur wants them to, he gets angry. Arthur's mother tells him to go ahead and be angry. So Arthur's anger gets bigger and bigger. His anger becomes a thunder storm, a hurricane, a typhoon, and finally a universe quake. Then Arthur's world becomes peaceful. He realizes that he is no longer angry, nor can he remember why he got so angry in the first place.

Hurt

The Hurt, T. Doleski, Ramsey Paulist Press, New York, 1983—When a friend hurts Justin's feelings he hides the hurt inside of himself. Other hurts happen and they too are held inside. As the hurts grow bigger and bigger they fill up his room and his insides and threaten any happiness he might have. One day Justin's father teaches him how he can get rid of his hurts before they can grow bigger.

Inspiration and Hope

Aarvy Aardvark Finds Hope, D. O'Toole, Mountain Rainbow Publications, Burnsville, North Carolina, 1989—See entry under Loss and Bereavement.

The Education of Little Tree, F. Carter, University of New Mexico Press, Albequerque, New Mexico, 1976—See entry under Death as a Part of Life.

The Little Engine That Could, retold by W. Piper, Putnam, New York, New York, 1991—This classic illustrates the power of positive thinking in overcoming great odds. It provides a metaphor of hope and determination that is linked to compassion and action.

RESOURCES FOR THERAPEUTIC STORY
MATERIAL RELATED TO DEATH
AND DYING, LOSS AND GRIEF

Directories of storytellers and information regarding storytelling conferences can be obtained from:

The National Storytelling Association
P.O. Box 309
Jonesborough, Tennessee, 37659

The Storytellers School of Toronto
412A College Street
Toronto, Ontario, M5T 1T3

The following organizations provide mail-order catalogues of their
materials:

Centering Corporation
1531 North Saddle Creek Road
Omaha, Nebraska 68104-5064

Childswork–Childsplay
Center For Applied Psychology, Inc.
P.O. Box 1568
King of Prussia, Pennsylvania 19406

Compassion Books
479 Hannah Branch Road
Burnsville, North Carolina 28714

Kids Rights
10100 Park Cedar Drive
Charlotte, North Carolina 28210

Psychotherapy Book Club
834 North 12th Street
Allentown, Pennsylvania 18102

Rainbow Connection
477 Hannah Branch Road
Burnsville, North Carolina 28714

About the Editors

David W. Adams, M.S.W., C.S.W. is a Professor, Department of Psychiatry, Faculty of Health Sciences, McMaster University and Executive Director, Greater Hamilton Employee Assistance Consortium. Over the past twenty-five years in his affiliation with Chedoke-McMaster Hospitals and McMaster University, he has concentrated much of clinical social work practice and teaching on life-threatening illness, dying, death and bereavement in childhood and the impact on children and families. He is the author of *Childhood Malignancy: The Psychosocial Care of the Child and His Family* and *Parents of Children with Cancer Speak Out: Needs, Problems, and Sources of Help*. David is co-author with Ellie Deveau of *Coping with Childhood Cancer: Where Do We Go From Here?* He is a charter member of the board and Chair, Professional Advisors of the Candlelighters Childhood Cancer Foundation Canada, Chair of the International Work Group on Death, Dying and Bereavement and past Chair of the Psychosocial Services Committee of the Pediatric Oncology Group of Ontario. David is a certified death educator and grief counsellor. He has contributed numerous chapters and articles and is internationally known as a speaker, program consultant and workshop facilitator.

Eleanor (Ellie) J. Deveau, R.N., B.Sc.N. is coordinator of program evaluation in the Educational Center for Aging and Health, Faculty of Health Sciences, McMaster University, Hamilton, Ontario, Canada. She is bereavement consultant and advisor to Friends in Grief, Inc., Hamilton, Ontario and a founding member of their board of directors. Ellie is a certified death educator through the Association of Death Education and Counseling (USA) and a member of the International Work Group on Death, Dying and Bereavement. Many years of experience as a nurse practitioner in the pediatric hematology/oncology program at McMaster University Medical Center led to her co-authorship of the award-winning book, *Coping with Childhood Cancer: Where Do*

349

We Go From Here? Ellie is a speaker and workshop facilitator and has contributed chapters and articles which focus on issues relating to children and adolescents' understanding of death, the impact of life-threatening illness and palliative care on children, siblings and parents, the pattern of grief in children and adolescents, and child and adult bereavement.

Contributors

DAVID W. ADAMS, M.S.W., C.S.W., Professor, Department of Psychiatry, Faculty of Health Sciences, McMaster University; Executive Director, Greater Hamilton Employee Assistance Consortium, Hamilton, Ontario, Canada.

JOAN M. AUDEN, B.A., M.S.W., Social Worker, Pediatric Oncology, Children's Hospital of Eastern Ontario; Consultant, Bereaved Families of Ontario, Ottawa, Ontario, Canada.

GERRY R. COX, Ph.D., Professor of Sociology, South Dakota School of Mines and Technology, Rapid City, South Dakota, United States.

BETTY DAVIES, R.N., Ph.D., Professor, School of Nursing, University of British Columbia; Investigator, Research Division, British Columbia's Children's Hospital; Board of Directors, Canuck Place: A Hospice for Children, Vancouver, British Columbia, Canada.

ELEANOR J. DEVEAU, R.N., B.Sc.N., Coordinator, Program Evaluation, Educational Centre for Aging and Health, Faculty of Health Sciences, McMaster University; Bereavement Consultant, Friends in Grief, Inc., Hamilton, Ontario, Canada.

L. L. (Barrie) deVEBER, M.D., FRCP(C), Department of Pediatrics, King Fahod National Guard Hospital, Rayadh, Saudi Arabia; former Director, Pediatric Hematology/Oncology, Children's Hospital of Western Ontario, London, Ontario, Canada.

BRENDA ENG, R.N., M.N., Clinical Nurse Specialist, British Columbia's Children's Hospital; Associate, Program and Development, Canuck Place: A Hospice for Children, Vancouver, British Columbia, Canada.

MARK L. GREENBERG, M.B., Ch.B., FRCP(C), Professor, Pediatrics and Surgery, University of Toronto; Chief, Division of Oncology, The Hospital for Sick Children, Toronto, Ontario, Canada.

PETRA HINDERER, Dipl. Psych., Director, Social Programs; Psychologist and Music Therapist, Community Center Konstanz, Brauneggerstrasse, Konstanz, Germany.

LEORA KUTTNER, Ph.D., Reg. Clin. Psych., Clinical Psychologist; Assistant Clinical Professor, Department of Pediatrics, Faculty of Medicine, University of British Columbia, Vancouver, British Columbia, Canada.

ANTOON A. LEENAARS, Ph.D., C. Psych., Psychologist, Researcher, Author, and Editor, Windsor, Ontario, Canada, and Ulvenhout, N.B., The Netherlands; Editor-in-Chief, Archives of Suicide Research, United States.

JOHN T. MAHER, M.A., M.D., Resident in Psychiatry, University of Ottawa; Former Director, Trillium Childhood Cancer Support Centre; Former Assistant Director, Cancer 2000 Task Force, Ottawa, Ontario, Canada.

SHARON M. McMAHON, R.N., B.Sc.N., B.A., M.Ed., Ed.D., Associate Professor, School of Nursing, University of Windsor; Founder, Pet Bereavement Support Services, Windsor, Ontario.

DONNA O'TOOLE, M.A., Counselor, Author, Trainer, and Storyteller, Rainbow Connection, Burnsville, North Carolina, United States.

ELEANOR G. PASK, R.N., B.Sc.N., M.Sc.N., Ed.D., Executive Director, Candlelighters Childhood Cancer Foundation Canada, Toronto, Ontario, Canada.

RUTH M. SNIDER, E.C.Ed., B.A., Chair, Pediatric Patient Services, Canadian Cancer Society, Ontario Division; Consultant, Sunshine Foundation of Canada; Former Director, Child Life Studies Diploma Program, Faculty of Health Sciences, McMaster University, Hamilton, Ontario, Canada.

MICHAEL M. STEVENS, M.B., B.S., FRACP., Senior Staff Specialist and Head, Oncology Unit, Royal Alexandra Hospital for Children, Camperdown, New South Wales, Australia.

ROBERT G. STEVENSON, Ed.D., Educator, River Dell Schools; Counselor, The Center for Help in Time of Loss, Westwood, New Jersey, United States.

CYNTHIA A. STUTZER, R.N., M.S., C.P.O.N., Clinical Nurse Specialist, Pediatric Oncology, British Columbia's Children's Hospital, Clinical Assistant Professor, University of British Columbia, School of Nursing, Vancouver, British Columbia, Canada.

SUSANNE WENCKSTERN, M.A., C. Psych. Assoc., Psychological Associate, Board of Education for the City of Windsor, Windsor, Ontario, Canada.

Index